Cardiovascular 3D Printing

Jian Yang • Alex Pui-Wai Lee • Vladimiro L. Vida
Editors

Cardiovascular 3D Printing

Techniques and Clinical Application

Chemical Industry Press Co., Ltd.

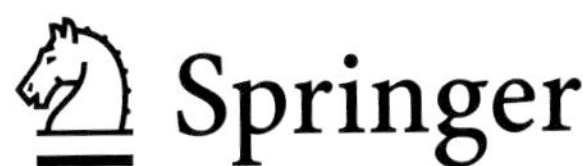

Editors
Jian Yang
Department of Cardiovascular Surgery
Xijing Hospital
Xi'an
China

Vladimiro L. Vida
Paediatric and Congenital Cardiac Surgery Unit
Department of Cardiac, Thoracic and Vascular Sciences and Public Health
University of Padua
Padua
Italy

Alex Pui-Wai Lee
Laboratory of Cardiac Imaging and 3D Printing
Li Ka Shing Institute of Health Science
Department of Medicine and Therapeutics
Faculty of Medicine
The Chinese University of Hong Kong
Hong Kong
China

ISBN 978-981-15-6959-3 ISBN 978-981-15-6957-9 (eBook)
https://doi.org/10.1007/978-981-15-6957-9

Jointly published with Chemical Industry Press
The print edition is not for sale in China (Mainland). Customers from China (Mainland) please order the print book from: Chemical Industry Press.

This Springer imprint is published by the registered company Springer Nature Singapore Pte Ltd.
The registered company address is: 152 Beach Road, #21-01/04 Gateway East, Singapore 189721, Singapore

Foreword

Medical three-dimensional (3D) printing, as an important part of the third industrial revolution, has been widely used in orthopedics and traumatology in recent years and shows great promise. However, for various reasons, its application in the cardiovascular field has lagged behind its uses in other areas.

The book *Cardiovascular 3D Printing Technology and Application*, edited by Professor Jian Yang, Department of Cardiovascular Surgery, Xijing Hospital, condenses his team's many years of clinical experience guided by 3D printing technology. It combines biomedical engineering with clinical medicine and builds a bridge between 3D printing and cardiovascular treatment, which conforms to the national developmental strategy of individualized treatment and precision medicine. It is the first professional book on cardiovascular 3D printing in China and includes practical clinical experiences from around the world. Of particular value is the fact that the case and imaging data are original. They provide valuable knowledge, rich experiences, and innovative practices from many well-known institutes and many top experts at home and abroad, which is of strong academic value.

Over the past two years, my research team has cooperated with the team led by Professor Jian Yang in the research of 3D printing using new hydrogel materials. At Professor Yang's invitation, I have participated in the revision of some of the chapters in this book, and I deeply feel his dedication, rigor, and high level of professionalism.

When closely combined with clinical needs, this book can effectively guide cardiovascular medical professionals, biomedical engineering experts, and medical students to better diagnose and understand cardiovascular diseases, thereby increasing the success rate of patients' surgery, improving the effect of cardiovascular disease diagnosis and treatment, and better benefiting the vast number of patients with cardiovascular diseases. It is recommended to readers.

Zhigang Suo
Allen E. and Marilyn M. Puckett
Professor of Mechanics and Materials
Harvard University
Cambridge, MA
USA

Preface

Cardiovascular disease is one of the most serious diseases that endangers human health. It places a heavy burden on families and society. Therefore, preventing it and treating it effectively are of utmost importance. With continuous progress in surgical techniques and interventional therapy technologies, the concepts and strategies for the treatment of cardiovascular diseases are constantly being updated, which have led to a massive transformation of the treatment of cardiovascular diseases in recent years. Together with the current trend toward precision medical therapy, the demand for individualized treatment has become the main theme of the contemporary medical era.

Three-dimensional (3D) printing is one of the representative technologies of the third industrial revolution that has been applied to fields such as aerospace, architecture, automobile, and medicine. In recent years, with continuous progress in digital modeling technology, information technology, imaging, material science, and chemistry, 3D printing technology has been applied more and more widely in the cardiovascular field: from personalized printing of cardiovascular models, determining surgical plans, and improving communication between doctors and patients to simulating intravascular surgery and improving the success rate and safety of surgery. The application of 3D printing technology in cardiovascular diseases is deepening, and it will continue to further reshape our definition, understanding, diagnosis, and treatment of cardiovascular diseases. The emergence of new therapeutic techniques, such as transcatheter aortic valve replacement, has opened up new horizons in the diagnosis and treatment of cardiovascular diseases. At the same time, new therapeutic techniques have put forward higher clinical demand for accurate diagnosis with multimodality imaging. The development of 3D printing technology may be a solution to potential deficiencies of traditional imaging technology in displaying complex anatomical structures. It brings new ideas for individualized and precise diagnosis and treatment of patients with heart disease.

This book assembles the works of international experts in the cardiovascular field to introduce the history, methods, material selection, and clinical applications of 3D printing in cardiovascular medicine, including 3D bioprinting. The authors combine their own extensive practical experiences in cardiovascular 3D printing with a thorough review of the literature on the use of 3D printing technique in various cardiovascular diseases. In-depth discussions can be found in the areas of congenital heart diseases, valvular diseases, left atrial appendage intervention, coronary artery disease, cardiomyopathy, cardiac tumors, and vascular diseases. Our goal is to provide a concise review on the clinical applications of 3D printing with the relevant physiologic and anatomic backgrounds of each cardiovascular disease.

The book is divided into 13 chapters, including 432 figures, most of which are original works from the Department of Cardiovascular Surgery of Xijing Hospital and many other centers. The authors have received strong support and help in pictures and models from Xi'an MAKE Medical Technology Co., Ltd. This book also includes excellent cases, valuable information, and careful guidance from well-known experts and scholars from Harvard University, Cambridge, MA, USA; Georgia Institute of Technology, Atlanta, GA, USA; Hong Kong Asian Heart Disease Center; Prince of Wales Hospital of the Chinese University of Hong Kong; University of Padua, Italy; National Center for Supplementary Manufacturing Innovation of Xi'an; and many major cardiovascular centers in China. It is expected that this book will be helpful to cardiovascular surgeons, cardiologists, anesthesiologists, radiologists, ultrasound imaging specialists, and cardiopulmonary bypass and critical care doctors at all levels, as well as to biomedical engineers, nurses, and other medical professionals in clinical practice. Hopefully, it will also serve as a reference for recent graduates, specialist trainers, refresher students, and senior students in medical colleges and universities. The authors hope that readers will find much that is useful in the book and will not hesitate to bring to their attention any shortcomings or inaccuracies.

Xi'an, China
Hong Kong, China
Padua, Italy
2020/3/1

Jian Yang
Alex Pui-Wai Lee
Vladimiro L. Vida

Disclosure

The figure sources involved in the book entitled *Cardiovascular 3D Printing- Techniques and Clinical Application* were approved by the Ethics Committee of Xijing Hospital (No. KY20150205-1), which was carried out in accordance with the Declaration of Helsinki (1996) and all relevant Chinese laws. There were no conflicts of interest in the figures.

As the clinical appearance and intraoperative pictures of patients are listed in this book, we have obtained the informed consent of the patients themselves and their families or their guardians.

Jian Yang, MD, PhD, FACC, FAHA

Contents

Editors and Contributors

Editors

Jian Yang, MD, PhD, FACC, FAHA Xijing Hospital, Xi'an, China

Alex Pui-Wai Lee, MBChB, MD, FRCP, FACC, FESC Laboratory of Cardiac Imaging and 3D Printing, Li Ka Shing Institute of Health Science; Department of Medicine and Therapeutics, Faculty of Medicine, The Chinese University of Hong Kong, Hong Kong, China

Division of Cardiology, Department of Medicine and Therapeutics, The Chinese University of Hong Kong, Hong Kong, China

Vladimiro L. Vida, MD, PhD Paediatric and Congenital Cardiac Surgery Unit, Department of Cardiac, Thoracic and Vascular Sciences and Public Health, University of Padua, Padua, Italy

Contributors

Matteo Andolfatto, MD Paediatric and Congenital Cardiac Surgery Unit, Department of Cardiac, Thoracic and Vascular Sciences and Public Health, University of Padua, Padua, Italy

Francesco Bertelli, MD Paediatric and Congenital Cardiac Surgery Unit, Department of Cardiac, Thoracic and Vascular Sciences and Public Health, University of Padua, Padua, Italy

Tiesheng Cao, MD, PhD Tangdu Hospital, Xi'an, China

Claudia Cattapan, MD Paediatric and Congenital Cardiac Surgery Unit, Department of Cardiac, Thoracic and Vascular Sciences and Public Health, University of Padua, Padua, Italy

Peng Ding, MD Xijing Hospital, Xi'an, China

Weixun Duan, MD, PhD Xijing Hospital, Xi'an, China

Yiting Fan, MD, PhD Laboratory of Cardiac Imaging and 3D Printing, Li Ka Shing Institute of Health Science, Hong Kong, China

Division of Cardiology, Department of Medicine and Therapeutics, The Chinese University of Hong Kong, Hong Kong, China

Zhenge Fan, MD Xijing Hospital, Xi'an, China

Fang Fang, MD, PhD Beijing Anzhen Hospital, Affiliated with Capital Medical University, Beijing, China

Alessandro Fiocco, MD Paediatric and Congenital Cardiac Surgery Unit, Department of Cardiac, Thoracic and Vascular Sciences and Public Health, University of Padua, Padua, Italy

Alvise Guariento, MD Paediatric and Congenital Cardiac Surgery Unit, Department of Cardiac, Thoracic and Vascular Sciences and Public Health, University of Padua, Padua, Italy

Zhenxiao Jin, MD, PhD Xijing Hospital, Xi'an, China

Yat-Yin Lam, MD Hong Kong Asian Heart Disease Center, Hong Kong, China

Alex Pui-Wai Lee, MBChB, MD, FRCP, FACC, FESC Laboratory of Cardiac Imaging and 3D Printing, Li Ka Shing Institute of Health Science; Department of Medicine and Therapeutics, Faculty of Medicine, The Chinese University of Hong Kong, Hong Kong, China

Division of Cardiology, Department of Medicine and Therapeutics, The Chinese University of Hong Kong, Hong Kong, China

Lanlan Li, PhD Xijing Hospital, Xi'an, China

Jiahe Liang, PhD Tangdu Hospital, Xi'an, China

Jincheng Liu, MD, PhD Xijing Hospital, Xi'an, China

Liwen Liu, MD, PhD Xijing Hospital, Xi'an, China

Yang Liu, MD, PhD Xijing Hospital, Xi'an, China

Fanglin Lu, MD, PhD Changhai Hospital, Naval Medical University, Shanghai, China

Yanyan Ma, PhD Xijing Hospital, Xi'an, China

Wenzhi Pan, MD, PhD Zhongshan Hospital Affiliated with Fudan University, Shanghai, China

Xiangbin Pan, MD, PhD Fuwai Hospital, Chinese Academy of Medical Sciences, Beijing, China

Xin Pan, MD, PhD Chest Hospital Affiliated with Shanghai Jiaotong University, Shanghai, China

Hang Qi, PhD Georgia Institute of Technology, Atlanta, GA, USA

Xiaoke Shang, MD, PhD Union Medical College Affiliated with Tongji Medical College, Wuhan, China

Guangyuan Song, MD, PhD Fuwai Hospital, Chinese Academy of Medical Sciences, Beijing, China

Jiayou Tang, MD, PhD Xijing Hospital, Xi'an, China

Paola Veronese, MD Paediatric and Congenital Cardiac Surgery Unit, Department of Cardiac, Thoracic and Vascular Sciences and Public Health, University of Padua, Padua, Italy

Vladimiro L. Vida, MD, PhD Paediatric and Congenital Cardiac Surgery Unit, Department of Cardiac, Thoracic and Vascular Sciences and Public Health, University of Padua, Padua, Italy

Jing Wang, PhD National Innovation Center for Additional Materials Manufacturing, Xi'an, China

Yongjian Wu Fuwai Hospital, Chinese Academy of Medical Sciences, Beijing, China

Chennian Xu Xijing Hospital, Xi'an, China

Jian Yang, MD, PhD, FACC, FAHA Xijing Hospital, Xi'an, China

Lifang Yang, MD, PhD Xi'an Children's Hospital Affiliated with Xi'an Jiaotong University, Xi'an, China

Meng Yang, PhD Aviation College of Xi'an Jiaotong University, Xi'an, China

Wei Yi, MD, PhD Xijing Hospital, Xi'an, China

Shiqiang Yu, MD, PhD Xijing Hospital, Xi'an, China

Lijun Yuan, MD, PhD Tangdu Hospital, Xi'an, China

Da Zhu, MD, PhD West China Hospital of Sichuan University, Chengdu, China

Haibo Zhang, MD, PhD Beijing Anzhen Hospital Affiliated with Capital Medical University, Beijing, China

Minwen Zheng, MD, PhD Xijing Hospital, Xi'an, China

History of Cardiovascular 3D Printing

1

Chennian Xu, Jiahe Liang, and Jian Yang

Three dimensional (3D) printing technology is also called additive manufacturing or rapid prototyping manufacturing (RPM). Traditionally, industrial "subtraction" products are carved from solid blocks of material, such as in CNC machining. However, 3D printing technology uses the method of "addition" to build a product layer by layer, which has high manufacturing accuracy and is more suitable for manufacturing complex or individualized products. 3D printing technology also enables manufacturers to print prototypes more quickly, making it easier to evaluate and test products before they are finalized. The first step of 3D printing is using computer-aided design (CAD) software to create a 3D model, followed by using a 3D printer to print the model itself.

As early as the 1960s, the Battelle Memorial Institute in Ohio, USA, researched the use of photopolymers to make 3D objects by crossing two laser beams of different wavelengths to polymerize resins. In 1984, Charles Hull in the USA invented stereolithography (SLA), a process that uses digital data and computer-controlled laser beams to build a structure layer by layer, solidifying a single layer of liquid polymers with ultraviolet light onto the previous one, to form what is basically a growing cross section of the 3D model. This technology was patented in 1986. In 1988, the world's first commercial SLA 3D printer was developed by 3D Systems [1]. Carl Deckard at the University of Texas proposed the concept of selective laser sintering (SLS), which uses laser beams to selectively solidify powders, instead of polymerizing a liquid resin. Deckard then founded the Desktop Manufacturing Corporation (DTM Corp), which produced the first SLS printer in 1992 and advanced SLS technology into the 3D printing industry. In 1989, S. Scott in the USA established Stratasys and filed a patent application for rapid prototyping technology called fused deposition modeling (FDM) in the same year. Plastic filaments or metal wires are heated and then extruded from the nozzle. The deposition process is guided by a preset digital model. Each layer is kept at a temperature just above the freezing point to achieve good interlaminar adhesion. Stratasys finally developed a thermoplastic consumable and a printer system for 3D printing. In the second half of 1989, Hans Langer in Germany developed a technology called Electro Optical Systems (EOS), which mainly involves metal laser sintering and directly manufactured 3D parts based on computer models. In this technology, metal powders are selectively sintered by lasers. All DTM's patents related to laser sintering were granted in 2004. In the 1990s, several other new 3D printing technologies were also being developed.

Since the 1990s, many well-known universities in China have carried out independent research on 3D printing technology. Research teams represented by Tsinghua University, Huazhong University of Science and Technology, Xi'an Jiaotong University, and other universities have begun to develop prototypes of rapid prototyping machines. For example, Huazhong University of Science and Technology has performed in-depth research on the manufacturing technology of 3D printed layered solids and successfully developed HRP series molding machines and molding materials; Tsinghua University had more extensive experience in modern molding theory, FDM technology, and layered solid research; the University of Science and Technology of China studied and successfully launched an eight-nozzle combination injection device, which has promoted the field of photoelectric devices and micromanufacturing. Xi'an Jiaotong University independently developed a three-dimensional printer nozzle and developed a light-curing forming system and corresponding suitable printing materials, which greatly improved the forming accuracy to 0.05 mm [2]. According to the "China's 3D Printing Industry Market Demand and Investment Potential Analysis Report 2015–2020" provided by the National Research Institute of 3D Printing Industry, there are more than two hundred 3D printing companies in the world, and more than a hundred of them are located in

C. Xu · J. Yang (✉)
Xijing Hospital, Xi'an, China

J. Liang
Tangdu Hospital, Xi'an, China

J. Yang et al. (eds.), *Cardiovascular 3D Printing*, https://doi.org/10.1007/978-981-15-6957-9_1

China. In 2014, the global 3D printing industry exceeded 30 billion RMB, and China accounted for approximately 1/10 of the industry. The scale of the global 3D printing industry is expected to exceed 200 billion RMB by 2020 [3, 4].

At the end of the twentieth century, digital precision medicine gradually became a focus in the medical field. CT and MRI scanning, together with 3D printing technology, have provided additional space for the development of the technology itself [5]. A growing number of operations have begun to use 3D printed medical models for preoperative planning and intraoperative navigation. Medical workers can now build a 3D model based on preoperative CT or magnetic resonance data and then create the required medical model through a 3D printer. Such models can provide clinicians with complex anatomical information and assist in surgical training, preoperative planning, and intraoperative guidance. Through 3D printing technology, surgeons can better understand the pathological characteristics of patients before an operation and formulate a more ideal surgical plan to minimize the occurrence of intraoperative accidents, shorten the operation time, and improve the clinical outcome. 3D printing technology is widely used to achieve precision and customization, and remarkable results have been achieved, especially in the fields of dentistry, maxillofacial surgery, orthopedics, plastic surgery, and other disciplines [6, 7]. However, in the cardiovascular field, because of the complex anatomical structure of the system itself and the soft tissue, the use of 3D printing technology has been limited [8–10]. Another important use of cardiovascular 3D printing is the creation of individualized models directly from the patient to assess the hemodynamics and performance of the heart [11]. Scholars are currently studying heart-specific implants but are faced with problems of blood compatibility and durability of materials. Therefore, 3D printing has not been used to make permanent cardiovascular implants.

With the continuous progress of 3D printing technology, 3D printing has proven to hold great value and potential in many fields. The emergence of 3D printing has provided new avenues for the diagnosis and treatment of many complex cardiovascular diseases, and it has become a bridge between traditional medical imaging and anatomy. Thus far, cardiovascular 3D printing technology has been used in surgical planning, medical research, medical education, and training tools, and it plays an indispensable role in the world's prospective tissue engineering research [12, 13]. The application of 3D printing technology in the diagnosis and treatment of cardiovascular diseases has recently matured. With the continued development of 3D printing technology and materials, it can be predicted that increasing progress will be made in the 3D printing of vascular scaffolds, stent grafts, and even organs [14, 15].

References

1. Beevisa D, Denisb GS. Rapid prototyping and the human factors engineering process. Appl Ergon. 1992;23:155–60.
2. Bing-heng L, Di-chen L. Development of the additive manufacturing (3D printing) technology. Machine Build Automat. 2013;42:1–4.
3. Wang Q, Jiang M, Guo S. Additive manufacturing industry development status and tendency analysis in China. Sci Technol Indus China. 2018:52–6. https://doi.org/10.1142/S2424862219300011.
4. Bingheng L. Smart manufacturing and 3D printing drive "made in China 2025". High-Technology & Commercialization 2018:22–25.
5. McGurk M, Amis AA, Potamianos P, Goodger NM. Rapid prototyping techniques for anatomical modelling in medicine. Ann R Coll Surg Engl. 1997;79:169–74.
6. Kewei L, Shuai R, Yong T, Hao L, Lian-tao L, Ke-pei Z, Feng L. Application of 3D printing technique in pediatric orthopaedics. Orthopedic J China. 2018;26:436–40.
7. Dan L, Wei C, Bing L. Application of 3D printing technology in medical field. China Medical Device. 2018;33:117–121+135.
8. Narutoshi Hibino M. Three dimensional printing: applications in surgery for congenital heart disease. World J Pediatr Congenit Heart Surg. 2016;7:351–2.
9. Fan Y, Hong Z. The application of 3D printing technology in cardiovascular diseases. J Cardiovasc Surg. 2015;04:93–6.
10. Kim MS, Hansgen AR, Wink O, Quaife RA, Carroll JD. Rapid prototyping: a new tool in understanding and treating structural heart disease (Review). Circulation. 2008;117:2388–94.
11. Yanxiang Z, Wei H, Ruiqiang G. Ultrasound-derived three-dimensional printing technology in cardiology: current applications. J Clin Ultrasound. 2018;20:547–50.
12. Li Z, Qing L. Applications of 3D printing technology in cardiovascular field. China Medical Device Information. 2017;23:16–21.
13. Haijun Y, Tianying F, Yaoxia G. Clinical progress of 3D printing technology applied to precise medical treatment of cardiovascular diseases. J Cardiovasc Pulmonary Dis. 2017;36:602–603+609.
14. Zhuer L, Liu-yuan G. Cytocompatibility study of 3D printing bioresorbable coronary stent. Biomed Eng Clin Med. 2018;22:232–5.
15. Rosu C, Demers P. Three-dimensional printing in cardiovascular surgery: logical next step after three-dimensional imaging. J Thorac Dis. 2017;9:2720–2.

The Methods of Cardiovascular 3D Printing

2

Peng Ding, Lanlan Li, Meng Yang, and Jian Yang

2.1 Acquisition of Cardiovascular Imaging Data

Obtaining appropriate imaging data is the first step in 3D model printing. The quality of the image itself is significantly related to the quality of the final 3D-printed model. Thus, improving image acquisition technology and quality are the most important and effective ways to improve the accuracy of 3D-printed models. Imaging data that are currently available for the manufacture of cardiovascular 3D-printed models include computed tomography angiography (CTA), echocardiography, 3D rotational angiography, and cardiac magnetic resonance (CMR) data. These imaging data are collected and stored in Digital Imaging and Communications in Medicine (DICOM) format, which is the international standard format for medical images and related information [1].

2.1.1 Computed Tomography Angiography (CTA)

Contrast-enhanced CTA is currently the most commonly used 3D printing data resource in clinical practice. The advantage of CTA over echocardiography is the obvious contrast between the lumen and the myocardium/vascular wall, which can distinguish vascular and nonvascular structures or coronary arteries [2]. CTA provides better spatial resolution, shorter imaging time, and easier access than MRI. However, CTA also has its shortcomings: First, CTA has a low time resolution. Second, it requires the use of contrast agents and exposure to ionizing radiation, and its application is often restricted in certain patient groups, such as those who are allergic to contrast agents, children, and pregnant women

To obtain high-quality CTA images, the following considerations should be highlighted:

1. Preparation
   (a) Scanning device: In theory, the smaller the layer thickness of the scan is, the more accurate the image. At present, the layer thickness of general 3D printers can reach as small as 0.02 mm–0.2 mm. The actual printing layer must be less than 1 mm, and CTA with 16 or more rows can meet these requirements. However, due to the advantages of the new generation of scanners in terms of imaging time, imaging accuracy, and radiation reduction, it is still recommended to use a scanner with at least 64 rows for CTA.
   (b) Contrast agent approach: Both the central venous approach and the peripheral venous approach can be used, such as in the PICC pathway, while the peripheral vein route is also widely used. Among those, injection of the contrast agent through the antebrachial vein is preferred because this route can reduce artifacts. However, for patients with abnormal cardiovascular structures, the approach needs to be chosen based on the specific anatomy.
   (c) Contrast protocols: Low- or iso-osmolar iodinated contrast agents are the current standard for CTA. The dose of the contrast agent is usually 1–2 ml/kg; if mixed with physiological saline, the dose can reach 2–3 ml/kg. The speed of injection is determined by time, the diameter of the vein, and the pressure limits [3]. Usually, as long as the position is correct and the pressure is properly controlled, the injection is safe [4]. By combining contrast agents and saline, the need for different anatomical structures can be met. For structural heart disease patients without any special shunts, a two-phase protocol is usually chosen,

P. Ding · L. Li
Department of Cardiovascular Surgery, Xijing Hospital, Xi'an, China

M. Yang
Aviation College of Xi'an Jiaotong University, Xi'an, China

J. Yang (✉)
Department of Cardiovascular Surgery, Xijing Hospital, Xi'an, China

J. Yang et al. (eds.), *Cardiovascular 3D Printing*, https://doi.org/10.1007/978-981-15-6957-9_2

namely, a compact bolus of contrast followed by a saline chaser. For cases requiring simultaneous display of the left and right cardiovascular structures, a three-phase protocol is available: an initial faster contrast injection followed by a slower contrast injection and a final saline flush, or contrast injection followed by injection of a mixture of contrast and saline and a final saline flush. In cases where it is necessary to simultaneously show the arteries and veins, a venous two-phase protocol can be performed, that is, performing 30–60 seconds of suspension after the initial injection of the contrast agent, and then a standard two-phase protocol, allowing the arteries and veins to be displayed separately.

2. Image acquisition
   (a) Breathing and heart rate control: Advanced scanners can achieve ideal image acquisition in less than one cardiac cycle. For these devices, the control of breathing and heart rate is of less importance. However, for other scanners that need to achieve image acquisition during multiple cardiac cycles, it is important to control breathing and heart rate to reduce artifacts caused by thoracic and cardiac motion. Children under seven often have difficulty cooperating with examinations, and therefore, it is sometimes necessary to distract their attention or allow their parents to accompany them. If necessary, a sedative drug can be used. When performing CTA examination of the coronary arteries, breathing control is often necessary to improve image quality, and general anesthesia may be required for patients who cannot cooperate. The image quality of coronary arteries is inversely related to heart rate. In the absence of contraindications, beta-blockers and/or sublingual nitroglycerin are usually used to increase coronary diameter and reduce heart rate to less than 80 bpm. For patients with a pacemaker or defibrillator, it is often necessary to reset the device parameters to ensure that the heart rate meets the requirements.
   (b) Image acquisition time: Timing of acquisition is determined by the arrival of contrast agent to the region of interest (ROI). In most cases, the ROI is located in the target chamber, and when the attenuation rises above a certain threshold, image acquisition starts automatically. Where the anatomy is unknown and the contrast agent path cannot be predicted, a small dose angiogram test can be performed first to determine when it reaches the target structure. Or the contrast agent can also be tracked, and the acquisition is manually performed as long as the contrast reaches the target anatomical region [5].
   (c) ECG gating: Currently, there are several ECG-synchronized scanning modes that allow comparable radiation exposure. There are currently four types of ECG-gated CTA available:

Retrospective ECG-gated helical scanning: Radiation is given throughout the cardiac cycle, and images are retrospectively reconstructed in the desired cardiac phase of the cardiac cycle. It has the advantages of allowing visualization of cardiac motion and being more robust to arrhythmias; however, it requires a higher radiation dose.

Prospective ECG-triggered axial scanning: Images are acquired in a single phase of the cardiac cycle over several heartbeats. Radiation exposure is significantly reduced, but this type of scanning is susceptible to arrhythmias and tachycardia.

Prospective ECG-triggered scanning with a wide detector array (volumetric target scan mode): With a wide enough detector array (typically 320 detectors), the heart can be covered in a single heartbeat. Similarly, in the previous mode, the cardiac phase needs to be predetermined, and quality is best with slow, regular heart rates.

Prospective ECG-triggered helical scanning: In scanners with two X-ray tubes, detection of the QRS can trigger a high-pitch helical scan that allows large anatomic areas to be covered in a short time. This technique also requires a slow, steady heart rate.

Currently, volume target scan mode and prospective ECG-triggered helical scanning with a lower radiation dose should be used as often as possible. On the opposite, unless it is necessary to evaluate cardiac or valve function, retrospective ECG-gated helical scans should be avoided.

2.1.2 3D Echocardiography

The use of 3D echocardiography for 3D printing became possible after the year 2000 based on the emergence of matrix array transducers. In recent years, 3D echocardiography has been widely used in the diagnosis and treatment of congenital heart abnormalities, valve assessment, ventricular septal defect, and complex intraventricular block. When using 3D echocardiography in combination with color Doppler techniques, its advantages in assessing chamber size, volume, partial or whole function, valve morphology, and valve function have also been widely recognized. 3D echocardiography mainly uses the gradation change to create a sense of depth to assist in spatial imagination, although the image acquired is still essentially two-dimensional. 3D printing technology can help the anatomy to be observed in a real three-dimensional way. To obtain high standard 3D echocardiography data, the following considerations are highlighted:

1. Preparation
   (a) Breathing and heart rate control: Like CTA, heart and thoracic motion can cause artifacts in imaging, and therefore, ensuring that the patient remains calm and comfortable and reducing heart rate and breathing

changes are the key to good imaging. In special cases, sedative drugs may be given.

(b) Method selection. Transthoracic echocardiography works through the acoustic window (the sternum, the parasternal, and the xiphoid), which provides the best far-field resolution and the least near-field noise, although artifacts are induced due to the chest wall and lungs. Transesophageal echocardiography can reduce artifacts and acoustics from the chest wall and lungs and provide better imaging quality, especially for the mitral and aortic valves, but its visual field is often not as broad as that of transthoracic ultrasound.

2. Image acquisition
   (a) Steps After the target structure appears, the sound window is first optimized in the 2D plane, and the grayscale is adjusted to create obvious contrast between the blood and the heart muscle. At the same time, care should be taken not to excessively increase the tissue contrast to avoid reducing the resolution. The 4D ZOOM function is then used to obtain raw 3D DICOM data of the ROI and converted to DICOM format on the workstation [6, 7].
   (b) Cardiac cycle: Data acquisition for a single cardiac cycle avoids artifacts, but its image resolution is often unsatisfactory. Therefore, to obtain higher resolution images, it is more common to perform image acquisition in multiple cardiac cycles.
   (c) Range optimization: Locating the target anatomy before image acquisition and focusing on the target area during imaging can avoid unnecessary full-volume imaging of the heart and improve imaging quality.

2.1.3 Cardiac Magnetic Resonance

There are two main advantages of magnetic resonance imaging: higher temporal resolution and less radiation. Disadvantages are that inspection takes a long time and that this type of imaging is contraindicated for some patients [8].

1. Preparation
   - The primary consideration is excluding patients who are contraindicated for magnetic resonance examination. Patients with a cardiac pacemaker, defibrillator, or other metal implant that may be subjected to thermal or mechanical forces in a strong magnetic field are prohibited from undergoing magnetic resonance examination. In addition, cardiac stents, coils, or sternum lines cause significant artifacts in the images, and although they are not absolute contraindications, patients with such devices are not recommended when the purpose of imaging is for 3D modeling. Finally, other imaging modalities should also be considered for patients with renal insufficiency and sputum contrast allergies.
2. Imaging acquisition
   (a) Breathing and heart rate control. Sufficient breath holding time should be ensured during image acquisition to avoid motion artifacts. For patients such as infants or young children who are unable to cooperate, general anesthesia can be given in conjunction with an anesthesiologist.
   (b) Sequence selection 3D balanced steady-state free precession (bSSFP) and magnetic resonance angiography (MRA) are commonly used CMR 3D sequences, both of which are gradient echo sequences, i.e., "white blood" sequence without contrast agent and 0.7–2.0 mm omnidirectional voxels. They have good blood pool-myocardial contrast and have fewer motion and respiratory artifacts. Hu Liwei et al. showed that 3D-SSFP has higher spatial resolution than contrast-enhanced magnetic resonance angiography (CE-MRA) with the same scanning parameters. The 3D model constructed with the 3D-SSFP sequence can more clearly show the space of the right atrial septal obstruction. 3D-SSFP can be used as the preferred magnetic resonance sequence for constructing 3D models.

2.2 Model Reconstruction and Postprocessing

After DICOM format image data resources are collected, professional computer software is needed to complete the model reconstruction and postprocessing. The most commonly used commercial software, Mimics and 3-Matic, are produced by Materialise (Leuven, Belgium) and are run on the Windows operating system. Mimics has advanced manual, automatic, and semi-automatic image segmentation capabilities and can export files in STL format. 3-Matic is computer-aided design (CAD) software for model postprocessing. Here, we provide a brief introduction of the basic process of computer modeling and postprocessing of cardiovascular 3D printing based on Mimics and 3-Matic.

2.2.1 Model Reconstruction of Cardiovascular 3d Printing

1. Image preparation
   - After the original DICOM data are imported into Mimics software, the data set is composed. In addition to the original axial plane, the software automatically reconstructs the sagittal and coronal planes. We can view the images in three orthogonal cross sec-

tions (axial, sagittal, and coronal) (Fig. 2.1). The software can also adjust the position of three orthogonal planes according to need (Fig. 2.2), as the planes are not limited to their original positions.

2. Image segmentation
   - Image segmentation is the basis and key of computer three-dimensional reconstruction. The so-called image segmentation is the process of distinguishing different regions in an image and can also be understood as the process of combining the pixels with the same meaning in the image [9]. Pixels representing specific tissues (blood pools, myocardium) can be collected together in a group called a mask. Each mask can be combined or segmented with other masks. Several software functions are used in the process of image segmentation.

(a) Thresholding: Thresholding is usually the first step of image segmentation. The purpose is to preserve the pixels between the upper and lower boundary sets by the operator (Fig. 2.3). When image segmentation of

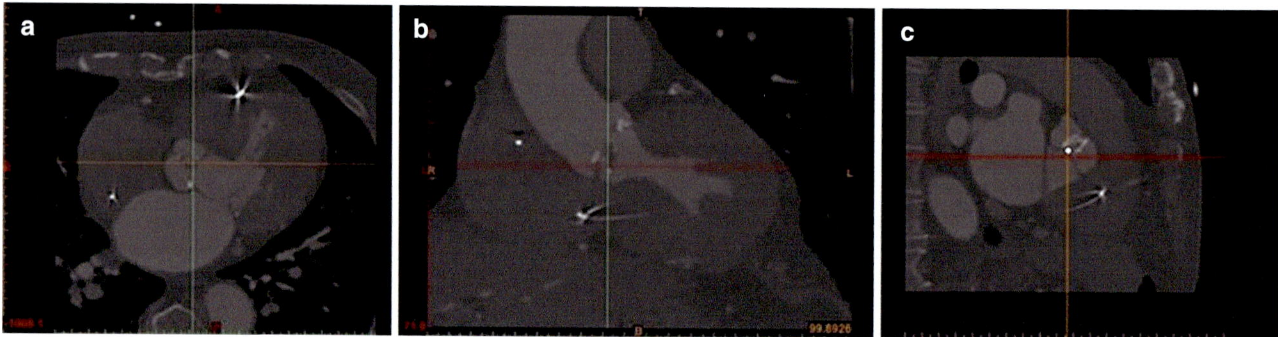

Fig. 2.1 After DICOM data are imported, three orthogonal sections can be viewed in the Mimics interface (**a**) axial plane; (**b**) coronal plane; (**c**) sagittal plane. Images were obtained from the Department of Cardiovascular Surgery of Xijing Hospital

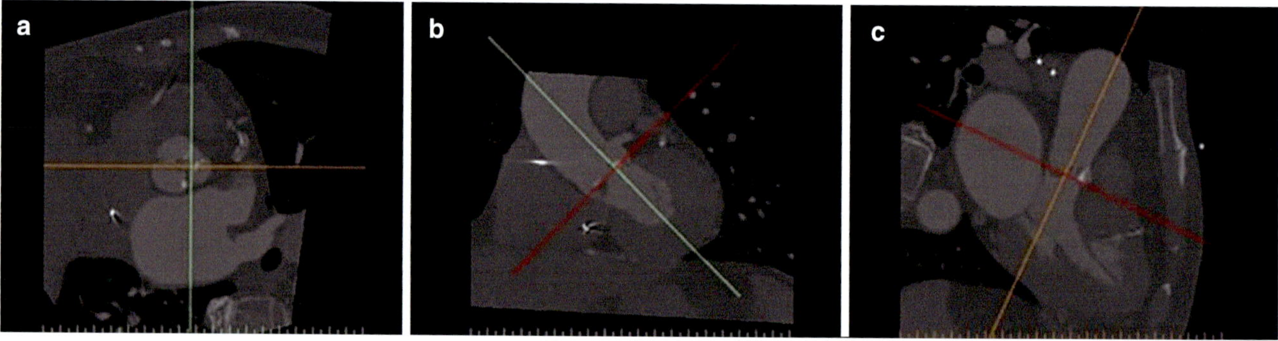

Fig. 2.2 To better display the structure of the aortic sinus, the image was reconstructed to obtain a new section. (**a**) axial plane; (**b**) coronal plane; (**c**) sagittal plane. Images were obtained from the Department of Cardiovascular Surgery of Xijing Hospital

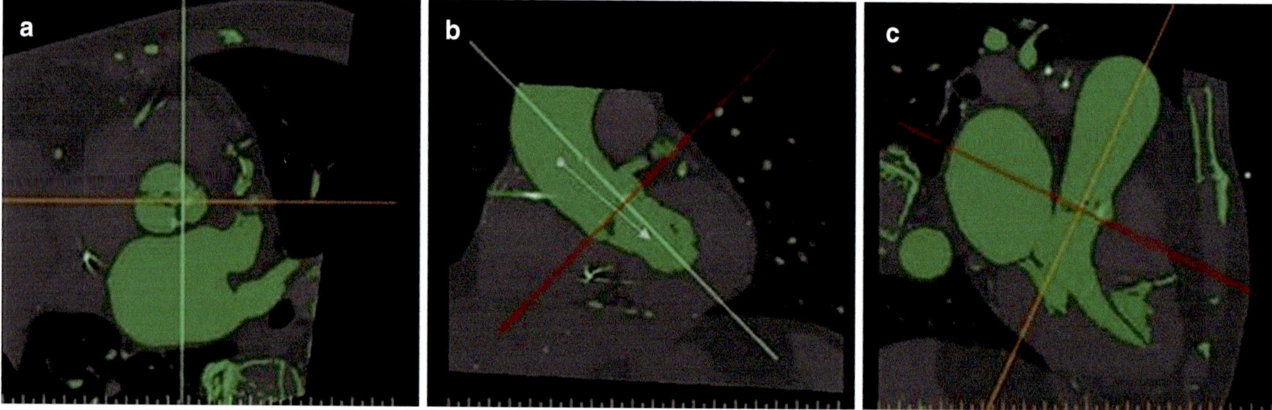

Fig. 2.3 All gray values between the upper and lower boundary are selected. (**a**) axial plane; (**b**) coronal plane; (**c**) sagittal plane. Images were obtained from the Department of Cardiovascular Surgery of Xijing Hospital

the heart is performed, the boundary is usually set according to the pixels of the blood pool or myocardium. Thresholding segmentation is easy to perform and can effectively segment tissues with different gray values. However, when the gray values of different tissues overlap with each other, such as myocardium and thymus, blood pool and bone, or blood pool and myocardium, the effect of thresholding segmentation is limited. At this time, the overlap can be eliminated by manually adjusting the range. Expanding the thresholding range can ensure that all target tissues are covered at the price of incorporating more unwanted ones. In contrast, narrowing the thresholding range will help exclude all unnecessary tissues but will also increase the risk of excluding target parts. Therefore, the adjustment should be performed by experienced operators to find the optimal threshold.

(b) Region growing: When the threshold processing is applied to an image, it will be selected regardless of whether each pixel is collected in the target organization. Region growing can divide the uncollected regions into subgroups and generate new masks. The basic principle is selecting the continuous part with the seed chosen by the operator. The "floating" pixels and discontinuous parts will be excluded from the mask (Fig. 2.4).

(c) Cropping: Cropping is used to remove redundant structures from image edges. For example, when only the heart image needs to be preserved, the arm, rib, and peripheral vascular can be removed laterally, the spine and sternum can be removed anteriorly and posteriorly, and the neck and abdomen can be removed up and down. Before cropping, the mouse must be carefully scrolled to observe the entire ROI to prevent the target structure from being cropped on an unviewed plane. Cropping can be performed on 2D images (see Fig. 2.5) or on virtual 3D reconstruction models.

(d) Mask splitting: The mask can be disassembled according to need, simplifying the following operation (Fig. 2.6).

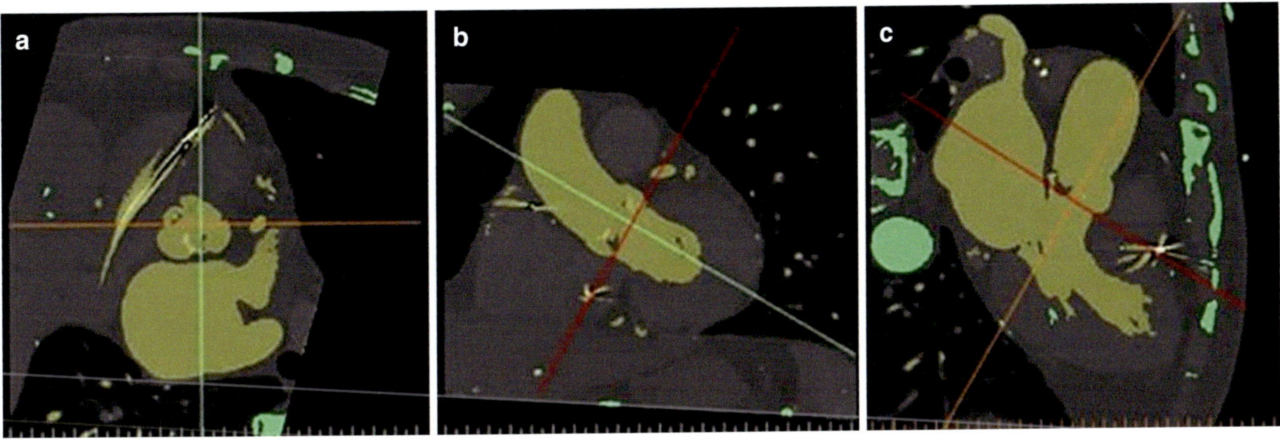

Fig. 2.4 Floating pixels and discontinuous parts (green parts) are excluded from the mask after region growth. (**a**) axial plane; (**b**) coronal plane; (**c**) sagittal plane. Images were obtained from the Department of Cardiovascular Surgery of Xijing Hospital

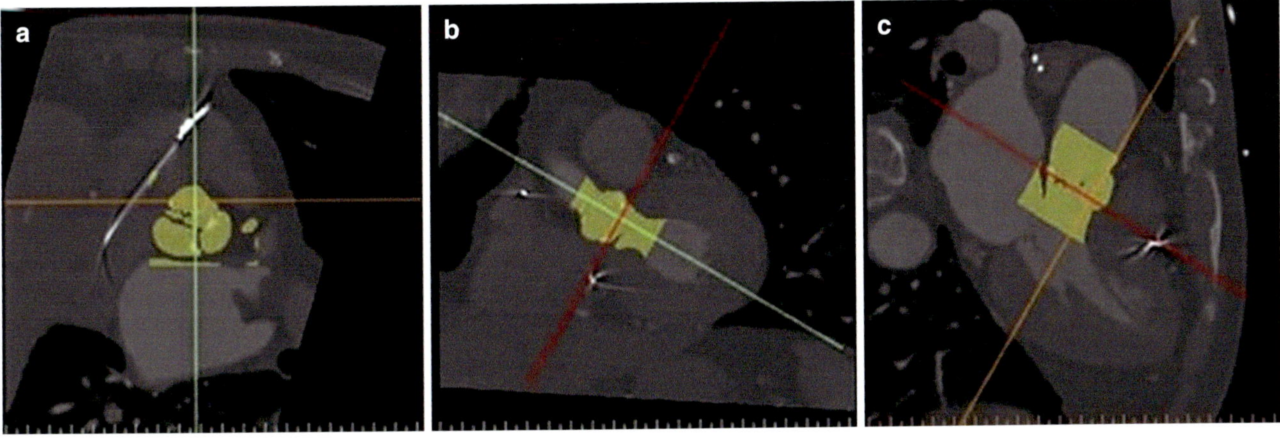

Fig. 2.5 Limit the target area to the aortic root structure by cropping. (**a**) axial plane; (**b**) coronal plane; (**c**) sagittal plane. Images were obtained from the Department of Cardiovascular Surgery of Xijing Hospital

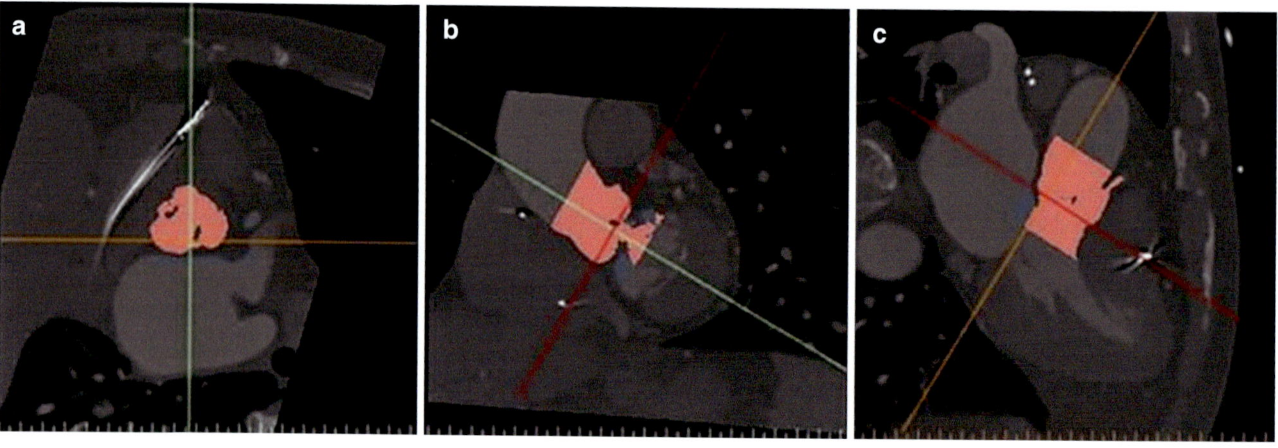

Fig. 2.6 The mask is divided into two parts: target structure (pink) and redundant structure (blue). (**a**) axial plane; (**b**) coronal plane; (**c**) sagittal plane. Images were obtained from the Department of Cardiovascular Surgery of Xijing Hospital

(e) Mask editing: After thresholding and region growing, further editing of the masks usually requires manual or semi-automatic operations. Due to the limitation of spatial resolution and the partial volume effect, the gray values of thin structures such as the atrial septum, septal membranes, valvular tissue, and surrounding tissues around strong artifacts such as calcification often lie between those of the myocardium and the blood pool. Automatic threshold segmentation technology cannot recognize these structures, and manual segmentation is usually needed at this time. In addition, due to the limited spatial resolution, the pixels of adjacent vascular tissues are usually similar. When the blood pool masks need to be distinguished, the role of regional growth is often limited, and the use of manual editing to remove the pixels of continuous areas can solve this problem very well. The most basic method of manual segmentation is to use cursors and shapes of different sizes as "brushes" or "erasers" to add or remove pixels directly from the mask (Fig. 2.7). A more complex method is to add threshold functions for these cursors, such as adding unmarked pixels whose gray values are within the threshold range, deleting marked pixels outside the threshold range of gray values, and so on.

(f) Multiple slice edit: Manual segmentation of slices is tedious and monotonous, especially for high-resolution images with many slices, as well as time-consuming and laborious. Multiple slice editing can extend the operation from a single slice to multiple adjacent slices, thus reducing the editing time. This operation can be performed on adjacent slices, or they can be edited by semi-automatic interpolation. The latter requires the operator to manually edit two discontinuous planes, and the software will automatically analyze the slices between them, which greatly reduces the workload. It should be noted that the multilayer editing operation can only be performed on the original orthogonal planes, not on the reconstructed section.

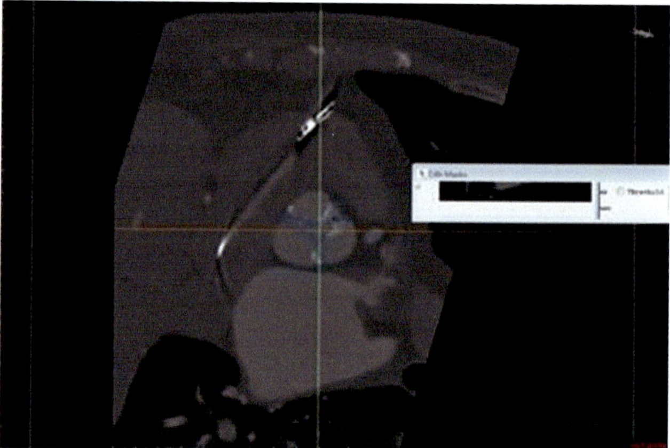

Fig. 2.7 Manual editing of the mask in the axial plane. Images were obtained from the Department of Cardiovascular Surgery of Xijing Hospital

(g) The segmented 3D mask can be visualized and edited (Fig. 2.8).

2.2.2 Postprocessing

After mask segmentation, data can be exported in the form of a 3D digital model through an STL file. STL is a file format that uses triangular meshes to represent 3D models. These files only contain the geometric shape of the 3D models but do not contain information about color or texture. STL files can theoretically be used for model printing, but in the actual operation process, STL files are usually imported into CAD software (such as 3-Matic, Magics, or other software) for postprocessing, such as for model repair or editing.

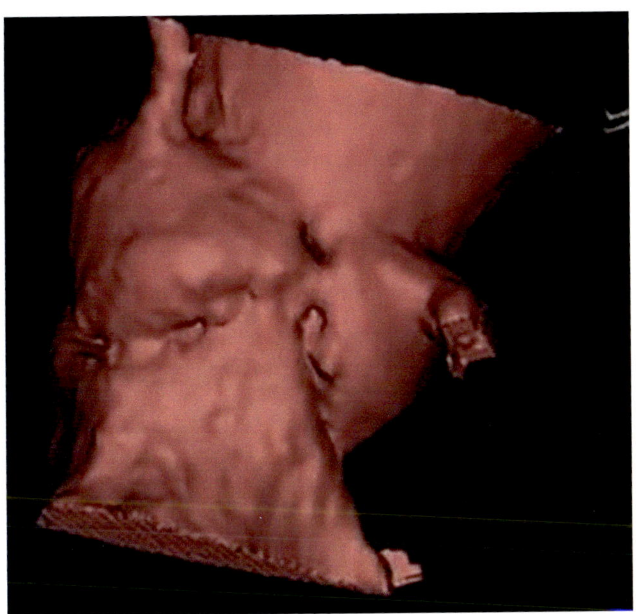

Fig. 2.8 Visualizes the segmented mask in 3D. Images were obtained from the Department of Cardiovascular Surgery of Xijing Hospital

The software functions needed in the postprocessing include editing or cutting the unnecessary parts of the graphics; beautifying and smoothing the details of the model; repairing the defects of the model; shelling the model to create a hollow cardiovascular model; splitting the model to observe the internal structure; combining models from different image sources; and adding text annotations to the model.

After the postprocessing of the STL file is completed, the final file can be reimported into Mimics software to confirm the accuracy.

2.3 3D Printing Technology of Cardiovascular Models

There are currently many printing technologies that can be used for 3D printing of cardiovascular models. Different technologies have their unique advantages and disadvantages in terms of accuracy, printing time, and material cost [10, 11]. Therefore, before 3D printing, the appropriate printer should be selected according to the nature of the model and the expected application. In recent decades, 3D printing technologies have made great progress and breakthroughs [12–18]. The following is an introduction to the technologies widely used in the cardiovascular field.

2.3.1 Fused Deposition Modeling (FDM)

By utilizing the thermoplastic materials that are melted after heating and solidified immediately after cooling, filamentous materials are melted and sprayed out through a micronozzle, which solidifies and deposits on the manufacturing platform. The product is formed by stacking the materials layer by layer. After the printer head is connected to the mechanical chassis, it can move quickly according to the required path under control of a computer to complete a layer of printing. Then, the head will move up by the height of one layer and continue to print the next layer. For a given model, the thicker the layer is, the less printing time needed and the rougher the printed model. In contrast, the thinner the layer height is, the longer the printing time and the more accurate the model. In the actual operation process, it is often necessary to compromise model accuracy for printing time [19, 20]. The mechanical strength of the model can be changed by adjusting the density of the thermoplastic filler to meet the requirements of different models.

Thermal factors dominate the FDM process. The temperature of the sprinkler should be set to at least 10 °C higher than the melting point of the material. For PLA and ABS, the temperature of the sprinkler should be approximately 30 °C higher. If the temperature is not high enough, the printing quality will be uneven. However, if it is too much higher than the melting point, the viscosity of the material will be reduced, and the resolidification time will be prolonged. Both of these factors affect the quality and reproducibility of products. The materials delivered to the nozzle in unit time depend on the printing speed. The faster the printing speed is, the shorter the residence time of materials in the nozzle and the shorter the heating time. Therefore, for machines that can set nozzle temperature, users should consider changing the nozzle temperature to avoid errors.

The resolution of FDM is usually proportional to the diameter of the nozzle orifice and the accuracy of shaft mechanical motion. The combination of these two factors results in a minimum print accuracy of 500 microns in entry-level FDM printers and an accuracy of 20–50 microns in professional printers. The minimum theoretical printable characteristic width is approximately the diameter of the nozzle hole. In practice, the characteristics of a single filament may be too subtle to be retained in the printing or postprocessing steps. The minimum layer thickness also corresponds to the diameter of the nozzle. Products generated by FDM have a visible surface ladder structure, and very fine details can be obtained without postprocessing. The common orifice diameter is 200–500 microns, but according to relevant reports, nozzle orifices of 50 microns or smaller have been produced.

For products with supporting materials, if a smoother, real surface or a more suitable size is needed, postprocessing is required [21]. Postprocessing mainly involves removing the supporting materials by mechanical manipulation (physically crushing, peeling, etc.) or dissolving the materials in solution. Thus, the model can be made more realistic by manual grinding, use of a cleaning agent, steam treatment, or postprocessing operations, and the model can be further refined by grinding or filing. The advantage of FDM printers is their ability to print a wide variety of materials, which differs from other 3D printing technologies that are limited to a single category of materials; any material with thermoplastic ability can be used by FDM printers. Second, the printing cost is relatively low, and the printing speed is not slow. The biggest disadvantage of this technology is that the accuracy of the printing model is not high, and the printed products only roughly exhibit the appearance of the model [22]. When high precision or complex anatomical structures need to be printed, its application is often limited.

2.3.2 Selective Laser Sintering (SLS)

Selective laser sintering (SLS) uses infrared laser as energy. Under the command of a computer control system, the powder materials sprayed on the operating platform are sintered layer by layer selectively to complete model printing. The powder to be sintered is placed on a heating bed, heated to a temperature slightly below the melting point, and then spread onto a flat surface through the powder roll. The path of laser sintering is transformed from the STL file, which is automatically recognized and optimized by the machine to achieve a uniform temperature distribution and a short construction time [23]. The laser beam is guided by a lens and a reflecting mirror, and the set path is directionally patterned by the laser beam to the powder bed so that the paved powder can be melted into a solid [24]. After the layer is finished, the platform descends a distance of one layer, and the supply bed connecting the material container is raised to provide the powder source for the next layer. The powder roller then lays the preheated powder onto the newly formed surface, and the powder layer is smoothed before the next pattern is printed so that the remaining powder can act as support for the next layer [25].

The resolution of SLS printers depends on the type of powder used, the sensitivity of laser optical device, the machine power, and the machine parameters. Compared with other 3D printing technologies, SLS has medium resolution [26, 27]. Resolution in the X–Y plane mainly depends on the laser optical device, which is determined by the spot size and the thermal conductivity of materials. The Z-direction resolution is determined by the thickness of the selected layer, usually in the range of 50 to 200 microns. The overall construction size is determined by the size of the powder bed. Sizes range from 200 mm × 250 mm × 300 mm to 700 mm × 400 mm × 600 mm. Because the printer bed must satisfy the actual size of the products, the actual expected size of the 3D-printed model must be considered in advance when selecting the printer. Of course, the larger the printer bed is, the more powder is consumed. Recycling and reuse of sintered powders has become a hot topic in recent research. Suppliers will provide this paid service to customers in need. Unsintered powders may have been exposed to high temperatures, resulting in deviations in material properties. Therefore, suppliers provide guidelines to avoid low resolution of printed products due to the use of recycled powders.

The length of printing time depends on the laser grating speed, powder resurfacing efficiency, printing layer thickness, geometric size, and direction. Recently developed SLS machines are able to print 700 cm^3/h, which has greatly improved the speed of printing products. The X–Y axis velocity depends on the laser grating, which is relatively fast because the laser speed is usually on the order of 2–6 m/s. In contrast, construction in the Z-direction is very slow, requiring the physical processes of supplying new consumable material and rolling the material into a smooth surface for printing the next layer of patterns. Progress in the Z-direction is a key factor, and thus, reducing the number of layers will greatly reduce the printing time. The shortest axial dimension of the parts to be printed should be placed on the Z axis to minimize the total number of layers required (such as horizontal printing of slender objects).

After printing, there is no need to deal with any supporting materials; only the loose powder attached to the surface needs to be removed. Usually, this process can be performed with a soft brush or pressurized air flow. The surface of the products discharged from the furnace is relatively rough and needs to be polished or chemically treated later. The surface layer may also be filled with microholes. If a nonporous surface is needed, it is usually filled with a thin by-product polymer layer, which can smooth the finished product surface and reduce the polishing workload. Baking is usually used to improve mechanical properties.

SLS printing costs are higher than those of FDM printing. Machine costs are medium to high levels ($100,000+ USD), while powder consumables are relatively low in cost ($50–150 per kilogram). The operation of the SLS printer must comply with the highest standard of safe operation of a high-power laser system.

2.3.3 Color Inkjet Printing (CJP)

Color inkjet printing technology is similar to laser sintering [28]. It is also a powder-based 3D printing technology. Gypsum particles or acrylate powder are first spread on the platform by a drum, and then, a transparent liquid binder is sprayed through the printing nozzle to bind the powder materials together [29]. At the same time, the color inkjet printing head selectively sprays the color binder on the material according to the settings. The principle is the same as that of ink deposited on paper. Printing is carried out layer by layer until the model is completed. Color inkjet printing technology is now available for complete printing of full-color models.

2.3.4 Stereolithography (SLA)

Stereolithography is the earliest and most mature 3D printing technology [30, 31]. SLA printers use a specific wavelength of ultraviolet laser to selectively solidify liquid resin for printing [32]. Liquid resins usually consist of three components: oligomers/monomers, crosslinkers, and photoinitiators. Different components endow materials with different properties: oligomers are usually some form of acrylate molecules, which mainly provide optical transmission, color, and chemical reaction characteristics of materials. Crosslinkers keep long chains of polymer molecules together and mainly provide mechanical properties; photoinitiators mainly act as catalysts. When materials are exposed to appropriate wavelengths of light, photoinitiators will catalyze transverse elongation and vertical crosslinking of oligomer/monomer precursors to complete curing. Among them, the level of photoinitiator is usually stable in the material to ensure the appropriate polymerization rate, while the level of the other two components can be properly adjusted to meet the different requirements for the mechanical strength and hardness of the model.

In the SLA process, resin grooves are prepared for liquid photopolymers, and when exposed to a sufficiently small wavelength, the photopolymer can be polymerized to form solids [33]. A UV laser or other light is guided to the surface of the liquid resin bath through the lens and a reflector, and the local resin is polymerized to form a solid 2D layer. Then, the construction platform drops one layer to the resin tank, and the depth of the solidified layer is equal to the thickness of one layer. At the end of each layer, the wiper passes through the resin surface to make it uniform and prepare for the printing of the next layer. This process is repeated until the model is printed. Recently, a low-cost and faster continuous liquid interface production (CLIP) printing method was developed. There is a projection window at the bottom of the resin groove, and the ultraviolet image is projected into the resin through the bottom of the resin groove to induce the polymerization reaction. Prints are constructed from the bottom up and are lifted vertically from the resin tank by the construction platform layer by layer, rather than descending to the resin tank layer by layer such as in SLA. CLIP has many advantages: It can create the next surface layer without scraper movement or printing platform compensation, and the printing speed becomes faster because it only needs to cover the thin layer rather than immersing in the resin bath as a whole; thus, the liquid resin needed for printing is also reduced.

The resolution of SLA is mainly affected by the lens accuracy of the guided laser, the optical characteristics of the light source, and the properties of the optical polymer [34]. The X–Y resolution is usually 75 microns, while the Z resolution is usually 25 microns. For the CLIP-based method, the total construction volume is determined by the volume of the bath block, the window area, and the traveling height of the base plate. The common SLA construction quantity is 1500 mm × 750 mm × 550 mm, while commercial CLIP is 190 mm × 120 mm × 325 mm.

SLA is considered to be the fastest 3D printing method due to the moving speed of SLA and the simultaneous projection and rapid aggregation of DLP [35]. In addition, although the projection pattern is still printed layer by layer, CLIP does not require wipers and works continuously, so the printing speed is increased. If lower resolution is acceptable, the larger laser spot can cover some detailed features in each level of the construction plane, and the construction time will be further reduced.

SLA posttreatment includes removal of support materials, surface modification, and postcuring [36]. In the traditional resin groove mode, the support is usually needed throughout the entire printing process to prevent excessive draping between layers. This is the same for CLIP. The platform supports the weight of the print when it pulls in the liquid. Chemical reagents such as isopropanol can be used to remove the excess resin adhering to the surface and make the surface smooth. Postcuring usually refers to exposing the newly formed cured material to strong ultraviolet radiation and/or placing it in an oven at an appropriate temperature (e.g., <120 C) to react with the residual reactive groups in the printed matter to enhance the mechanical properties and long-term durability of the printed product. Postcuring mainly depends on the chemical properties of the materials.

In terms of cost and other factors, the average price of SLA printers is more than that of FDM printers. Photopolymer resin materials are also relatively expensive and have a shorter quality guarantee period. Storing in a dry environment and avoiding light exposure can prolong the service life of the resin. SLA machines are widely used in the cardiovascular field because of their simple operation and high accuracy. The advantages of SLA printers include a high printing accuracy and the excellent surface smoothness of the product, but the application of SLA for printing complex models is limited because of its inability to combine other types of materials.

2.3.5 Material Jetting (MJ)

MJ printers use a technology that selectively deposits droplet materials on the construction bed to create 3D structures. Polyjet (PJ) is a subtype of MJ. The resin used in PJ is a photopolymer [37]. Non-optical polymers such as low melting point wax can be added to the common MJ consumables palette, whereas PJ can only use liquid optical polymer consumables. The technology is known for its high resolution, complex details, smooth surfaces, multimaterial and multicolor printing, and diversity in mechanical properties of products from rigid to flexible and tough. However, similar to SLA, the mechanical properties of products may degrade over time. The toner and resolution of materials, i.e., the color and hardness of products, are the most distinctive features of this process in bio-tissue printing, and they are also the most critical features in medical applications. The printer can deposit many types of materials at the same time so that this type of printer can not only maintain model accuracy but also print various complex geometric models. By changing the proportion of materials with different properties, the mechanical strength of the model can also be adjusted [38].

MJ/PJ process: MJ printers use two input materials: the construction material and a low melting point wax support material. PJ printers can use two or more types of input materials, one or more construction materials, and again a support material. In MJ, the construction material is heated and sprayed onto the construction platform with a cooling function and then solidified. In PJ, the printing head sprays photopolymer droplets onto an X–Y platform with UV light, and the layer is cured by the light. The platform descends the thickness of one layer, prepares for deposition of the next layer, and coordinates the movement of the droplet spraying with the platform.

The resolution of MJ depends on the resolution of the inkjet printing head, the physical properties of the droplets, and the curing kinetics of the photopolymer. Inkjet printers are similar to commercial paper printers and can reach up to 600 dots per inch. The physical properties, viscosity, and surface tension of the resin determine the diffusion mode of droplets in contact with the constructed bed or the upper deposited surface. The melt resin in MJ will cool rapidly during deposition, but the photopolymer in PJ remains liquid until it is exposed to UV light, leading to uncontrollability of droplet diffusion and loss of resolution. Some professional equipment will roll out the photopolymer layer before UV curing to make the Z plane more uniform and improve the resolution of the next layer. Some upgraded professional printers and consumable systems have a resolution of 40 μm in the X–Y direction, a resolution of 15 μm in the Z-direction, and a total construction volume of 520 mm × 380 mm × 300 mm.

Although MJ has a good resolution, its printing speed is the slowest among all three-dimensional printing methods. The construction time depends on the geometry and direction of the object, the selected resolution, and the kinds of materials. To obtain high X–Y resolution, the droplet layer thickness is usually only approximately 15 microns. Although this high Z-direction resolution has advantages, numerous layers lead to very slow vertical construction speeds. Therefore, it is recommended that users place the shortest axial dimension in the Z-direction to reduce the construction time. However, there are exceptions: additional supporting materials needed to replace direction printing will also increase the construction time.

Postprocessing of the products developed using this printing technology is relatively easy. If the profile of the supporting material is required, the supporting material is mechanically removed either by melting (for MJ) or by a solution bath (for PJ). The surface quality of the product is usually fine enough without polishing. The surface of the area that contacted the supporting material will not be lustrous, in sharp contrast to the surfaces of the other parts. It is recommended that most PJ materials be cured under an ultraviolet lamp or in a moderately heated oven.

MJ or PJ is the most expensive of all three-dimensional printing methods, and the machine is also the most expensive. Its advantages lie in its easy operation, high resolution, and ability to incorporate complex details. In addition, multimaterial and multicolor printing is especially suitable for displaying the local structure of the cardiovascular system. The large diversity of mechanical properties from rigid to flexible and tough objects is also useful for in vitro simulation and testing of cardiovascular models, which has broad application prospects. New materials for this technology are still being developed, and the price is gradually reducing to more acceptable levels.

2.4 Scientific Selection of 3D Printers

The three-dimensional printing techniques listed above can be used to print heart models. However, a certain printer technology may be more suitable than others for specific printing purposes. When deciding which to use, several factors must be considered, including the cost of printers and materials, printing accuracy, the method of adding supporting materials, and printing speed. Although the accuracy of FDM printers is poor, the cost is low. FDM is suitable for model printing with low resolution. The printing accuracy and resolution of SLA printers are ideal, and transparent model printing can also be carried out. Disadvantages of SLA are its high printing cost and the method for adding supporting materials, which limits the printing of complex heart models. Photopolymer inkjet printers retain a high resolution similar to SLA while overcoming the disadvantage of being unable to print complex structures; however, their cost is the highest among all printing technologies. An advantage of the ColorJet printer is its ability of color printing, which can help highlight the special parts of the model, such as the surgical incision path, the anatomy of arteries and veins, congenital defects, and infarct areas. Importantly, 3D printing of multi-materials and multicolors has broad applications for use in in vitro tests and in the cardiovascular field.

References

1. Wang L, Feng Y. Research and implementation of DICOM data for 3D printing. China Med Equip. 2015;30:79–81.
2. Halliburton S, Arbab-Zadeh A, Dey D, Einstein AJ, Gentry R, George RT, Gerber T, Mahesh M, Weigold WG. State-of-the-art in CT hardware and scan modes for cardiovascular CT. J Cardiovasc Comput Tomogr. 2012;6:154–63.
3. Buijs SB, Barentsz MW, Smits MLJ, Gratama JWC, Spronk PE. Safety and efficacy of pressure-limited power injection of iodinated contrast medium through central lines in children. Am J Roentgenol. 2007;188:726–32.
4. Han B, Lindberg J, Overman D, Schwartz R, Grant K, Lesser J. Safety and accuracy of dual-source coronary computed tomography angiography in the pediatric population. J Cardiovasc Comput Tomogr. 2012;6:252–9.
5. Han BK, Rigsby CK, Leipsic J, Bardo D, Abbara S, Ghoshhajra B, Lesser JR, Raman SV, Crean AM, Nicol ED, Siegel MJ, Hlavacek A. Computed tomography imaging in patients with congenital heart disease, Part 2: technical recommendations. An expert consensus document of the society of cardiovascular computed tomography (SCCT): endorsed by the society of pediatric radiology (SPR) and the North American Society of Cardiac Imaging (NASCI). J Cardiovasc Comput Tomogr. 2015;9:493–513.
6. Lang RM, Badano LP, Tsang W, Adams DH, Agricola E, Buck T, Faletra FF, Franke A, Hung J, LPd I, Kamp O, Kasprzak JD, Lancellotti P, Marwick TH, ML MC, Monaghan MJ, Nihoyannopoulos P, Pandian NG, Pellikka PA, Pepi M, Roberson DA, Shernan SK, Shirali GS, Sugeng L, FJT C, Vannan MA, Zamorano JL, Zoghbi WA. EAE/ASE recommendations for image acquisition and display using three-dimensional echocardiography. Eur Heart J Cardiovasc Imaging. 2012;13:1–46.
7. Lang RM, Badano LP, Tsang W, Adams DH, Agricola E, Buck T, Faletra FF, Franke A, Hung J, Pérez De Isla L, Kamp O, Kasprzak JD, Lancellotti P, Marwick TH, ML MC, Monaghan MJ, Nihoyannopoulos P, Pandian NG, Pellikka PA, Pepi M, Roberson DA, Shernan SK, Shirali GS, Sugeng L, Ten Cate FJ, Vannan MA, Zamorano JL, Zoghbi WA. EAE/ASE recommendations for image acquisition and display using three-dimensional echocardiography. J Am Soc Echocardiogr. 2012;25:3–46.
8. Hundley WG, Bluemke DA, Finn JP, Flamm SD, Fogel MA, Friedrich MG, Ho VB, Jerosch-Herold M, Kramer CM, Manning WJ, Patel M, Pohost GM, Stillman AE, White RD, Woodard PK. ACCF/ACR/AHA/NASCI/SCMR 2010 expert consensus document on cardiovascular magnetic resonance. A report of the American College of Cardiology Foundation Task Force on Expert Consensus Documents. J Am Coll Cardiol. 2010;55:2614–62.
9. Byrne N, Forte MV, Valverde AT, Hussain T. A systematic review of image segmentation methodology, used in the additive manufacture of patient-specific 3D printed models of the cardiovascular system. JRSM Cardiovasc Dis. 2016;5:1–9.
10. Xinling L. 3D printer and its working principle. Netw Inf. 2012;26:30.
11. Changzheng W, Xiaolong L. Principle and application of 3D printing. Digit Technol Appl. 2014:93.
12. Tumbleston JR, Shirvanyants D, Ermoshkin N, Janusziewicz R, Johnson AR, Kelly D, Chen K, Pinschmidt R, Rolland JP, Ermoshkin A, Samulski ET, DeSimone JM. Continuous liquid interface production of 3D objects. Science. 2015;347:1349–52.
13. Xie B, Parkhill RL, Warren WL, Smay JE. Direct writing of three-dimensional polymer scaffolds using colloidal gels. Adv Funct Mater. 2006;16:1685–93.
14. Billiet T, Vandenhaute M, Schelfhout J, Van Vlierberghe S, Dubruel P. A review of trends and limitations in hydrogel-rapid prototyping for tissue engineering. Biomaterials. 2012;33:6020–41.
15. Wan Y. Principles and prospects of 3D printing construction technology. J Beijing Univ Architec. 2015;4:1081–3.
16. Janusziewicz R, Tumbleston JR, Quintanilla AL, Mecham SJ, DeSimone JM. Layerless fabrication with continuous liquid interface production. Proc Natl Acad Sci U S A. 2016;113:11703–8.
17. Tian X, Liu T, Yang C, Wang Q, Li D. Interface and performance of 3D printed continuous carbon fiber reinforced PLA composites. Compos Part A Appl Sci Manuf. 2016;88:198–205.
18. Yap YL, Wang C, Sing SL, Dikshit V, Yeong WY, Wei J. Material jetting additive manufacturing: an experimental study using designed metrological benchmarks. Precis Eng. 2017;50:275–85.
19. Mohamed OA, Masood SH, Bhowmik JL. Optimization of fused deposition modeling process parameters: a review of current research and future prospects. Adv Manuf. 2015;3;42–53.
20. Turner BN, Gold SA. A review of melt extrusion additive manufacturing processes: II. Materials, dimensional accuracy, and surface roughness. Rapid Prototyp J. 2015;21:250–61.
21. Cunico MWM, Cunico MM, Cavalheiro PM, Carvalho JD. Investigation of additive manufacturing surface smoothing process. Rapid Prototyp J. 2017;23:201–8.
22. Pandey PM, Venkata Reddy N, Dhande SG. Improvement of surface finish by staircase machining in fused deposition modeling. J Mater Process Technol. 2003;132:323.
23. Lexow MM, Drexler M, Drummer D. Fundamental investigation of part properties at accelerated beam speeds in the selective laser sintering process. Rapid Prototyp J. 2017;23:1099–106.
24. Kruth J-P, Mercelis P, Van Vaerenbergh J, Froyen L, Rombouts M. Binding mechanisms in selective laser sintering and selective laser melting. Rapid Prototyp J. 11:26–36.
25. Yadroitsev I, Shishkovsky I, Bertrand P, Smurov I. Manufacturing of fine-structured 3D porous filter elements by selective laser melting. Appl Surf Sci. 2009;255:5523–7.
26. Guo J, Bai J, Liu K, Wei J. Surface quality improvement of selective laser sintered polyamide 12 by precision grinding and magnetic field-assisted finishing. Mater Des. 2018;138:39–45.
27. Shen F, Yuan S, Chua CK, Zhou K. Development of process efficiency maps for selective laser sintering of polymeric composite powders: modeling and experimental testing. J Mater Process Technol. 2018;254:52–9.
28. Derby B. Inkjet printing of functional and structural materials: fluid property requirements, feature stability, and resolution. Annu Rev Mater Res. 2010;40:395–414.
29. Hardin JO, Ober TJ, Valentine AD, Lewis JA. Microfluidic printheads for multimaterial 3D printing of viscoelastic inks. Adv Mater. 2015;27:3279–84.
30. Greil GF, Wolf I, Kuettner A, Fenchel M, Miller S, Martirosian P, Schick F, Oppitz M, Meinzer H-P, Sieverding L. Stereolithographic reproduction of complex cardiac morphology based on high spatial resolution imaging. Clin Res Cardiol. 2007;96:176–85.
31. Melchels FPW, Feijen J, Grijpma DW. A review on stereolithography and its applications in biomedical engineering. Biomaterials. 2010;31:6121–30.
32. Zheng X, Lee H, Weisgraber TH, Shusteff M, DeOtte J, Duoss EB, Kuntz JD, Biener MM, Ge Q, Jackson JA, Kucheyev SO, Fang NX, Spadaccini CM. Ultralight, ultrastiff mechanical metamaterials. Science. 2014;344:1373–7.
33. Stansbury JW, Idacavage MJ. 3D printing with polymers: challenges among expanding options and opportunities (conference paper). Dent Mater. 2016;32:54–64.

34. Watters MP, Bernhardt ML. Curing parameters to improve the mechanical properties of stereolithographic printed specimens. Rapid Prototyp J. 2018;24:46–51.
35. Campbell I, Combrinck J, Beer DD, Barnard L. Stereolithography build time estimation based on volumetric calculations. Rapid Prototyp J. 2008;14:271–9.
36. Kazemi M, Rahimi A. Supports effect on tensile strength of the stereolithography parts. Rapid Prototyp J. 2015;21:79–88.
37. Kumar K, Kumar GS. An experimental and theoretical investigation of surface roughness of poly-jet printed parts. Virtual Phys Prototyp. 2015;10:23–34.
38. Yang H, Lim JC, Liu Y, Qi X, Yap YL, Dikshit V, Yeong WY, Wei J. Performance evaluation of project multi-material jetting 3D printer. Virtual Phys Prototyp. 2017;12:95–103.

Selection of Cardiovascular 3D Printing Materials

3

Meng Yang, Jing Wang, Lanlan Li, and Alex Pui-Wai Lee

3D printing materials are an important factor in the development of 3D printing technique in the cardiovascular field; however, the type and quality of materials for 3D printing remain a challenge. At present, polymeric materials and biomaterials are the ones mainly applied in the 3D printing cardiovascular field [1]. Of them, polymeric materials are mainly used currently to make cardiovascular demonstration models, preoperative planning models, and training tools, and their tissue mechanical property fidelity is the key [2–4]. The bio-printing materials are mostly used to manufacture the consumable items, such as stent, valve, tissue engineered scaffold, and other consumable items that can mimic physiological function of the heart [5, 6]. Therefore, the future development direction of cardiovascular medical 3D printing will focus on bio-printing that can generate the circulatory system, which can transport blood and nutrients.

3.1 Synthetic Materials

So far, synthetic materials have met the majority of requirements for cardiovascular medical 3D printing; for instance, they are used to make the preoperative visual 3D model and the models used in in vitro testing, and most of them can be realized using the commercially available polymers. The mechanical properties of cardiovascular 3D printing materials are mainly measured through the elastic modulus (E), which can determine the materials more suitable for preparing the tissue structure. The mechanical property (except for calcification) of most cardiac tissues lies within the range of 0.01 MPa–100 MPa, and soft materials, especially those with an elastic modulus within such range, have then become the most applied among all synthetic materials at present. The mechanical properties of cardiac tissue are extremely complicated (nonlinearity and anisotropy); besides, age, past medical history, and tissue condition vary from different individuals. Therefore, the mechanical features of each patient's cardiac tissue should be taken into consideration to prepare the most realistic heart model. Generally, healthy myocardial tissue is thicker and softer ($E \approx 0.02$ MPa −0.5 MPa), whereas the pathological tissues may become harder. In addition, the artery is slightly harder ($\approx$0.1 MPa–10 MPa), and its property is different at various positions (namely, carotid artery is usually softer than coronary artery). Moreover, chordae tendineae and valve leaflet are harder, with the secant elastic modulus of about 100 MPa under tension [7]. Finally, calcifications have the greatest hardness, which ranges from 100 MPa up to 10GPa depending on the composition.

3.1.1 Commercial Material System

The products printed by rigid polymer materials are mainly used for visualization or preoperative examination, and numerous commercial materials are suitable. In the fused deposition modeling (FDM) printer, the classical materials, such as acrylonitrile-butadiene-styrene (ABS), polylactic acid (PLA), and polyvinyl alcohol (PVA), are used, which are the non-elastic materials with considerable rigidity.

As for the photo-curing technique, such as material jetting (MJ) or stereolithography apparatus (SLA) printer, the specific property of each resin may be slightly different, but on the whole, the consumable item is generally a certain type

M. Yang
Aviation College of Xi'an Jiaotong University, Xi'an, China

J. Wang
National Innovation Center for Additional Materials Manufacturing, Xi'an, China

L. Li
Xijing Hospital, Xi'an, China

A. P.-W. Lee (✉)
Division of Cardiology, Department of Medicine and Therapeutics, The Chinese University of Hong Kong, Hong Kong, China

Laboratory of Cardiac Imaging and 3D Printing, Li Ka Shing Institute of Health Science; Department of Medicine and Therapeutics, Faculty of Medicine, The Chinese University of Hong Kong, Hong Kong, China
e-mail: alexpwlee@cuhk.edu.hk

J. Yang et al. (eds.), *Cardiovascular 3D Printing*, https://doi.org/10.1007/978-981-15-6957-9_3

of acrylic ester/methacrylate. Such materials are eligible and can even realize multi-color printing if the printer has enough resolution. A small fraction of printers use tough materials (also referred to as the stress, $\varepsilon > 10\%$), which are appropriate for printing 3D models with stronger function. For instance, the thermoplastic polyurethane (TPU) powder is suitable for the selective laser sintering (SLS) printer.

Other materials, such as the carbamate-acrylic ester material system (like Stratasys tango), are mainly used in the PolyJet printer. They also have compatibility with the rigid acrylic ester material system, so these two materials can be mixed with each other for multimaterial printing. The carbamate-acrylic ester material system and the rigid acrylic ester material system are the best to prepare realistic cardiac anatomical models, and the models printed by mixing these two materials have been applied in demonstrating various cardiovascular physiological processes. These models suggest that the commercial 3D printing systems can construct some complicated heart models, yet they have some drawbacks. When printing at the wall thickness of <1.5 mm, the obtained products may be associated with the problems of poor mechanical stability, hardly removable supporting material, and rough grain on surface. These problems are added to the already difficult process of printing a realistic model, especially for the vascular ones. Recently, a novel 3D printing technique utilized the carbon elastomeric polyurethane and silicone to overcome these limitations using a single lens reflex (SLR), which can attain superb durability even at a wall thickness of only hundreds of micrometers. In addition, this method requires no removal of the supporting material and has a smooth internal wall. Nonetheless, its major disadvantage is that it does not allow for multimaterial printing, and thereby the model cannot manifest the complexity of the complete and realistic cardiac tissue.

The abovementioned material systems have some really useful features, but soft materials (low elastic modulus, $E < 1$ MPa) should be used to realize the complex mechanical properties, as well as the superb sensing-execution system and realistic cellular function of a real living tissue. Typically, a large number of sophisticated exclusive devices are required, which is the hot topic in current academic research [8–10].

3.1.2 Elastomers

Elastomers are a kind of polymeric network materials with low crosslinking density, this peculiar molecular structure enables them to have high scalability (ultimate strain, εult = 100%–1500%), and the material can also easily recover its initial shape after removing the external force [11]. Such polymers have extremely low glass transition temperature (GTT, Tg <25 °C), and thus, they can be soft and tough under room temperature. The elastic modulus of soft cardiac tissue can range from KPa to MPa, and the elastomer materials are the hot materials for printing cardiac tissue. Most elastomers for biomedical printing are based on polyurethane (PU), poly-dimethyl siloxane (PDMS), or hydrogel. The chemical property, printing method, and environmental factor of the resin selected have a great influence on the network elasticity of the obtained polymer, and as a result, the mechanical properties of elastomeric material products obtained under different conditions have an extremely large span.

PU is generally formed by the reaction between polyols and isocyanate, and multiple properties can be produced depending on the number of side chain introduced during reaction. PU can be classified as thermoplastic PU and thermosetting PU according to the molecular interaction in the PU structure. For instance, Ninjaflex is a kind of FDM-compatible thermoplastic PU (TPU) filament, which can be fused and extruded. Direct ink writing (DIW) can print PU particles in an aqueous dispersion, which when used in combination with SLA can satisfy the requirements of softness ($\approx$2.5 MPa) and thin wall (<200 mm) simultaneously. Moreover, the products can even be integrated into cells or tissues as long as the used PU material is non-cytotoxic. On this account, the PU products are generally used in manufacturing catheter sheaths, medical balloons, and other blood-contacting medical devices.

PDMS (siloxane) is another common elastomer, which tends to maintain elasticity within a large deformation band, while PU is inclined to plastic deformation. In brief, PDMS is softer and has greater elasticity than PU. PDMS resin is formed through an hydroxylation and condensation reaction in the presence of catalyst, and, for this reason, many bi-component mixtures containing liquid siloxane will mix and cure within several hours. PDMS cannot be used in FDM, but PDMS resin materials are quite suitable for DIW and SLR. Taking the above factors into consideration, the main feature of PDMS resin material is to form a thin-walled soft model through dip coating or to replicate a 3D printing template used for molding, so as to manufacture both a heart model and a flow model.

Hydrogel is a very versatile material, and it is possible to adjust its crosslinking density, molecular bonding, and swelling degree to customize its mechanical property within a wide range [12, 13]. For example, the elastic modulus of hydrogel can be as low as several KPa and hydrogel can also be used as a cell transport agent. Typically, the commonly used chemicals used to prepare the hydrogel are acrylic ester/methacrylate, as they can easily develop the polymerization reaction with the free radicals [14]. In this way, it is possible to manufacture a light-cured resin compatible with DIW and SLR printers. Recently, scientists have invented a novel hydrogel with high toughness based on the "ion-covalent linkage technique" and "dual-network" method, but its sensitivity to humidity has resulted in its more demanding working conditions, and additional packaging is usually needed [15].

3.1.3 Layer Materials

The cardiac tissue printed using the abovementioned homogeneous materials can get only close to the physical property of a real cardiac tissue, but the real tissue itself is far more complicated. For instance, arterial wall can be divided into three layers, namely, endothelial cell layer, muscle cell layer, and elastic and collagen fiber layer. Difference in interlayer structure, together with the directionality of collagen fiber in tunica externa, results in the asymmetry and nonlinearity of atrial tissues, which are closely related to the arterial function. It is noteworthy that an artery can minimize the tissue injury under some excessive dilation conditions, and the underlying mechanism has been described in related research on nonlinear "J-shaped strain stress curve." Currently, most 3D printers can only construct the macroscopic multilayer structure, but the hierarchical structure unit dimension of cardiac tissue is lower than the resolution of most 3D printers (submicron to millimeter scale). Therefore, for layered materials, attention should be paid to materials whose physiochemical properties are suitable for printing or to those that can be printed in the multiscale hierarchical structure, modifying the printing manner if necessary.

However, many printing methods at present can already generate the complicated microstructure; moreover, some "regulatory methods" can be used to reproduce the fine tissue structure. The simplest method is to use a composite material containing embedded micro/nanomaterials and to control the operation through the printing process itself or with some external means during the process. Under the first condition, the particles and fibers can be oriented simply through the fluid force produced when extruding the ink or resin from the jet nozzle; in the latter, acoustic or magnetic stimulation-sensitive additive (such as magnetic nanoparticles) can be added in the ink or resin to guide the orientation. Additionally, the freeze casting technique has been utilized to print the most complicated layer structure. Other methods include the addition of phase-separable polymer into the raw material and removal of one phase during the postprinting processing. A cardiac tissue model can become quite soft with the addition of elastomer foam into the raw material. All the abovementioned methods are powerful techniques to prepare a complicated 3D microstructure, and more efforts should be made to develop more materials close to cardiac tissue, paying particular attention to these techniques.

3.1.4 3D Printing Actuator

Mimicking the physiological motion process of cardiac tissue is one of the greatest challenges in preparing heart model with high fidelity. The best example is the left ventricle, the blood volume of which at each systole will be reduced to 50%–60% of that at diastolic state. At present, a mobile, soft material, passive fluid model can be produced under the drive of a jerk pump. But it is greatly different from the real cardiac motion, due to the fact that the model contracts to the original volume after removing the external force, since it is dilated under the action of external force. Consequently, the minimal volume of left ventricle is at diastole stage, which is opposite to the normal cardiac cycle. Developing the materials and systems that allows autonomous motion is the key to manufacture a truly realistic heart model.

Soft robotics is one of the simplest methods to overcome such problems. Adding a watertight pneumatic material into the printing material system, the model can produce an autonomous motion under a pressurized state. For example, some seal cavities are created outside the left and right ventricles of the heart flow model, and the two can produce a contraction when driven (pressurized). Another method is to add a porous foam material into the ventricular wall, and this also allows a contraction when pressurized. The few methods above can realize myocardial contraction-like motion to a certain degree, but the real ventricular contraction mechanism involves the complicated combined action of linear and rotational motion. The most ideal setup is to use a simple muscle actuator when constructing the model, just like the myocardial band embedded into the soft "tissue-like" ventricular wall, which can exert its function close to the real ventricular wall. Recently, some researchers have utilized PU and hydrogel materials to develop a more realistic myocardial robot actuator using FDM, DIW, and SLA as printing techniques, and this actuator has been utilized to produce the novel resin printing material or directly adopted to manufacture a high-fidelity model, but it still depends on a pneumatic transmission system, which has restricted its transportability.

Multiple materials can produce drive through the intrinsic mechanical response to external stimulation. For instance, 3D printing materials like hydrogel and other swelling materials can produce complex mechanical response to swelling. Similarly, there are thermosensitive polymers such as acrylic ester-based shape memory materials, liquid crystal elastomers, and silicone embedded with volatile liquid. The above material have interesting properties, but the drawback of swelling and thermosensitivity is that they are slow. Thus, it is impossible to use them to mimic the systolic cycle in terms of motion frequency. The electrical driven actuators can overcome such a difficulty, but it has its own defect of insufficient braking force, which generally requires high current or high voltage. Finally, the 3D-printed metal-ion polymer composite materials can produce drive under low voltage, but they require complicated liquid cooperation.

3.2 Bio-Printing Materials

3D bio-printing technique is a new technology that uses computer 3D model as the "template" and is equipped with the tailored "bio-ink," so as to finally manufacture artificial organs and biomedical products. At the current stage, bio-printing is mainly used in two research fields, namely, tissue and organ regeneration and repair, and manufacturing the in vitro model to investigate biological development, disease progression, and drug interaction. A bio-printing material library has been constructed 15 years ago, but there are still some major technical obstacles in constructing the viable tissues, including (1) the inability to print cells of multiple types simultaneously due to the resolution and printing density; (2) the lack of an extracellular matrix (ECM) capable of transporting the necessary physical and chemical signals to cells; and (3) the inability to match with the vascular system to deliver nutrients and oxygen and to remove the metabolic waste [16].

3.2.1 Characteristics of Bio-Ink

The following factors should be taken into consideration when selecting the bio-ink for tissue manufacturing. The ideal bio-ink has to match specific needs such as printability, biocompatibility, degradation kinetics, and mechanical and swelling property. In addition, other application properties should also be considered, such as blood compatibility and degradation by-products [17].

The fidelity of the bio-print depends on the capacity of the ink to maintain its biological structure after printing; for this reason, the viscosity, surface tension, and crosslinking mechanism of the bio-ink should be suitable for the selected printing method. At present, the major bio-printing methods include Inkjet, DIW [18, 19], and laser-assisted printing [20]. Among them, Inkjet works by spraying numerous tiny (1–100 pL) droplets onto the surface to agglomerate them into the printing layer. The viscosity of bio-ink used in Inkjet must be extremely low ($\eta < 10$ mPa s). The generally used materials are hydrogel, colloid suspensions, and cell suspensions, and gel should be formed immediately after the bio-ink leaves the jet nozzle. DIW is a kind of extrusion-based pneumatic or mechanically driven printing method. Its advantage lies in the optimized material viscosity, as low viscosity results in a low fidelity of the printed structure after the deposition, while high viscosity leads to restricted cell migration and proliferation environments after printing. In the presence of cells in the ink, cells at high density can be obtained, but the printing resolution is lower (200–1000 μm) due to the high shear stress at the jet nozzle, along with lower cell activity. The method to reduce such shear stress is to increase the jet nozzle size at the expense of resolution. Another method is to use a non-Newtonian fluid with shear thinning property [21]. For instance, sodium alga acid has strong shear thinning property, and its viscosity is reduced with the increase in the shearing rate in the jet nozzle during the printing process, but it is rapidly increased at the time of deposition, thus preserving the printed structural integrity. Currently, DIW has been used to print polymeric solutions, hydrogels, colloid suspensions, decellularized ECM, and cell sphere. Biological adhesive with moderate viscosity (1–300 mPa s) is used in laser-assisted printing, and this method can avoid the problems of jet nozzle blocking and high shear stress since no jet nozzle is needed. The rapidly crosslinking biomaterials, such as alginic acid for ion crosslinking and fibrinogen for enzymatic crosslinking, have superb effect when used in combination with the laser-assisted printing system.

The crosslinking of biomaterial can be divided into physical crosslinking and chemical crosslinking. Among them, physical crosslinking is not permanent; thus, the crosslinking involved in polymer gelatination can be destroyed and reformed repeatedly. Crosslinking is a process to connect the macromolecule through ion interaction, Van der Waals's (VDW) force, hydrogen bond, or even polymeric chain to form a covalent bond. DIW printers are capable of constructing a structural network through physical crosslinking. However, the network structure is usually destroyed under the action of high shear stress, which at the same time facilitates the polymer materials to flow through the micro-jet nozzle, and it is reformed under low shear stress. The permanent chemical crosslinking material is recommended for printed structure that should maintain certain long-term physical intensity. Chemical crosslinking refers to the crosslinking between the polymer chain/network to form the covalent bond through photo-polymerization, thermal polymerization, Michael-type addition reaction, click chemistry, enzymatic reaction, or pH changes.

According to reports, the Young modulus (tensile modulus) of human soft tissue and organ ranges from 0.1 kPa to 1000 kPa. When designing the tissue model, the original mechanics in cell microenvironment should be kept in great consideration, since cells will obtain important regulatory signals (namely, adhesion, migration, proliferation, and differentiation) from their surrounding environment. For example, when myocardial cells are cultured in the synthetic hydrogel (polyacrylamide, PAM, $E \approx 10$ kPa) with close biological rigidity, they display the striated myofibrils and exhibit favorable contractibility, but they behave in a completely different manner when cultured on the hard substrate. Additionally, the mechanical property of hydrogel has a key influence on the stem cell growth and differentiation. For instance, when human mesenchymal stem cells (MSCs) are cultured in the hard hydrogel ($E \approx 0.1$–1 kPa), they will differentiate into neuroblasts, but they will differentiate into myogenic and osteogenic cells at $E \approx 8$–17 kPa, and into new bones when placed in the $E > 34$ kPa environment. The polymer tangent modulus distribution can be adjusted through the medium changing the chemical concentration, polymer concentration, and crosslinking degree in the hydrogel, so as to simulate various soft tissues. For example, the Young modulus (E) of polyethylene glycol (PEG)-based hydrogel can change within the range of 60–500 kPa just increasing the polymer concentration from 10% to 20%. It is suggested in another study that a simultaneous increase (5.4–11.8 kPa) in elastic modulus (E) can be observed increasing the crosslinking degree in the hyaluronic acid (HA)-tyramine hydrogel.

3.2.2 Bio-Ink

The existing bio-printing material library is developing, including cellular hydrogel, non-hydrogel cell suspension, cell [22]/tissue sphere, decellularized ECM, and acellular polymers. The decellularized ink can use cytotoxic reagents in the process involving high temperature or high shear stress method, because it is not necessary to be compatible with cells after printing and postprocessing. On the contrary, a cellular bio-ink requires to keep biocompatibility also in the processing technology, because it should always provide a suitable environment for viable cells. Hydrogel is the most commonly used in bio-printing, since it is easily editable and applicable to various printing methods and diverse materials. The synthetic and naturally derived hydrogels have been used as cell-loading inks, and these macromolecules possess an hydrophilic polymer skeleton capable of swelling in water. Hydrogel has high water content and good mechanical properties, and this makes it a promising material to be applied in cell encapsulation; moreover, it can also be used to create the 3D microenvironment so that the original ECM reappears.

The most common materials used as bio-inks can be classified into two types: the naturally derived hydrogels and synthetic polymers.

3.2.3 Natural Bio-Ink

Natural polymers (hydrogels) are generally polysaccharidic chain polymers, which can also contain peptides and proteins. These natural polymers can provide the suitable ECM and biological factors for cell growth, proliferation, and migration, and as a result, they are particularly suitable for biological engineering. The most commonly seen natural hydrogels include alginate, gelatin, collagen, fibrin, and HA.

Alginate is extracted from algae or seaweed, which gives it the advantages of low price, great yield, natural extraction, biocompatibility, and non-toxicity. When coming into contact with calcium chloride, the alginate can interact with Ca^{2+} ions to rapidly form the physical gel [23]. Subsequently, Ca^{2+} can be removed by using chelating agent like sodium citrate or ethylenediaminetetraacetic acid (EDTA) to rinse the alginate gel, which can also promote gel liquidation. Alginate has biocompatibility but not bioactivity; therefore, it should be mixed with other natural polymers to promote cell adhesion and proliferation [24]. For instance, some researchers have prepared the alginate/gelatin mixture to print a high-fidelity aortic valve using bio-printing technique after adding swine aortic valve mesenchymal cells and smooth muscle cells [25].

Collagen is one of the major components of natural ECM, and its separation and purification technique is quite mature. Collagen is a kind of natural derivative, but pure collagen is not the ideal biopolymer, since it may induce unexpected biological signal when used alone (not containing other ECM material). Therefore, the mixed use of collagen or other ECM materials such as elastin, glycosaminoglycan (GAG), fibrinogen, and laminin is more suitable for bio-printing [26].

Gelatin is produced through the partial hydrolysis of the three-screw structure of collagen into smaller molecules. In a < 30–35 °C environment, gelatin is a solid due to physical crosslinking, but it melts into a flowing liquid under its physiological temperature. Consequently, bio-printing containing gelatin should use permanent chemical crosslinking. When printing the heart valve and vascular system, physical gelatin can be used as supporting material, and transglutaminase (TG) can be used subsequently to promote the crosslinking between gelatin and brinase, to form the tissue ECM.

Fibrin is a kind of protein formed through the action (enzymatic reaction) of thrombin on fibrinogen (FIB), and such crosslinking mechanism in human body plays a key role in blood clot formation and wound healing. Histological engineers have utilized such rapid crosslinking to manufacture the hydrogel with high mechanical strength, which is called the natural ECM [27].

HA is another major component of natural ECM, and it is an unvulcanized GAG constituted by repeated disaccharide units. HA has high polarity and absorbs water, making it the in vivo lubricant. HA modification using the methacrylate group can form an hydrogel capable of photo-crosslinking [26].

3.2.4 Synthetic Bio-Ink

Some synthetic hydrogels can accommodate cells during bio-printing, but numerous of these synthetic materials are processed at high temperature, or use the toxic solvent in printing; as a result, cells can only be inoculated in the printed structure when it is already formed. Synthetic materials do not have the biocompatibility of natural hydrogel; nonetheless, their molecular weights can be easily controlled, and their molecular weight distribution and cross-linking densities can be mechanically modified (namely, elastic modulus) to adapt to specific conditions; therefore, their existence is valuable. Besides, synthetic materials have bioinertia, that is, they lack the cell adhesion-specific binding sites. In this way, they can be used in combination with naturally derived materials containing specific biofactors mimicking ECM. Polycaprolactone (PCL) is a commonly used synthetic polymer in tissue engineered scaffold, since it has good biocompatibility and can provide solid mechanical support. The melting point of such polyester-based polymer is about 60 °C, and it is biodegradable. PCL lacks the cell adhesion-specific binding sites; therefore, it is generally binded with bioactive materials to promote cell adhesion and proliferation. Moreover, PCL can be rapidly cooled, and it is implemented with natural hydrogels (gelatin, HA, and fibrin) by the Atala Group, so as to produce the cell-loading tissue construct. They have developed a kind of multi-nozzle extrusion printer to simultaneously print the cell-loading hydrogel, supportive PCL, and Pluronic hydrogel as the supporting material. Typically, PCL is selected since it is degraded in two years, which can thereby provide long-term mechanical support for the printed tissue or organ structure.

3.3 Summary

At present, the commercial 3D printing systems can complete basic heart model preparation, and these visualized models are usually used to formulate surgical guidelines, as a preoperative planning aid and as blood flow models. The current development of material science has laid the solid foundation for manufacturing more realistic models, and the new models promise to mimic the heart histological mechanics based on the complicated tissue structure, which can provide the complex and high-fidelity flow models for clinical surgical training, thus replacing animal experiments or other simulated surgical modes. Moreover, the bio-printed realistic tissue models can be utilized to test drugs and other complicated physiological responses, finally realizing the objective of 3D printing living organs. However, to realize these objectives, more efforts should be made in material science and the development of more precise printers.

References

1. Duan B. State-of-the-art review of 3D bioprinting for cardiovascular tissue engineering. Ann Biomed Eng. 2017;45:195–209.
2. Luhui F. Research on ABS 3D printing materials based on FDM. 2016:83.
3. Homan KA, Kolesky DB, Skylar-Scott MA, Herrmann J, Obuobi H, Moisan A, Lewis JA. Bioprinting of 3D convoluted renal proximal tubules on perfusable chips. Sci Rep. 2016;6:34845.
4. Ahn BY, Duoss EB, Motala MJ, Guo X, Park S-I, Xiong Y, Yoon J, Nuzzo RG, Rogers JA, Lewis JA. Omnidirectional printing of flexible, stretchable, and spanning silver microelectrodes. Science. 2009;323:1590–3.
5. Mingming W, Zifeng L, Delin C, Haobo P, Changshun R. Progress in 3D bioprinting for tissue and organ regeneration. J Integr Technol. 2018:59–71.
6. Wang KWC-CHCZB. A review of the application of 3D printing technology in medical molds and regenerative tissues and organs. Engineering. 2017;5:173–93.
7. Kolesky DB, Homan KA, Skylar-Scott MA, Lewis JA. Three-dimensional bioprinting of thick vascularized tissues [engineering]. Proc Natl Acad Sci. 2016;113:3179.
8. Kim K, Zhu W, Qu X, Aaronson C, McCall WR, Chen S, Sirbuly DJ. 3D optical printing of piezoelectric nanoparticle–polymer composite materials. ACS Nano. 2014;8:9799–806.
9. Miller JS, Stevens KR, Yang MT, Baker BM, Nguyen D-HT, Cohen DM, Toro E, Chen AA, Galie PA, Yu X, Chaturvedi R, Bhatia SN, Chen CS. Rapid casting of patterned vascular networks for perfusable engineered three-dimensional tissues. Nat Mater. 2012;11:768–74.
10. Mironov V, Visconti RP, Kasyanov V, Forgacs G, Drake CJ, Markwald RR. Organ printing: tissue spheroids as building blocks. Biomaterials. 2009;30:2164–74.
11. Anderson IA, Gisby TA, McKay TG, O'Brien BM, Calius EP. Multi-functional dielectric elastomer artificial muscles for soft and smart machines. J Appl Phys. 2012;112:041101.
12. Malda J, Visser J, Melchels F, Jungst T, Hennink W, Dhert W, Groll J, Hutmacher D. 25th anniversary article: engineering hydrogels for biofabrication. Adv Mater. 2013;25:5011–28.
13. Bryant SJ, Bender RJ, Durand KL, Anseth KS. Encapsulating chondrocytes in degrading peg hydrogels with high modulus: engineering gel structural changes to facilitate cartilaginous tissue production. Biotechnol Bioeng. 2004;86:747–55.
14. Robinson SS, O'Brien KW, Zhao H, Peele BN, Larson CM, Murray BCM, Meerbeek IMV, Dunham SN, Shepherd RF. Integrated soft sensors and elastomeric actuators for tactile machines with kinesthetic sense. Extreme Mech Lett. 2015;5:47–53.
15. Liu J, Zheng H, Poh PSP, Machens H-G, Schilling AF. Hydrogels for engineering of perfusable vascular networks. Int J Mol Sci. 2015;16:15997–6016.
16. Skardal A, Atala A. Biomaterials for integration with 3-D bioprinting. Ann Biomed Eng. 2015;43:730–46.
17. Ji S, Guvendiren M. Recent advances in bioink design for 3D bioprinting of tissues and organs, Front Bioeng Biotechnol. 2017;5:23.
18. Bertassoni LE, Cardoso JC, Manoharan V. Direct-write bioprinting of cell-laden methacrylated gelatin hydrogels. Biofabrication. 2014;6:12.
19. Williams SK, Touroo JS, Church KH, Hoying JB. Encapsulation of adipose stromal vascular fraction cells in alginate hydrogel spheroids using a direct-write three-dimensional printing system. BioResearch. 2013;2:448–54.
20. Gudapati H, Dey M, Ozbolat I. A comprehensive review on droplet-based bioprinting: past, present and future. Biomaterials. 2016;102:20–42.

21. Ozbolat IT, Hospodiuk M. Current advances and future perspectives in extrusion-based bioprinting. Biomaterials. 2016;76:321–43.
22. Yuxue W, Xiaoqiu L, Di L, Shanshan L, Zhen W. Application and development of 3D printing technology in cell printing. Hainan Med J. 2017;28:801–4.
23. Jia J, Richards DJ, Pollard S, Tan Y, Rodriguez J, Visconti RP, Trusk TC, Yost MJ, Yao H, Markwald RR, Mei Y. Engineering alginate as bioink for bioprinting. Acta Biomater. 2014;10:4323–31.
24. Rong R, Jianfei Z, Jia-wen S, Jia-sheng W, Wei L, Jun S. Preliminary study of alginate/gelatin composite hydrogel used for 3D bioprinting. China J Oral Maxillofac Surg. 2017;15:402–7.
25. Wen X. Charging performance and bio-3D printing of cell-alkali alginate bio-inks. 2018:109.
26. Pati F, Jang J, Ha D-H, Kim SW, Rhie J-W, Shim J-H, Kim D-H, Cho D-W. Printing three-dimensional tissue analogues with decellularized extracellular matrix bioink. Nat Commun. 2014;5:3935.
27. Kolesky DB, Truby RL, Gladman AS, Busbee TA, Homan KA, Lewis JA. 3D bioprinting of vascularized, heterogeneous cell-laden tissue constructs. Adv Mater. 2014;26:3124–30.

4 Clinical Applications of Cardiovascular 3D Printing

Haibo Zhang, Wenzhi Pan, Shiqiang Yu, and Alex Pui-Wai Lee

Using imaging data of human anatomy, 3D printing technology can be used for computer reconstruction. The data are the input for a 3D printer, and a structural model is constructed, which is convenient for direct visual inspection and operation [1]. Through more than twenty years of development, outstanding progress has been made in oral, maxillofacial, orthopedic, and plastic surgery and other disciplines. Moreover, 3D printing technology has been widely used in implant and tissue design, surgical planning, medical research, and medical education and as a training tool [2, 3]. Because it has broad development prospects, 3D printing has become an important new technology in the manufacturing industry of "Strategic Emerging Industries Classification (2018)" issued by the National Bureau of Statistics.

Because the heart is a flexible muscular organ with pulsatility, 3D printing technology has been developed and applied to the heart later than other organs. Compared with other disciplines, its application scope is also limited. However, the China Cardiovascular Disease Report 2017 reported that cardiovascular diseases are already the leading cause of death, with a rate greater than 40%. This rate is higher than that for tumors and other diseases. In general, the prevalence and mortality for cardiovascular diseases in China are increasing. A report of the National Health Committee revealed more than 290 million patients with cardiovascular disease in China only. Among them, there are 11 million patients with coronary heart disease, 5 million patients with pulmonary heart disease, 4.5 million patients with heart failure, 2.5 million patients with rheumatic heart disease, 2 million patients with congenital heart disease, and 270 million patients with hypertension. Due to the huge patient population and market application prospects, the continuous and vigorous development of 3D printing technology in the cardiovascular field has been promoted. The application of 3D printing technology in cardiovascular diseases has already begun to play an increasingly important role in the following aspects: aiding in clinical diagnosis for guiding surgical treatment, improving communication between doctors and patients, simulating endovascular surgery, advancing cardiovascular research in vitro and in animal experiments, and promoting other aspects. Cardiovascular applications of 3D printing are based on the following aspects: (1) 3D printing of individualized models can help doctors develop a surgical plan for complex structural heart diseases, improve the communication between doctors and patients, and improve the curative effect of surgery [4]. (2) Simulation of intravascular surgery, through computer simulation, in vitro simulation [5], animal experiments, and other methods, can further assist in formulating individualized surgical plans for treating heart diseases, improving the success rate and safety of surgery, and promoting the realization of accurate medical plans. (3) 3D printing medical models can be applied to train medical professionals and students to improve the overall quality of cardiovascular disease education. (4) Cardiovascular implants, such as vascular stents, artificial heart valves, catheters, etc., as well as cells and tissues, such as blood vessels, tissue-engineered heart valves, artificial hearts, etc., can be 3D printed as well.

H. Zhang
Beijing Anzhen Hospital Affiliated with Capital Medical University, Beijing, China

W. Pan
Zhongshan Hospital Affiliated with Fudan University, Shanghai, China

S. Yu
Xijing Hospital, Xi'an, China

A. P.-W. Lee (✉)
Division of Cardiology, Department of Medicine and Therapeutics, The Chinese University of Hong Kong, Hong Kong, China

Laboratory of Cardiac Imaging and 3D Printing, Li Ka Shing Institute of Health Science; Department of Medicine and Therapeutics, Faculty of Medicine, The Chinese University of Hong Kong, Hong Kong, China
e-mail: alexpwlee@cuhk.edu.hk

J. Yang et al. (eds.), *Cardiovascular 3D Printing*, https://doi.org/10.1007/978-981-15-6957-9_4

4.1 Education of Patients and Doctor–Patient Communication

The cardiovascular system, as a complex circulatory system, involves the internal structure of the heart, conduction system, systemic blood vessels, coronary arteries, valves, and other aspects. In addition, its structure varies from person to person. Moreover, the means of diagnosis and treatment are gradually expanding, and the treatment methods for many cardiovascular diseases have changed. Because cardiovascular diseases have gradually become the biggest health problem faced by humans, the key and urgent matters include the following: how to implement surgical programs for patients with cardiovascular diseases, how to educate patients regarding the treatment methods, and how to ensure good doctor–patient communication. These factors are directly and indirectly related to the quality, efficiency, and benefits of medical care. Therefore, the dynamics of social, spiritual, and material civilizations are further affected. During the continuous evolution of medical technology, cardiovascular diseases have been treated with surgery, hybrid surgery, interventional therapy, and other procedures. Under the background of advocating accurate medical treatment, the demand for high levels of treatment has been increasing. Individualized treatment programs for patients with cardiovascular diseases have become the theme of the era of cardiovascular medicine.

In the past, patient education was usually embodied by the distribution of paper-based health education materials, watching videos, etc. However, these methods target diseases, not individuals. Due to individual differences, it is easy for patients to have deviations in terms of their understanding, learning, and compliance. It is also difficult for some patients to achieve the expected results. 3D printing technology is continuously developing, and some studies have reported that methods of 3D printing-assisted perioperative education intervention can effectively control anxiety in patients with acute trauma, relieve pain, and improve sleep satisfaction.

Medical technology is continuously improving, and medical models have become increasingly important. 3D printing can be used to create models that conform to patient characteristics, and it does not require the patient to be present with the doctor, while it can help the doctor carefully plan the operation [6]. 3D printing technology is also a valuable teaching aid, and 3D-printed models have been applied to facilitate doctor–patient communication for many patients with cardiovascular diseases. Such models enable patients and their families to more intuitively understand individual cardiovascular diseases and relative treatment methods. The technique also has significant effects on the evaluation of surgical risks, prevention of complications, and other aspects [7]. However, cardiovascular 3D printing technology is still in its infancy in China. Only a few medical institutions and enterprises have the ability to build 3D models related to cardiovascular diseases. The minimally invasive treatment team of the "Department of Cardiovascular Surgery" of Xijing Hospital, where the author of this book is employed, focuses on patients with complex aortic stenosis and insufficiency. Before conducting transcatheter aortic valve replacement (TAVR), 3D modeling and printing cardiovascular models are used for communication. Through this technique, patients and their families can more quickly understand the diseases they suffer from. They also can gain an in-depth understanding of the new minimally invasive technique in terms of surgical methods, treatment principles, clinical efficacy, etc., and mutual trust is enhanced (Fig. 4.1). In addition, through the application of 3D-printed cardiovascular models, more harmonious doctor–patient communication is achieved. These models not only convey information regarding the treatment of diseases, promote the improvement of diseases, and improve the cure rate of them but also resolve doctor–patient misunderstandings and contradictions in time, which reduces the occurrence of doctor–patient disputes and medical accidents.

4.2 Surgical Simulation and Surgical Planning

Another important area of application for cardiovascular 3D printing is surgical simulation. Cardiovascular doctors can carry out computer-aided 3D virtual surgery based on individualized medical image data to identify the best surgical plan for individual patients by simulated analysis, taking advantage of the characteristics of computer hemodynamics. Dr. Hasan Jilaihawi at New York University's Lagoon Hospital managed, using computer modeling, to perform a structural stress analysis of different types of valves on the aortic root. For individual cases, the patient's information is first transformed into three-dimensional imaging models using computer software, and then, the STL data files of different types of interventional valve stents are input to simulate the surgical scene. According to the structural stress analysis of different types of valves on the aortic root, the appropriate size of the valve can be chosen, and the effects of release from different parts can be compared; the possibility of complications can also be evaluated (Fig. 4.2).

Through virtual surgery design and computational hemodynamic simulation, 3D printing technology can also perform and predict quantitative changes in hemodynamic parameters and blood flow trajectories during surgery and reduce surgical risks by providing more reliable information. Researchers at the Shanghai Children's Medical Center have applied this technology to provide accurate treatment plans for patients undergoing Fontan surgery, pulmonary artery banding, and modified pulmonary shunt placement. Combining 3D digital medical technology, computer simu-

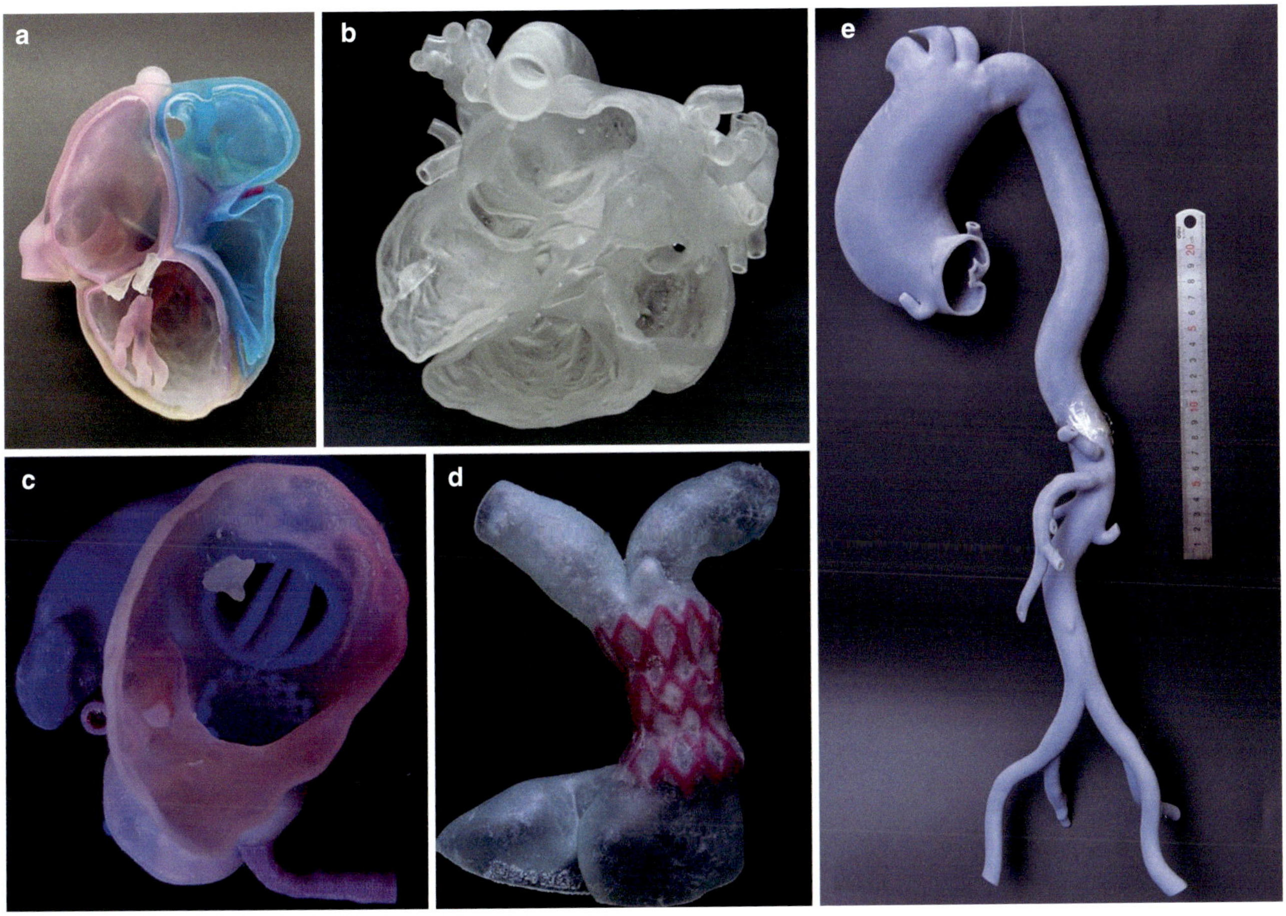

Fig. 4.1 Doctors at Xijing Hospital communicate with patients' relatives before surgery by using 3D-printed cardiovascular models. (**a**) 3D-printed hypertrophic cardiomyopathy model; (**b**) 3D-printed congenital heart disease model; (**c**) 3D-printed TAVR model; (**d**) 3D-printed pulmonary stented-valve model; (**e**) 3D-printed aorta model. Image data and 3D printed models from the Department of Cardiovascular Surgery of Xijing Hospital

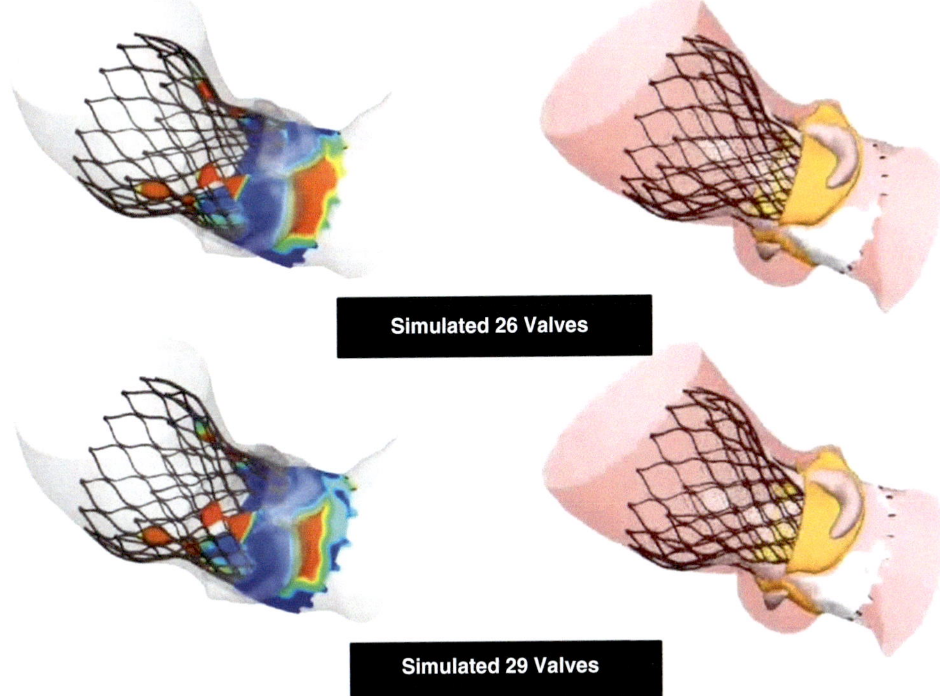

Fig. 4.2 The scientists at New York University perform structural stress analyses of different types of valves on the aortic root through computer modeling

lation, and clinical assessments not only can promote individualized and precise medical treatments but also greatly improve the success rate of complex surgeries for congenital heart disease and the patients' quality of life.

For many medical centers, computer simulation is not easy, requiring a multidisciplinary framework and cooperation and the application of cardiovascular implant model files by enterprises. Thus, an additional advantage of 3D printing is that surgical simulations can be performed in vitro by printing cardiovascular model samples. The patient's individualized anatomical model printed by computer reconstruction technology can help doctors more intuitively understand the individualized cardiovascular anatomy before surgery, such as the shape, size, location, degree of the heart defect, and structure of surrounding tissue [8, 9]. These models provide great clinical value for determining the patient's treatment plan.

With the help of 3D printing technology, clinicians can complete complicated surgery through simulated surgery, especially when handling challenging interventional cases. Because 3D printing technology can accurately reflect the heart structure, 3D models in preoperative planning and surgical planning have been widely used in cardiovascular therapy [10]. Olivieria et al. [11] reported that one patient was diagnosed with complete aortic transposition with right pulmonary venous obstruction by ultrasound testing. They attempted to use different types of catheters and stents on the 3D-printed heart model before surgery to clearly identify the advantages of large vessel position, leading to successful treatment by choosing the appropriate catheters and stents. At the TCT meeting in 2018, researchers from the Mayo Clinic in the USA reported the application of 3D printing technology to construct a paravalvular leak model. They used the model to accurately measure the internal diameter of the heart, to select the proper occluder in advance, to apply the appropriate type and size of the Plug for simulated surgery in vitro, and to ultimately select the surgical approach and develop the surgical plan (Fig. 4.3). On the basis of 3D printing technology, an interventional operation of a complicated transapical paravalvular leak was completed in only half an hour, which greatly shortened the treatment time and improved the effectiveness and safety of the operation. In addition, 3D printing technology has also made it possible to construct a special type of heart disease model. Hermsen et al. [12]. used a 3D model of hypertrophic obstructive cardiomyopathy to compare simulated surgery with real surgery. The excellent consistency was not only due to successful modeling but also due to the facilitation of new ideas for surgical technique training.

Chinese researchers have also made beneficial attempts in this regard. The Chinese University of Hong Kong and the University of Hong Kong applied 3D printing technology to complex left atrial appendage surgery. The 3D reconstruction of the data collected by transesophageal echocardiography of the patient resulted in a highly simulated 3D silica gel model of a complex cardiac structure. Preoperative simulation of the relevant treatment procedures was performed to design individualized interventional treatment options for patients. Yang Fan [13] at Fuwai Hospital used 3D printing technology to create a heart model for patients with inferior atrial septal defects. He tried to use a patent ductus arteriosus (PDA) occluder to successfully perform surgery and to avoid the failure of thoracotomy or interventional surgery. The individualized optimal treatment plan was then brought to the patient. Yan Yankun [14] of Fuwai Hospital reported a case in which a 3D printing technique assisted a transcatheter

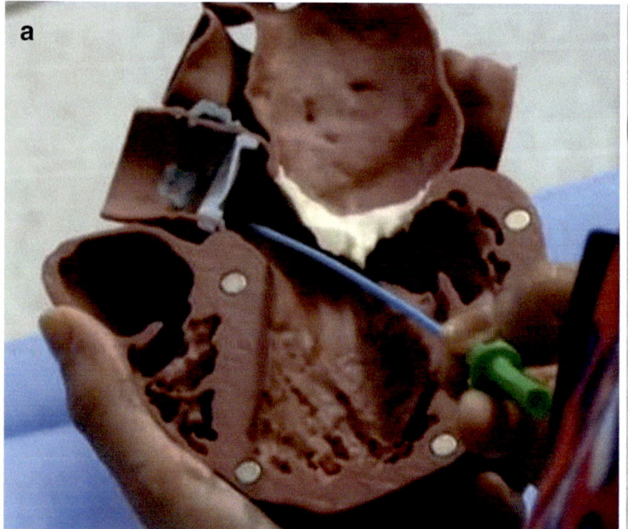

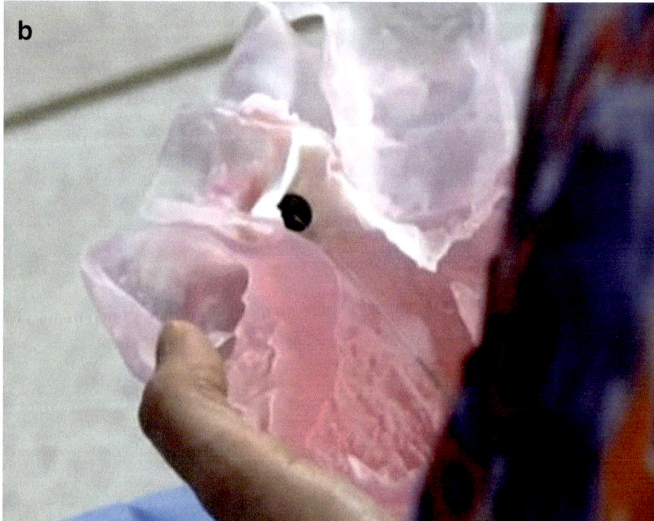

Fig. 4.3 The 2018 TCT meeting reported the application of 3D printing technology to assist in the treatment of paravalvular leaks. (**a**) Apply the first generation of a hard 3D-printed model to accurately locate the position of the paravalvular leak; (**b**) Apply the second generation of a soft and colorful composite 3D-printed model to select the apical approach and choose the plug occluder for simulated surgery in vitro

closure of an aortic sinus aneurysm rupture in 2014. Based on the relevant data of the patient's CTA, the heart model was 3D printed. Application of an 8/6 mm PDA occluder was tested for occlusion, and a perfect therapeutic effect was achieved. The minimally invasive treatment team of the Department of Cardiovascular Surgery at Xijing Hospital presented at the China Structural Week Conference in 2018. The 3D-printed aortic root model was used to accurately display the patient's lesion type, severity, and local anatomy and to simulate TAVR surgery in vitro by balloon expansion. This method was used to assess the risk of complications of coronary occlusion in the patient, and TAVR was successfully performed (Fig. 4.4).

3D printing technology can also be used to establish a whole-heart and profile model to observe the shape and position of a stent valve after surgery (Fig. 4.5).

In addition to computer software simulations and in vitro simulations, medical professionals can also verify the safety and effectiveness of cardiovascular surgery techniques and implants through animal experiments. Animal experiments are an important medium for directly studying various phenomena in life. The importance of understanding the various laws of the organic world is indisputable, and such knowledge is irreplaceable. By combining 3D printing technology with animal experiments, the development cycle of cardiovascular devices and drugs can be greatly shortened, and the cost of

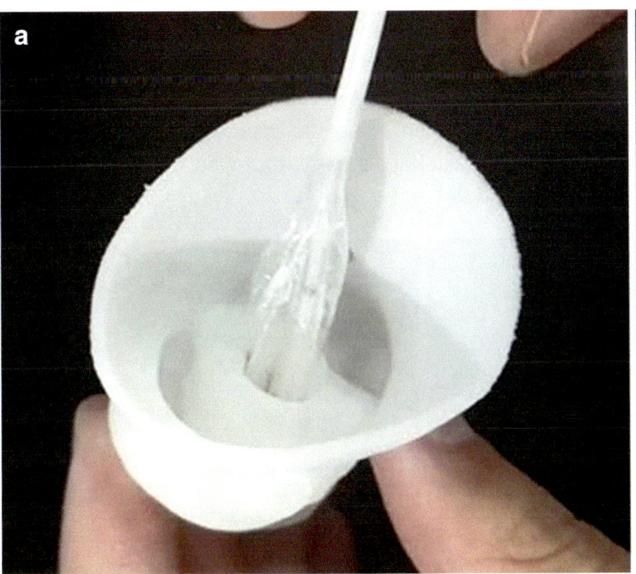

Fig. 4.4 The minimally invasive treatment team of the Department of Cardiovascular Surgery at Xijing Hospital used 3D printing technology to assist transcatheter aortic valve replacement. (**a**) composite 3D-printed aortic root model inserted into the balloon; (**b**) balloon expansion was simulated in TAVR surgery in vitro to assess the risk of coronary occlusion in the patient. Image data and 3D-printed model from the Department of Cardiovascular Surgery of Xijing Hospital

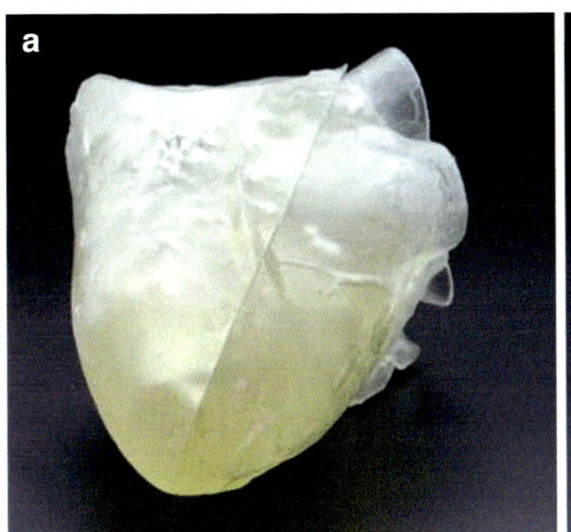

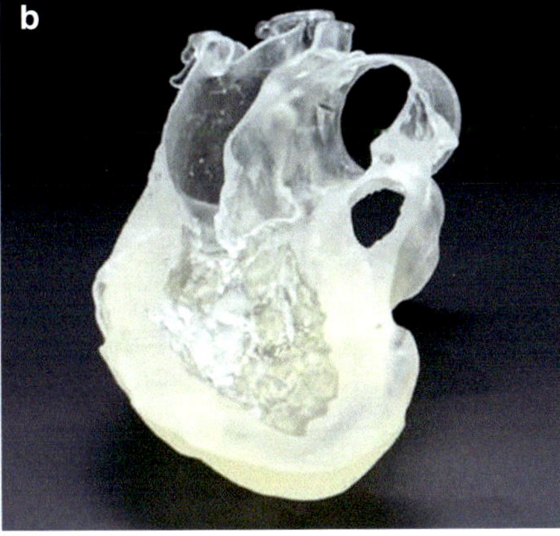

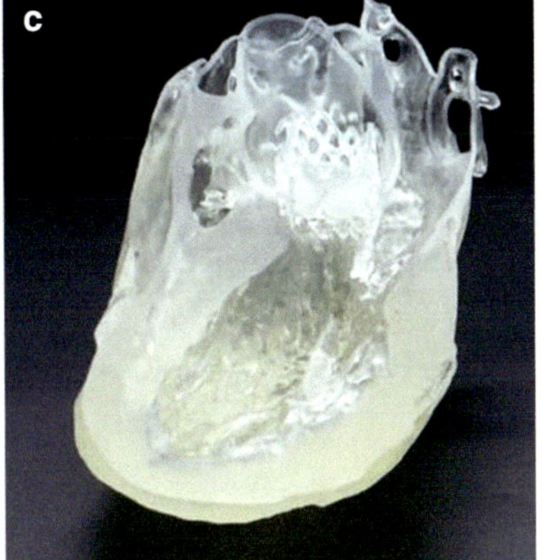

Fig. 4.5 3D printing technique to evaluate the effect of transcatheter aortic valve replacement. (**a**) 3D-printed whole-heart model; (**b**) 3D-printed half-heart model showing the intracardiac structure; (**c**) 3D-printed half-heart model showing the stent valve. Image data and 3D-printed model are from the Department of Cardiovascular Surgery of Xijing Hospital

research and development can be greatly reduced. The number of required experimental animals can also be reduced, and the quality of laboratory animal management can be improved. Animal welfare can also be maintained, and the harmonious development of man and nature can be promoted. The author of this book at the Department of Cardiovascular Surgery of Xijing Hospital has been engaged in the development and experimental research of cardiovascular implant devices. 3D printing technology has been combined with animal experiments to develop 3D cardiovascular models of different animal species, such as sheep, pigs, and dogs, and printed cardiovascular models of different populations of animals in vitro (Fig. 4.6). According to the anatomical characteristics of different animals, a dog was selected as the experimental animal for the implantation of a multibranched aortic stent, which revealed that endovascular repair of the whole aorta could be completed by intervention. The result was published in J Thorac. Cardiovasc Surg. 2016;151 (4): 1203–12 [15], and received a remark during the same period (Fig. 4.7). We selected the Bama Xiang pig as a laboratory animal for TAVR, and the results showed that the implanted aorta valve was in a good position, which laid a solid foundation for the clinical application of transcatheter aortic valve (Fig. 4.8). Furthermore, Xijing Hospital Cardiovascular Surgery and Shanghai Numed Medical Technology developed a domestic transcatheter interventional mitral valve replacement device to simulate the path and shape of the conveyor into the ventricle through a 3D-printed heart model. Observing the morphology of the valve after release can aid in determining whether it affects important adjacent anatomical structures, such as the coronary artery or the left ventricular outflow tract. Therefore, 3D-printed heart models provide a basis for further animal experiments and clinical research and have important reference value (Fig. 4.9). Sheep were selected as experimental animals for successful transcatheter mitral valve replacement (Fig. 4.10). Through refined animal species selection and accurate size measurement, path selection, program strategy formulation, etc., the success rate of animal experiments and the accuracy of cardiovascular implant equipment have greatly improved.

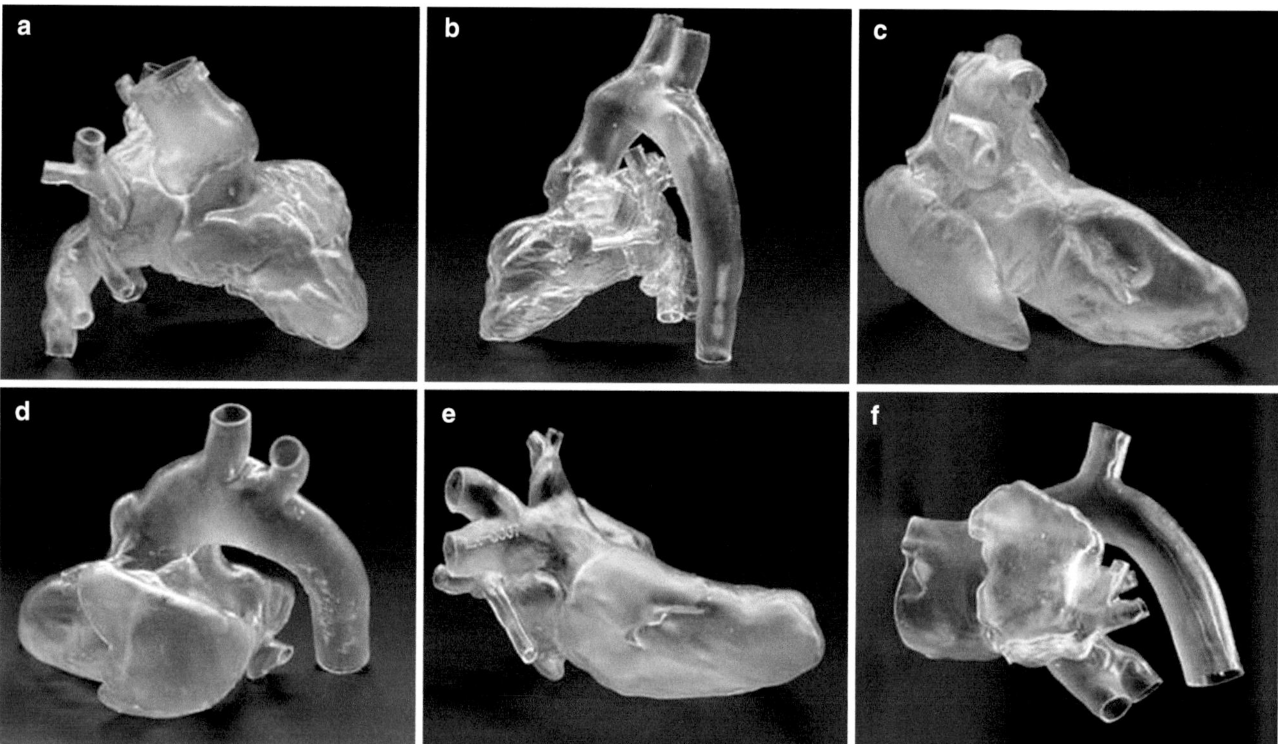

Fig. 4.6 Cardiovascular models of different types of animals printed by Xijing Hospital Cardiovascular Surgery. (**a**) 3D-printed canine heart model; (**b**) 3D-printed canine aortic model; (**c**) 3D-printed pig heart model; (**d**) 3D-printed pig aortic model; (**e**) 3D-printed sheep heart model; (**f**) 3D-printed sheep aortic model. Image data and 3D-printed models from the Department of Cardiovascular Surgery of Xijing Hospital)

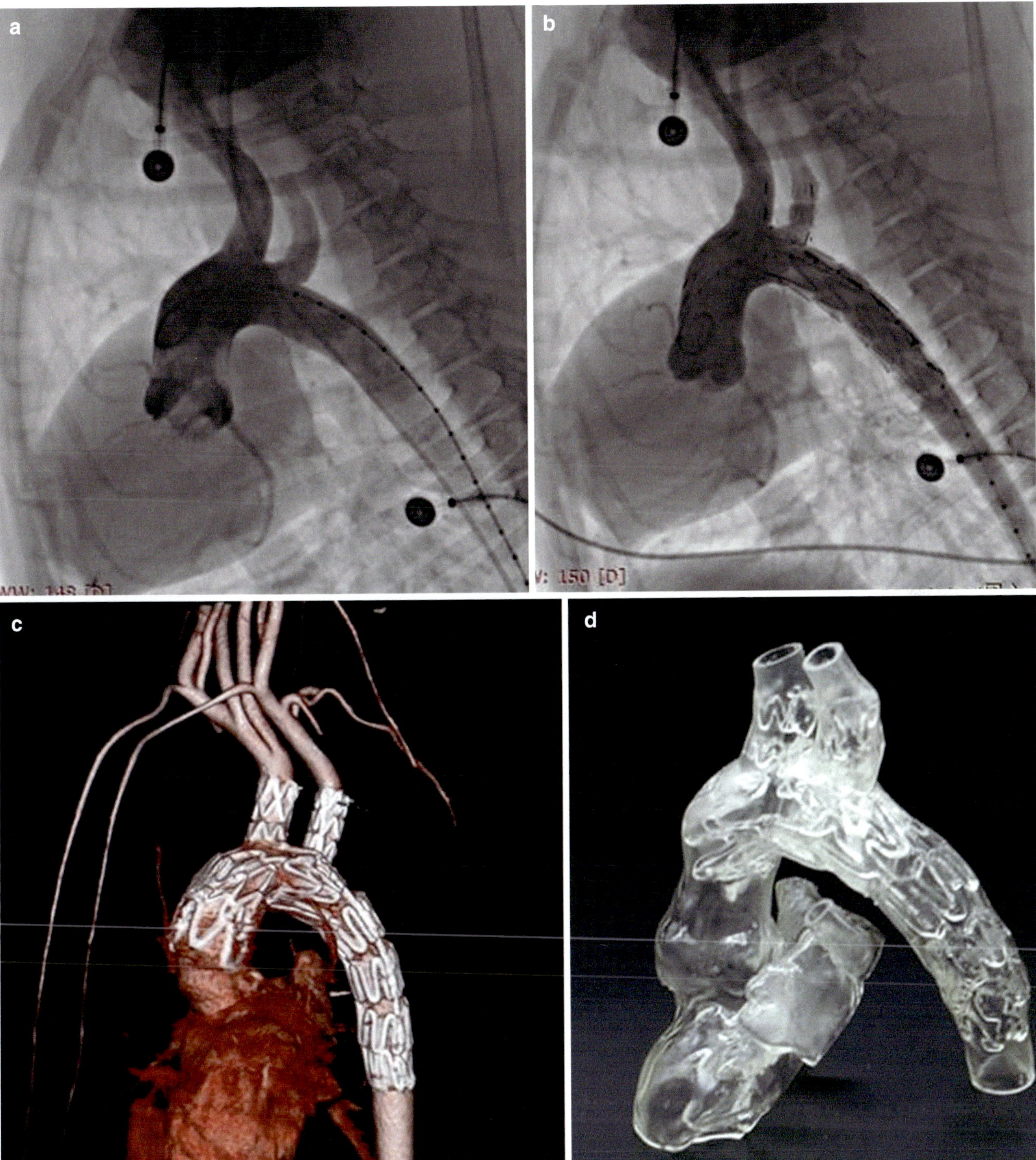

Fig. 4.7 Implantation experiment of a multibranched aortic stent printed by using 3D printing technology in a dog as the experimental animal. (**a**) preoperative angiography of the canine aorta; (**b**) angiography after multibranch aortic stenting; (**c**) CTA image after branch aortic stenting; (**d**) The canine aortic model that was 3D printed after multibranch aortic stenting. Image data, computer 3D reconstruction, and 3D-printed model from the Department of Cardiovascular Surgery of Xijing Hospital

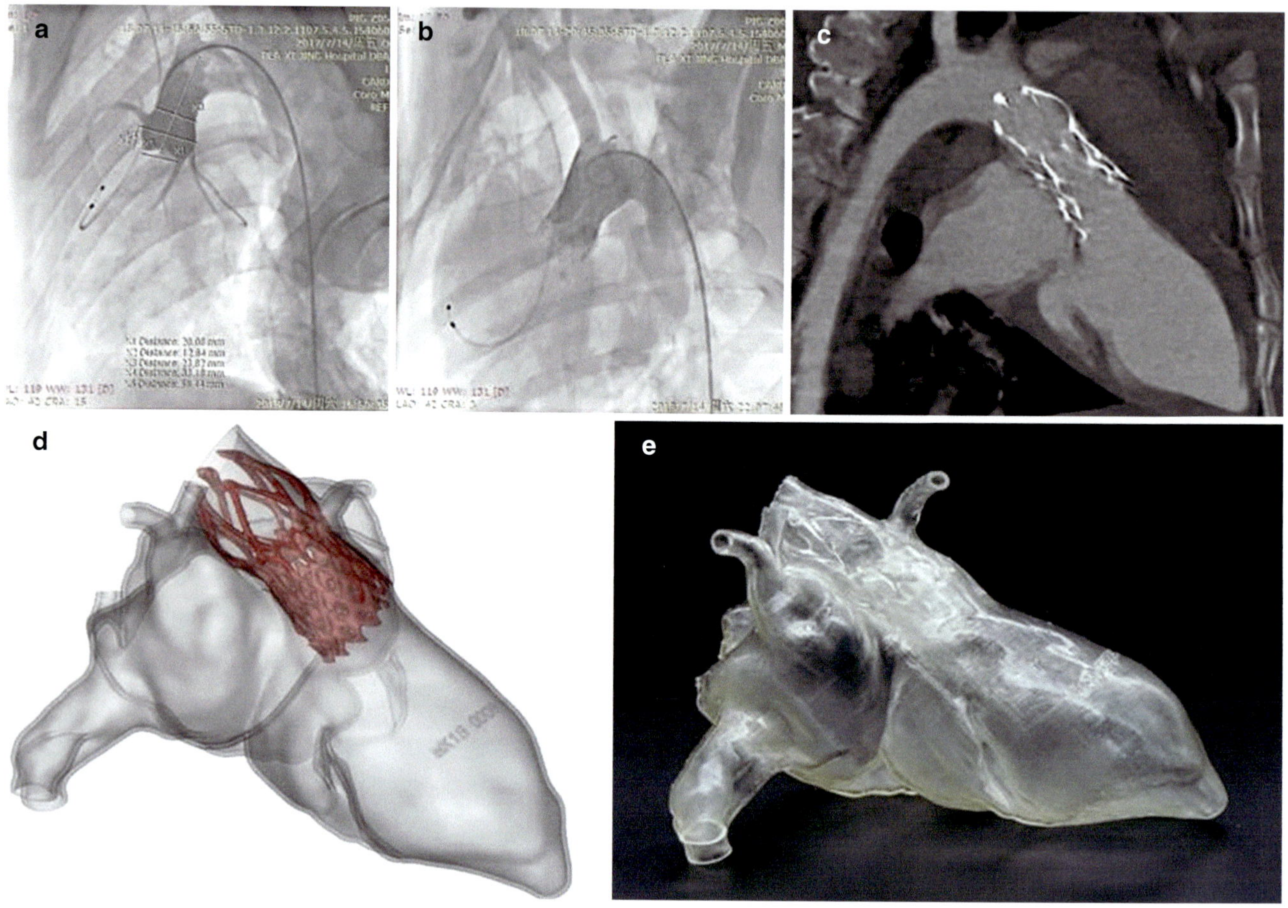

Fig. 4.8 The Department of Cardiovascular Surgery of Xijing Hospital applied 3D printing technology and selected the pig as an experimental animal for a transcatheter aortic valve replacement experiment. (**a**) Preoperative angiography of the aortic valve; (**b**) Post-transcatheter aortic valve implantation angiography; (**c**) CTA imaging after transcatheter aortic valve replacement; (**d**) 3D reconstruction model of transcatheter aortic valve replacement by a 3D printing computer; (**e**) 3D-printed model of the pig aorta after implantation of a transcatheter aortic valve. The image data, the 3D computer reconstruction, and the 3D-printed model were obtained from the Department of Cardiovascular Surgery of Xijing Hospital

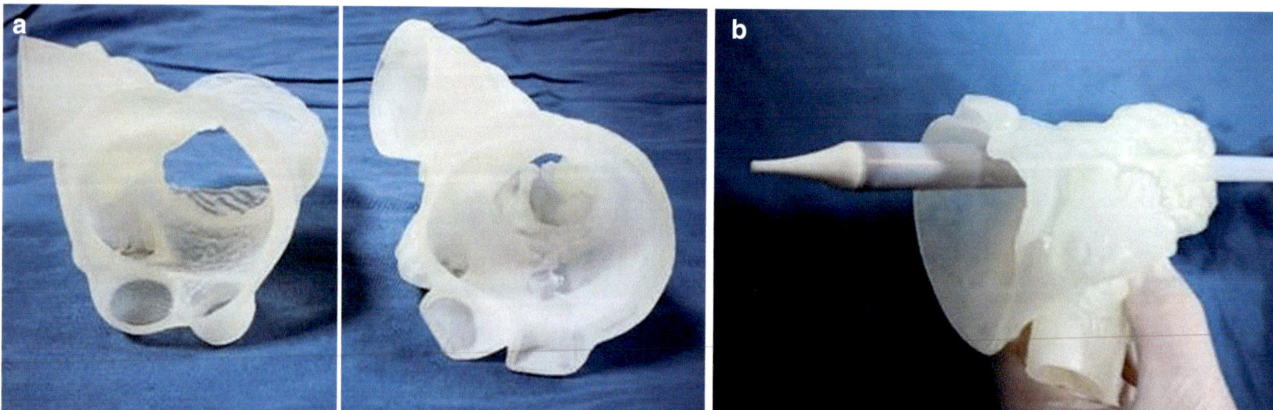

Fig. 4.9 The use of 3D printing technology in vitro to simulate transcatheter mitral valve replacement. (**a**) 3D-printed soft and hard sheep heart model; (**b**) The delivery system of the interventional mitral valve replacement device through the mitral valve into the left atrium was simulated in vitro; (**c**) Morphology after release via mitral valve replacement (left ventricular view); (**d**) Morphology after release via transcatheter mitral valve replacement (left atrial view); (**e**) Morphology of the transcatheter mitral valve replacement (aortic valve lateral view) for observing whether the left ventricular outflow tract was affected. Imaging data, 3D computer reconstruction, and 3D-printed models from the Department of Cardiovascular Surgery of Xijing Hospital

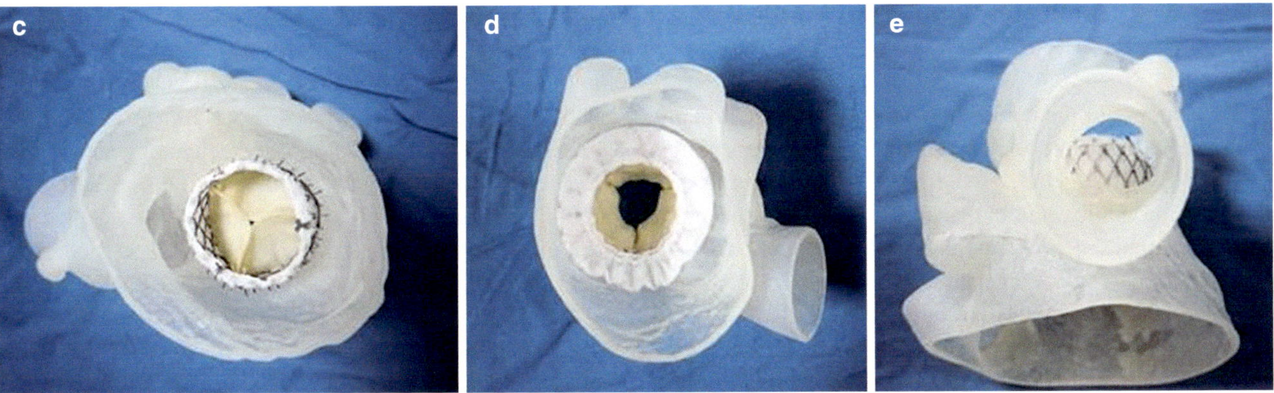

Fig. 4.9 (continued)

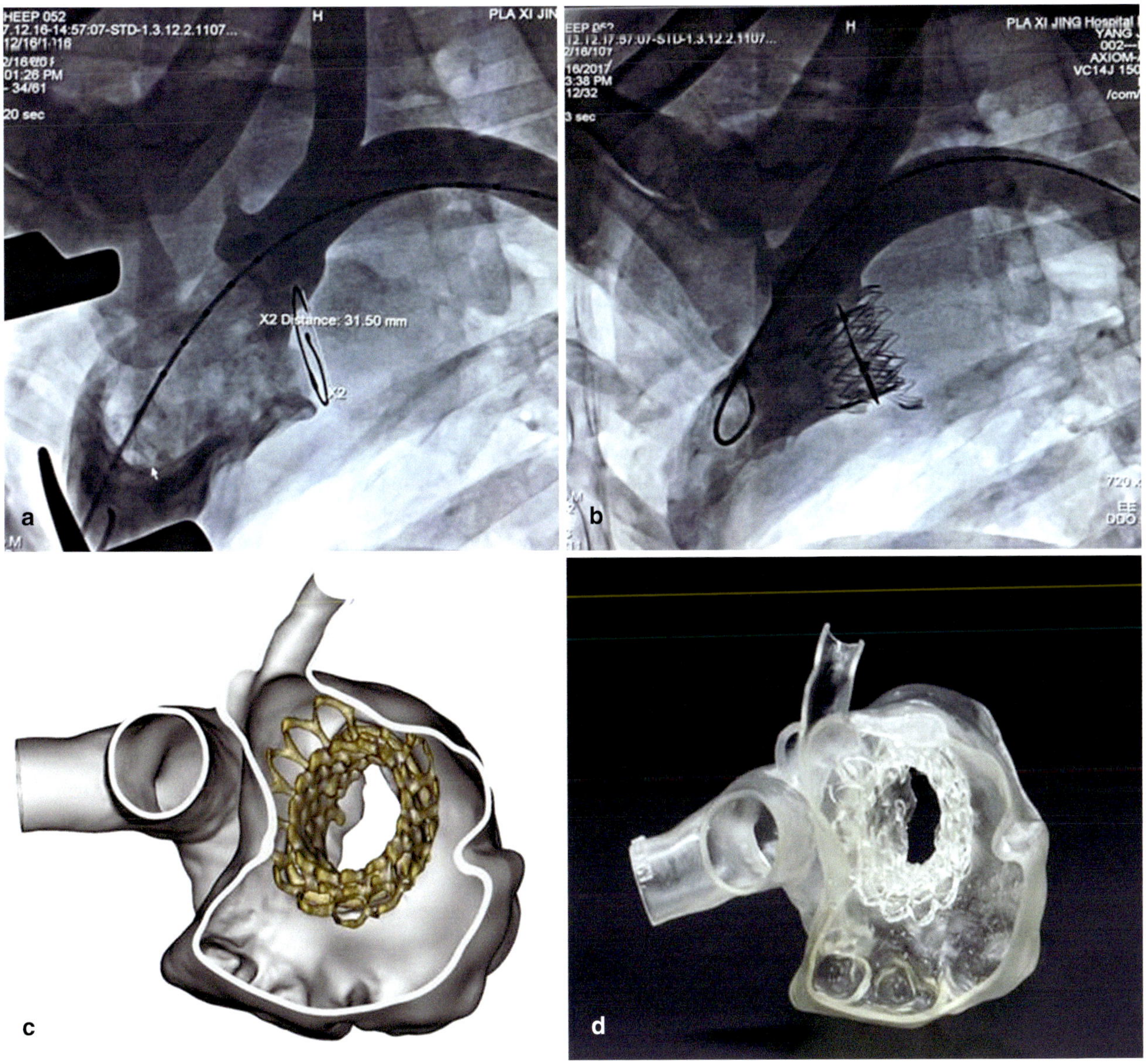

Fig. 4.10 The Department of Cardiovascular Surgery of Xijing Hospital applied 3D printing technology and selected sheep as experimental animals for transcatheter mitral valve replacement. (**a**) Preoperative angiography of the left ventricle of a sheep; (**b**) Ventriculography after transcatheter mitral valve replacement; (**c**) 3D-printed computer image after transcatheter mitral valve replacement; (**d**) 3D-printed heart model of sheep after transcatheter mitral valve replacement. Imaging data, computer 3D reconstruction, and 3D-printed models from the Department of Cardiovascular Surgery of Xijing Hospital

4.3 Medical Professionals and Medical Student Training

In the anatomy of the human body, the anatomical structure of the heart is delicate and complicated [16]. Understanding the anatomical structure of the heart requires strong spatial thinking ability, and the lack of a satisfactory teaching method remains a problem. With the introduction of 3D printing technology, clinicians can now visually display the heart, and 3D models are advantageous for their ability to display the spatial structure. An accurate 3D-printed cardiovascular anatomical model is a good training tool for medical students [17]. Anatomical models can help nurses, medical students, and surgeons interact and engage in surgery simulation to improve the success rate and accuracy of operations [18]. They can not only help reduce costs but also reduce the time spent in the catheterization room and operating room. In particular, 3D-printed cardiovascular anatomical models are excellent learning tools for structural heart disease education and can help medical professionals and medical students understand the changes of the heart and its connected large blood vessel structure under different disease states [19]. Breaking through traditional teaching paradigms relies on space imagination and thinking cultivation; 3D-printed models can visually demonstrate the real disease state, allowing medical professionals and medical students to better observe the true state of the disease and make up for the abstract space in routine teaching. These models can make up for the abstract mode of thinking that is required to understand the stereoscopic spatial structure of the heart in conventional teaching by instead allowing physical demonstrations. Thus, medical professionals and medical students can study structural heart diseases in a more simple, intuitive, interesting, and authentic manner.

Recent studies have shown that heart models made by 3D printing technology can be used for the training of cardiovascular specialists, which can lead to good results and a deeper understanding of the anatomical and pathophysiological characteristics of heart disease. Zhang of the Department of General Surgery of the Forth Military Medical University Tangdu Hospital [20] reported that students in a 3D printing teaching group gained superior professional knowledge to students in a traditional teaching group in terms of written test scores, basic operation test scores, anatomical structure mastery, and endovascular instrument familiarity. The application of 3D printing technology in clinical teaching can significantly improve educational programs of aortic diseases and has good application prospects. Yuan Liangxi, a subsidiary of Changhai Hospital affiliated with the Second Military Medical University [21], discussed the application of 3D printing technology in the clinical teaching of vascular surgery for aortic dilatation. He believes that 3D printing technology has important significance for the clinical teaching of endovascular treatment of aortic dilatation disease. Fan Fenling of the First Affiliated Hospital of Xi'an Jiaotong University [22] discussed the application of 3D printing technology in the clinical teaching of structural heart disease. He suggested that 3D printing technology can be used to display various types of structural heart diseases in visual three-dimensional models to help students develop good spatial thinking of the heart and large vessels. These models can aid in the observation of rare disease models, understanding the pathological results of the mechanism and hemodynamics, enriching professional knowledge, and improving analytical, diagnosis, and treatment ability. Furthermore, a variety of flexible materials can be used for 3D printing of in vitro models that can facilitate the training of medical students in procedures such as performing operations, cutting, and suturing. Complete surgeries can even be simulated to greatly improve surgical planning and training.

4.4 3D Printing of Cardiovascular Implants, Cells, and Tissues

3D printing technology is one of the most important technological breakthroughs in this era. The characteristics of individualized customization make 3D printing technology beneficial for the manufacture of cardiovascular implants. 3D printing technology has the ability to mimic the precise geometry and biological characteristics of patient blood vessels and to minimize the risk of complications.

In 2016, the research team of Delft University of Technology in the Netherlands developed a new multifunctional Sigma catheter based on a 3D-printed heart model, which has a complex curved shape. The tip of the model can move in a serpentine shape to take S- and Z-shaped curves or multiplanar curves. Because the 3D-printed heart is transparent, the design and route of the catheter can be clearly observed from many different angles, and necessary adjustments can be performed at any time during the experiment.

In 2017, Guillermo Ameer at Northwestern University developed a 3D printing technology for projection microstereolithography (PMSL) and printed a new vascular stent based on a citric acid-based polymer. The stent can be manufactured with the same radial compression stiffness and the same support size as nickel–titanium alloy supports.

In recent years, new breakthroughs have been made in the application of 3D-printed cardiovascular implants. The team of artificial hearts from the Swiss Federal Institute of Technology in Zurich developed the first 3D-printed silicone soft heart in the world, which is similar to the human heart. An external pump drives the beating of the heart. The model heart can beat more than 3000 times in approximately half an hour. In April 2019, Israeli scientists printed a miniature heart with complete atria and ventricles by using human cells. The use of human cardiomyocytes to print artificial 3D-printed hearts with heart function is expected in the future.

Biological printing is another application of 3D printing in the cardiovascular field, mainly including the printing of cardiovascular cells and tissues with biological ink instead of traditional material [23, 24]. After differentiating stem cells from the human body into other cell types, the researchers sealed them as "toner" and printed them in vitro in combination with hydrogel matrix. It should be noted that printing living cells, tissues, and organs using 3D printing technology is one of the most challenging tasks because the following technical difficulties need to be overcome: (1) The problem of whether cells can survive and can develop or whether mutations or tumors develop during the printing process. (2) The 3D biological printer must meet the strict standard of biological mimetic manufacturing accuracy. (3) The tissues and organs are nonhomogeneous systems composed of a variety of materials and cells, which have high requirements for manufacturing science.

It was reported that Jonathon Leipsic's team of Sao Paulo Hospital applied biological printing to construct tissue-engineered valves, and the survival rate of cells reached 89% in 21 days. Pati et al. used biological ink of decellularized extracellular matrix (DECM) to print a 3D structure that could provide a suitable microenvironment for cell growth.

Although breakthroughs have been made in laboratories, 3D biological printing is limited to simple organizational structures and is far from being able to be industrialized. Many experimental verification steps are needed to ensure its safety and effectiveness.

4.5 Limitations of 3D Printing

Given its rapid process and the intuitive nature of the resulting models, 3D printing plays a key role in the surgical process of cardiovascular diseases. However, there are still limitations in cardiovascular 3D printing: (1) All cardiovascular 3D printing is ultimately based on imaging techniques (including CTA, magnetic resonance, and ultrasonic Doppler layers), and the precision of different imaging techniques limits the accuracy of printing tiny structures. (2) Cardiovascular 3D printing requires the collaboration of multiple disciplines, including computer postprocessing technology. The experts who perform postprocessing not only need to understand cardiovascular anatomy and disease but also need to master computer software to fully coordinate with clinical communication to truly reflect the reality of the disease. (3) 3D printing, especially cardiovascular 3D printing, has demanding requirements for materials, which must combine a variety of soft and hard materials and multifunctional materials. There are very few types of materials that can currently be used in cardiovascular models, and thus, further research and development in materials science is crucial. (4) The high cost limits the application and development of cardiovascular 3D printing technologies. (5) Cardiovascular 3D bioprinting is still in the early stage and is far from clinical application.

4.6 Summary and Prospect

With the rapid development of imaging and computer technology, the accuracy and simulations of cardiovascular 3D printing are constantly improving. 3D printing can make up for deficiencies of traditional imaging technology regarding the precise display of complex structures, while 3D computer reconstruction can enable cardiovascular doctors to more intuitively understand the pathological changes of human tissues, thus representing a new method for the precise treatment of heart disease. Although the application of 3D printing in the cardiovascular field is still in the early stage, it can allow in vitro information to be visualized and patients' individualized 3D models to be printed. These features can allow doctors to better determine the optimal surgical procedures and promote communication between doctors and patients. 3D printing can also simulate surgeries and interventions, improve the success rate and safety of surgery, and help train medical professionals and medical students. Many breakthroughs have been made in 3D printing regarding cardiovascular cells and tissues. With the further development of 3D printing technology, the advantages of customized and individualized manufacturing will enable a better understanding of cardiovascular diseases. In the future era of 3D plus, with the development of biological engineering technology, materials science, biology, computer science, and other disciplines, additional materials will be developed that can be implanted in the human body and lead to new breakthroughs in the treatment of diseases and medical device development. The tissues and organs fabricated by biological 3D printing will also be able to be applied in the treatment of cardiovascular diseases. 3D printing will continue to change traditional treatment methods, improve the diagnosis and treatment effects of cardiovascular diseases, and better benefit patients with cardiovascular diseases in the future [25].

References

1. Kim MS, Hansgen AR, Wink O, Quaife RA, Carroll JD. Rapid prototyping: a new tool in understanding and treating structural heart disease. Circulation. 2008;117:2388–94.
2. Schmauss D, Gerber N, Sodian R. Three-dimensional printing of models for surgical planning in patients with primary cardiac tumors. J Thorac Cardiovasc Surg. 2013;145:1407–8.
3. Bagur R, Cheung A, Chu MWA, Kiaii B. 3-dimensional–printed model for planning transcatheter mitral valve replacement. JACC Cardiovasc Interven. 2018;11:812–3.

4. Anwar S, Singh GK, Varughese J, Nguyen H, Billadello JJ, Sheybani EF, Woodard PK, Manning P, Eghtesady P. 3D printing in complex congenital heart disease across a spectrum of age, pathology, and imaging techniques. JACC Cardiovasc Imaging. 2017;10:953–6.
5. Valverde I, Sarnago F, Prieto R, Zunzunegui JL. Three-dimensional printing in vitro simulation of percutaneous pulmonary valve implantation in large right ventricular outflow tract. Eur Heart J. 2017;38:1262–3.
6. Kurup HK, Samuel BP, Vettukattil JJ. Hybrid 3D printing: a game-changer in personalized cardiac medicine? Expert Rev Cardiovasc Ther. 2015;13:1281–4.
7. Biglino G, Capelli C, Wray J, Schievano S, Leaver LK, Khambadkone S, Giardini A, Derrick G, Jones A, Taylor AM. 3D-manufactured patient-specific models of congenital heart defects for communication in clinical practice: feasibility and acceptability. BMJ Open. 2015;5:e007165.
8. Reed GW, Tuzcu EM, Kapadia SR, Krishnaswamy A. Catheter-based closure of paravalvular leak. Expert Rev Cardiovasc Ther. 2014;12:681–92.
9. Ruiz CE, Jelnin V, Kliger C, Kronzon I, Leipsic J, Maisano F, Millan X, Nataf P, O'Gara PT, Pibarot P, Rodes-Cabau J, Ramee SR, Rihal CS, Sorajja P, Hahn RT, Leon MB, Suri R, Tuzcu EM, Swain JA, Turi ZG, et al. Clinical trial principles and endpoint definitions for paravalvular leaks in surgical prosthesis: an expert statement. J Am Coll Cardiol. 2017;69:2067–87.
10. Bramlet M, Olivieri L, Farooqi K, Ripley B, Coakley M. Impact of three-dimensional printing on the study and treatment of congenital heart disease. Circ Res. 2017;120:904–7.
11. Olivieri L, Krieger A, Chen MY, Kim P, Kanter JP. 3D heart model guides complex stent angioplasty of pulmonary venous baffle obstruction in a mustard repair of d-tga. Int J Cardiol. 2014;172:E297–8.
12. Hermsen JL, Burke TM, Seslar SP, Owens DS, Ripley BA, Mokadam NA, Verrier ED. Scan, plan, print, practice, perform: development and use of a patient-specific 3-dimensional printed model in adult cardiac surgery. J Thorac Cardiovasc Surg. 2017;153:132–40.
13. Fan Y, Hong Z, Jianhua L. A case of inferior atrial septal defect treated by patent ductus arteriosus sealer under the guidance of 3D printing technology. Chin J Cardiol. 2015;43:631–3.
14. Yankun Y, Hong Z, Zhengming X. A case of ruptured aortic sinus tumor assisted by 3D printing. Chin J Intervent Cardiol. 2014;22:135–6.
15. Yang J, Liu Y, Duan W, Yi D, Yu S, Ma R, Ren J. A feasibility study of total endovascular aortic arch replacement: from stent-graft design to preclinical testing. J Thorac Cardiovasc Surg. 2016;151:1203–12.
16. Wang J, Zuo J, Yu S, Yi D, Yang X, Zhu X, Li J, Yang L, Xiong L, Ge S, Ren J, Yang J. Effectiveness and safety of transcatheter closure of perimembranous ventricular septal defects in adults. Am J Cardiol. 2016;117:980–7.
17. Valverde I. Three-dimensional printed cardiac models: applications in the field of medical education, cardiovascular surgery, and structural heart interventions. Rev Esp Cardiol (Engl Ed). 2017;70:282–91.
18. Biglino G, Capelli C, Koniordou D, Robertshaw D, Leaver LK, Schievano S, Taylor AM, Wray J. Use of 3D models of congenital heart disease as an education tool for cardiac nurses. Congenit Heart Dis. 2017;12:113–8.
19. Cai T, Cheezum MK, Giannopoulos AA, Blankstein R, Rybicki FJ, Steigner ML, Mitsouras D. Accuracy of 3D printed models of the aortic valve complex for transcatheter aortic valve replacement (TAVR) planning: comparison to computed tomographic angiography (CTA). Circulation. 2015;132
20. Zhang Z, Lei W, Songlin G, Dong W, Jikai Y. Application of 3D printing technology in clinical teaching of aortic diseases. China Med Educ Technol. 2018;32:555–7.
21. Liangxi Y, Guangqin L, Zhiqing Z. Application of 3D printing technology in clinical teaching of aortic distension disease in vascular surgery. Health Vocat Educ. 2016, 34:119–21.
22. Fenling F, Gesheng C, Songlin Z. Application of three-dimension printing in teaching of structural heart disease. China Med Educ Technol. 2017;31:583–8.
23. Qian Z, Wang K, Chang YH, Zhang C, Wang B, Rajagopal V, Meduri C, Kauten J, Polsani V, Zhou X, Martin R, Houle H, Vannan M, Mansi T. 3-D printing of biological tissue-mimicking aortic root using a novel meta-material technique: potential clinical applications. J Am Coll Cardiol. 2016;67:7.
24. Borovjagin AV, Ogle BM, Berry JL, Zhang J. From microscale devices to 3D printing: advances in fabrication of 3D cardiovascular tissues. Circ Res. 2017;120:150–65.
25. Vukicevic M, Mosadegh B, Min JK, Little SH. Cardiac 3D printing and its future directions. JACC Cardiovasc Imaging. 2017;10:171–84.

5 3D Printing of Congenital and Prenatal Heart Diseases

Jian Yang, Xiangbin Pan, Wenzhi Pan, Meng Yang, Jincheng Liu, and Jiayou Tang

5.1 3D Printing of Congenital Heart Disease

Jian Yang, Xiangbin Pan, Wenzhi Pan

Congenital heart disease (CHD) refers to abnormalities in the cardiovascular anatomical structure caused by an abnormal cardiovascular development in the embryonic period. The incidence of neonatal disease is 0.8%–1.2%, which makes it the most common congenital malformation. Most patients need surgical treatment. There are many kinds of CHDs with complex anatomical structure and individual variability. The three-dimensional anatomy of lesions is especially complex for certain types of CHDs. At present, the diagnosis and treatment of CHDs currently remain a critical issue.

With the development of echocardiography, most congenital heart diseases can be diagnosed by transthoracic or transesophageal echocardiography. Echocardiography can clearly show the abnormal structure of the heart, including the development of ventricular chamber and valves, the condition of the atrial septum, blood flow and reflux, and the gradient of stenosis. It has a good diagnostic value for most congenital heart diseases (Fig. 5.1).

For complex congenital heart disease, angiography, as a common invasive method, plays an active role in identifying intracardiac connection, anatomy, and alignment, showing the direction of blood flow and the blood supply of collateral vessels (Fig. 5.2).

Although dynamic three-dimensional echocardiography, multislice spiral CT, magnetic resonance (MR), and other imaging techniques have increasingly matured in their ability to diagnose such complex CHDs, it is still difficult to obtain intuitive anatomical details by observing three-dimensional images on a two-dimensional screen; thus, a three-dimensional anatomical model for simulation is desirable before operation. 3D printing is the link between imaging and physical objects. A 3D-printed model can help to accurately, precisely, and intuitively understand the spatial relationship of congenital heart diseases. 3D printing is being increasingly applied in various fields of medicine [1]. Its fast and accurate advantages will help in making more exact diagnoses, creating 1:1 heart models, preoperative surgical and interventional planning, simulation of cardiac surgery operations, and so on. In the diagnosis and treatment of CHDs, especially complex CHDs, 3D printing technology is becoming a hotspot of current research. Data from 3D-printed cardiac models are realistic and reliable. Individualized 3D-printed cardiac models can be used to assist doctors in planning and predicting surgery and in designing the optimal surgical path. Such models are especially important for the surgical treatment of some complex congenital heart diseases and transcatheter interventional therapy for some special CHD patients. In addition, individualized heart models printed in 3D can display the complex heart structure of patients more vividly and intuitively and help medical teaching and communication between doctors and patients.

5.1.1 Application of 3D Printing Technology in the Diagnosis and Treatment of Complex CHDs

The diagnosis of CHDs currently mainly depends on imaging examinations. Echocardiographic diagnosis of CHDs is easy to perform, requires a short examination time, is noninvasive to the human body, can show abnormal internal structures of the heart, and can reflect the development of

J. Yang (✉) · J. Liu · J. Tang
Xijing Hospital, Xi'an, China

X. Pan
Fuwai Hospital, Chinese Academy of Medical Sciences, Beijing, China

W. Pan
Zhongshan Hospital Affiliated with Fudan University, Shanghai, China

M. Yang
Aviation College of Xi'an Jiaotong University, Xi'an, China

J. Yang et al. (eds.), *Cardiovascular 3D Printing*, https://doi.org/10.1007/978-981-15-6957-9_5

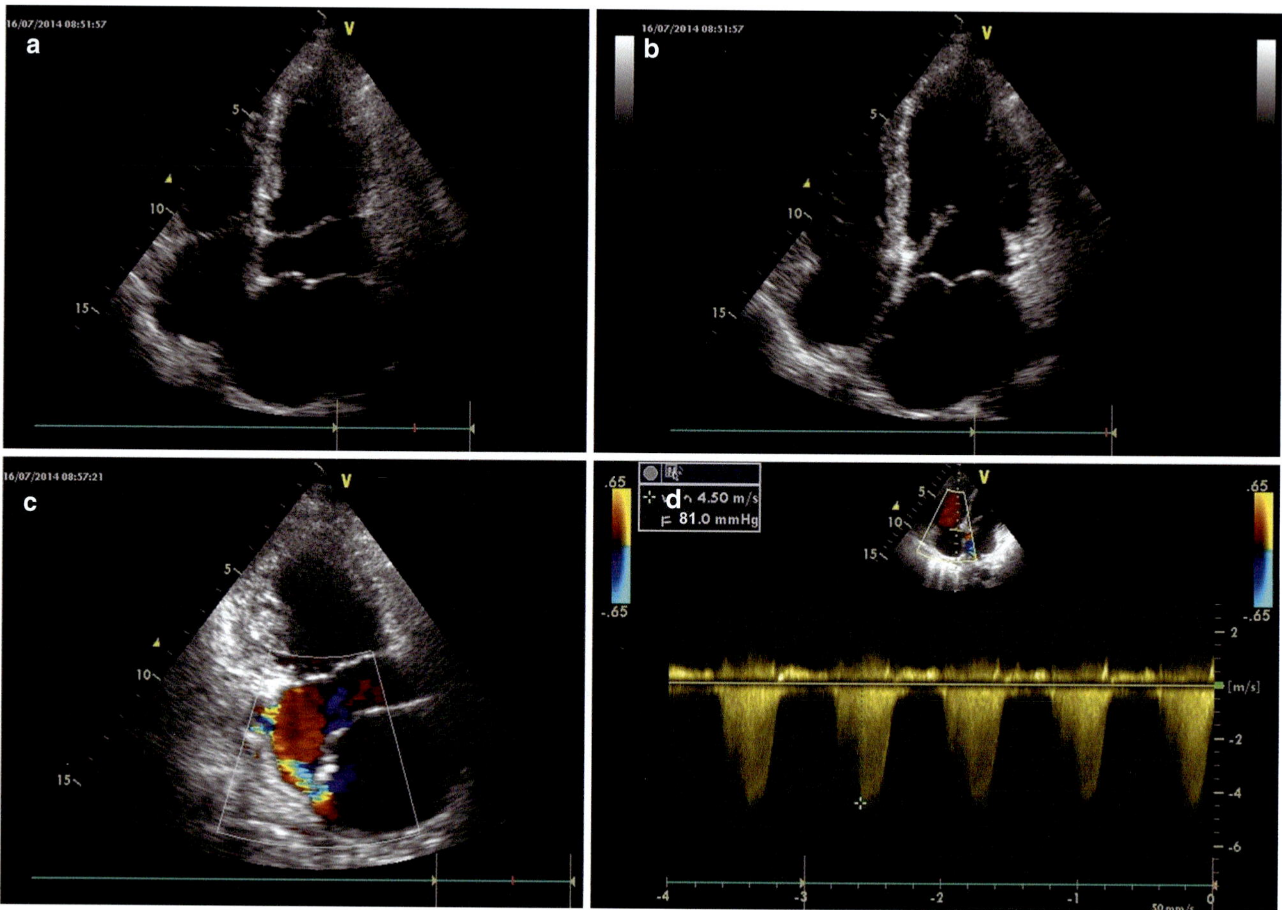

Fig. 5.1 Echocardiographic images of the cor triatriatum. (**a**) Mitral valve closure and left atrial septum in the systole phase; (**b**) Mitral valve opening and left atrial septum in the diastole phase; (**c**) Color Doppler shows spaces in the septum connecting the true and false atria and accelerated internal blood flow; (**d**) Doppler spectrum of the blood flow velocity and gradient in the stenosis. Images were obtained during cardiovascular surgery at Xijing Hospital

ventricular cavity and valves, etc. Echocardiographic diagnosis has important guiding significance for the diagnosis and treatment of CHD. Cardiac CTA and MRI can help depict the relationships among cardiac and macrovascular structure, shape, and development. Although two-dimensional imaging, such as echocardiography, CTA, and MRI, has important clinical value in the diagnosis and surgical planning of CHD, imaging data cannot provide detailed cardiac spatial structure for patients with complex CHD. With the development of imaging techniques, computer three-dimensional reconstruction technology makes the cardiac spatial structure more intuitive and clearer. By selecting cardiac CTA, MRI, and echocardiography data [2, 3], 3D printing technology can be used to create individual cardiac models, transform imaging data into physical models, reproduce pathological structures, and truly reflect the internal and external spatial structure of the heart to provide the basis for accurate diagnosis [4]. Operators can more intuitively understand heart disease, operate on heart models, formulate surgical pathways and strategies, and provide individualized treatment for CHDs, which can effectively shorten the operation time and reduce complications and mortality. The application of 3D printing technology in the diagnosis of complex CHDs is briefly described by considering the double outlets of the right ventricle as an example.

Double-outlet right ventricle (DORV) is a complex cyanotic congenital heart disease, the incidence of which accounts for approximately 0.5% of congenital heart disease. The morphological manifestation is that the aorta and pulmonary artery originate completely or mostly from the right ventricle. There is no fibrous connection between the two groups of semilunar valves and atrioventricular valves. Ventricular septal defect (VSD) is the only outlet of the left ventricle. Due to the incomplete rotation of the conical trunk septum during embryonic development, the trunk itself deviates from the corresponding connections of the left and right ventricles to varying degrees. Cones occur during the formation of the embryonic apex. After fusion of the right dorsal

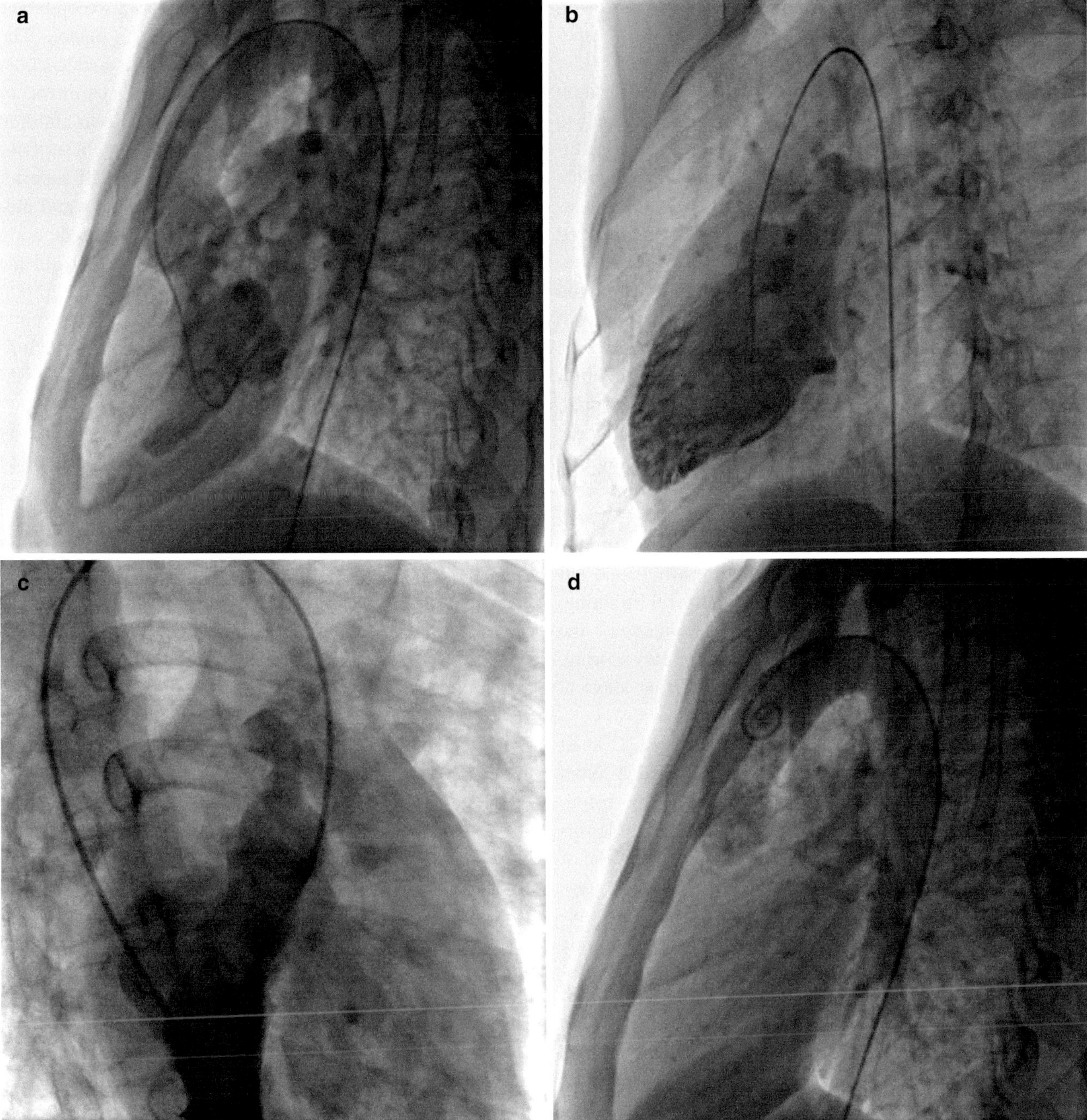

Fig. 5.2 Angiography of complex congenital heart disease. (**a**) Double outlets of the right ventricle can be seen by systolic ventriculography, as both the aorta and pulmonary vessels are visible; (**b**) Pulmonary angiography can be seen by left anterior oblique diastolic ventriculography; (**c**) Pulmonary angiography can be seen by right anterior oblique diastolic ventriculography. (**d**) Aortography showing collateral vessels. Images were obtained from the Department of Cardiovascular Surgery, Children's Hospital Affiliated to Xi'an Jiaotong University and Xijing Hospital

and left ventral ridges, they are separated into two cones, anterolateral and posteromedial, which connect the trabecular primordia of the right ventricle. The posteromedial cone fuses into the left ventricle and becomes its outflow tract. The formation of double outlets of the right ventricle is related to the abnormal rotation and absorption of the cone.

The anatomical structure and hemodynamics of DORV are complex and changeable. There are still controversies and challenges in the surgical treatment of DORV. Echocardiography, cardiac catheterization, CTA, and MRI can objectively display the anatomical structure of DORV, which is of guiding significance for the diagnosis, preoperative evaluation, and surgical planning of DORV. However, these modalities have limitations in evaluating DORV, especially for the development imbalance of atrioventricular valve and judging the different types of DORV. It is difficult to display precise anatomical information of DORV and to implement anatomical correction. Three-dimensional printing technology can transform two-dimensional imaging data into a solid heart model, can clearly display the cardiac anatomy of DORV patients, and can be used for individualized treatment of patients.

Shafkat Anwar [5] of the Medical College of Washington University used 3D printing technology to create a right ventricular double-outlet heart model, which can evaluate the feasibility of left ventricular-aortic tunnel repair in vitro. Khaled Hadeed et al [6]. of Toulouse Children's Hospital, France, used 3D printing technology to create a heart model for a double-outlet neonate. Through evaluation, internal tunnel repair was successfully performed at the age of 5 months. Shi-Joon Yoo [7] of Toronto Children's Hospital reported using 3D printing technology to make complex CHDs models, such as double-outlet right ventricle and left ventricular dysplasia syndrome, for surgical training. According to multidisciplinary expert evaluation, the 3D-printed model scored higher than imaging data scoring, which is an effective assistant method for surgical evaluation.

Huadong [8] et al. of Fuwai Hospital produced 12 heart models of VSD patients with noncommitted double-outlet right ventricle by using 3D printing technology and evaluated the effect of using 3D printing technology to guide surgical decision making, simulation, and surgical operation of noncommitted double-outlet right ventricle. Practice suggests that the 3D-printed model provides a precise anatomical structure for surgeons and a basis for the extent of muscle excision around VSD. 3D-printed models can be very helpful for surgical decision making in cases of double outlet far from the right ventricle, thus reducing the operation time and complications and improving the surgical results by providing preoperative evaluation of surgical simulation. Zhao Liyun [9] et al. of Henan People's Hospital evaluated the application value of 3D-printed heart models in the preoperative evaluation of double-outlet right ventricle and formulation of the surgical plan. The 3D-printed heart model was constructed using 3D printing technology, and the coincidence between the 3D-printed heart model and the intraoperative exploration results was compared. It was concluded that the 3D-printed cardiac model could accurately display the spatial structure of the heart and had a high coincidence with intraoperative exploration. The model could well display the structural relationship between the aorta and the pulmonary artery, the location of the ventricular septal defect and the great artery, the distance between the VSD and the pulmonary valve, etc. The model could also evaluate the feasibility of biventricular correction, and it was also conducive for the establishment of an intraoperative tunnel. The 3D-printed model of the right ventricle before double-outlet operation at the Cardiovascular Surgery Department of Xijing Hospital showed that the right ventricle in children with double outlet was anterior to the heart, the right superior vena cava flowed back to the right atrium, the left superior vena cava flowed back to the left atrium, the aorta and pulmonary artery originated from the right ventricle, the aorta was anterior, the pulmonary artery was posterior, and the ventricular septal defect was located from the perimembranous region to the inflow tract of right ventricle. The septal defect was far from the two major arteries. A clear anatomical relationship provides a sufficient basis for the establishment of surgical procedures (Fig. 5.3).

The cardiac models of CHDs were constructed in vitro by computer three-dimensional reconstruction and 3D printing technology for patients with double-outlet right ventricle in the Cardiovascular Surgery Department of Xijing Hospital. The models can be used to educate patients and to evaluate their surgical plans. With the help of a 3D-printed model, heart malformations, important surrounding structures, and the operation process of complex CHDs can be visualized, and young surgeons can be trained to recognize diseases and better understand surgery. Through simulated surgery, the operator can fully grasp the cardiac anatomical structure of CHD patients, reduce surgical exploration and operation time and costs, and achieve more certain results (Fig. 5.4).

In addition to the double-outlet right ventricle, researchers worldwide have made different attempts to use 3D printing technology on other complex types of CHD: Harikrishnan et al [10]. of Westchester Medical Center, New York, used MRI and transesophageal echocardiography data to print a heart model of a patient with pulmonary atresia combined with a single ventricle and successfully guided the completion of one-and-one-half single ventricle corrective surgery. The Spanish researcher Israel Valverde et al [11]. created a 3D heart model for a child with transposition of the great artery, ventricular septal defect, and severe pulmonary valve stenosis by using 3D printing technology. The location and size of the ventricular septal defect and its spatial structure relationship with the great artery were clearly displayed on the model. The surgeon successfully performed a Nikaidoh operation for the child according to the heart model. Isao Shiraishi [12] et al. of Osaka National Cardiovascular Center made models of patients with left ventricular dysplasia, double-outlet right ventricle, and total anomalous pulmonary venous drainage by using 3D printing technology and simulated the corrective operation of left ventricular dysplasia using the heart model. It was noted that 3D printing technology had important value in the surgical treatment of patients with complex CHD. In October 2017, Guangdong Provincial People's Hospital, Guangdong Institute of Cardiovascular

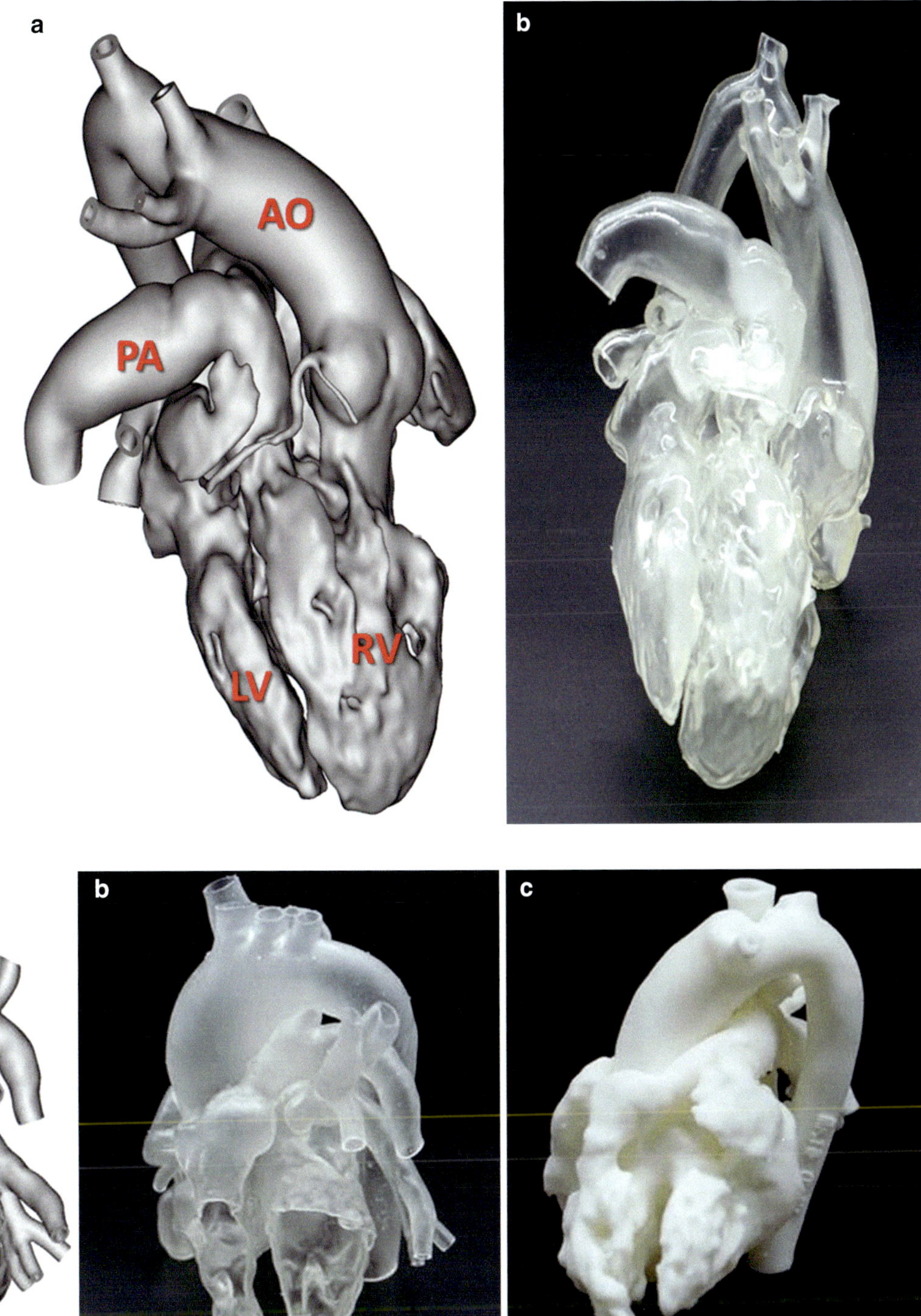

Fig. 5.3 Three-dimensional printing model of double outlets of the right ventricle. (**a**) Computer three-dimensional reconstruction model; (**b**) 3D-printed physical model. The image data, the three-dimensional computer reconstruction, and the 3D-printed model are from the Cardiovascular Surgery Department of Xijing Hospital

Fig. 5.4 Right ventricular dual-outlet 3D-printed model. (**a**) Computer three-dimensional modeling, profile showing the internal structure of the left and right ventricular cavity; (**b**) Transparent material 3D printing, profile showing the internal structure of the left and right ventricular cavity; (**c**) White material 3D printing showing the external structure of the heart cavity and blood vessels in patients with DORV. The image data, the computer three-dimensional reconstruction, and the 3D-printed model are from Qilu Hospital of Shandong University

Diseases, and Zhuhai Senna Printing Technology Co., Ltd. established the first domestic joint laboratory for 3D printing in cardiovascular medicine. With the help of 3D models, the laboratory repaired many different CHDs such as pulmonary atresia, complete transposition of the great artery, double outlet of right ventricle, coarctation or disconnection of aorta, vascular ring, abnormal coronary artery, persistent trunk of artery, etc. Surgery was performed on more than 100 patients with extremely complex congenital heart disease. The operation time was greatly shortened, and the effects were good. In recent years, the author's Department of Cardiovascular Surgery of Xijing Hospital has also carried out 3D printing of complex CHDs. Through 3D printing of the physical model, the treatment team obtained a clearer understanding of the internal space structure of complex CHDs. At the same time, operation plans could be individually formulated, especially for patients with complex CHDs who underwent Glenn's operation, cor triatriatum, and left ventricular double-chamber heart (Figs. 5.5, 5.6, and 5.7).

In April 2019, Tangdu Hospital of Air Force Military Medical University used echocardiographic data to print the first 3D fetal heart model. The volume of the model was eight times larger than the volume of an actual the fetal heart. The length, width, and height of the model were approximately 33 mm, 25 mm, and 24 mm, respectively. Three-dimensional modeling lasted 3 h, coloring lasted 6 h, and 3D printing and postprocessing lasted approximately 8–9 h. The key point of this technology is the accurate reconstruction of the fetal heart and the surrounding aortic and tracheal structures by a computer and multicolor printing in 3D. In some congenital heart diseases (such as vascular rings, which have great individual differences, and complex anatomical structures, which cause different degrees of pressure on the trachea and seriously endanger the life of the fetus),

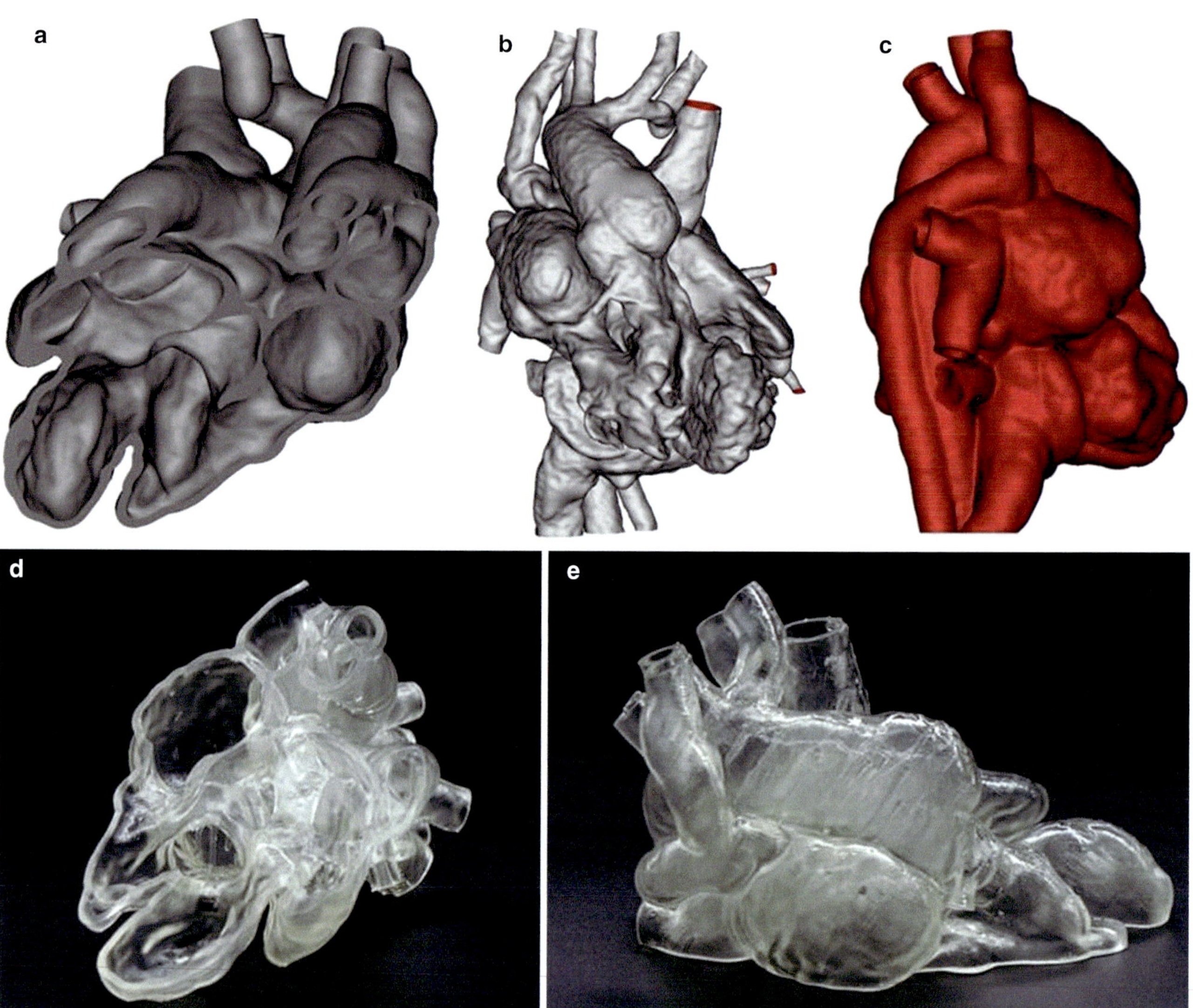

Fig. 5.5 A 3D-printed model was constructed by the Cardiovascular Surgery Department of Xijing Hospital after Glenn's operation for patients with complex CHDs. (**a**) Computer modeling shows the internal profile structure of complex CHDs; (**b**) Computer modeling shows the external structure of a complex CHD showing that the superior vena cava connects to the right pulmonary artery; (**c**) Computer modeling shows the external structure of a complex CHD and the inferior vena cava in the rear view. (**d**) The 3D-printed model shows the internal structure of a complex CHD; (**e**) The 3D-printed model shows the external structure of a complex CHD. The image data, the three-dimensional computer reconstruction, and the three-dimensional printing model are from the Cardiovascular Surgery Department of Xijing Hospital

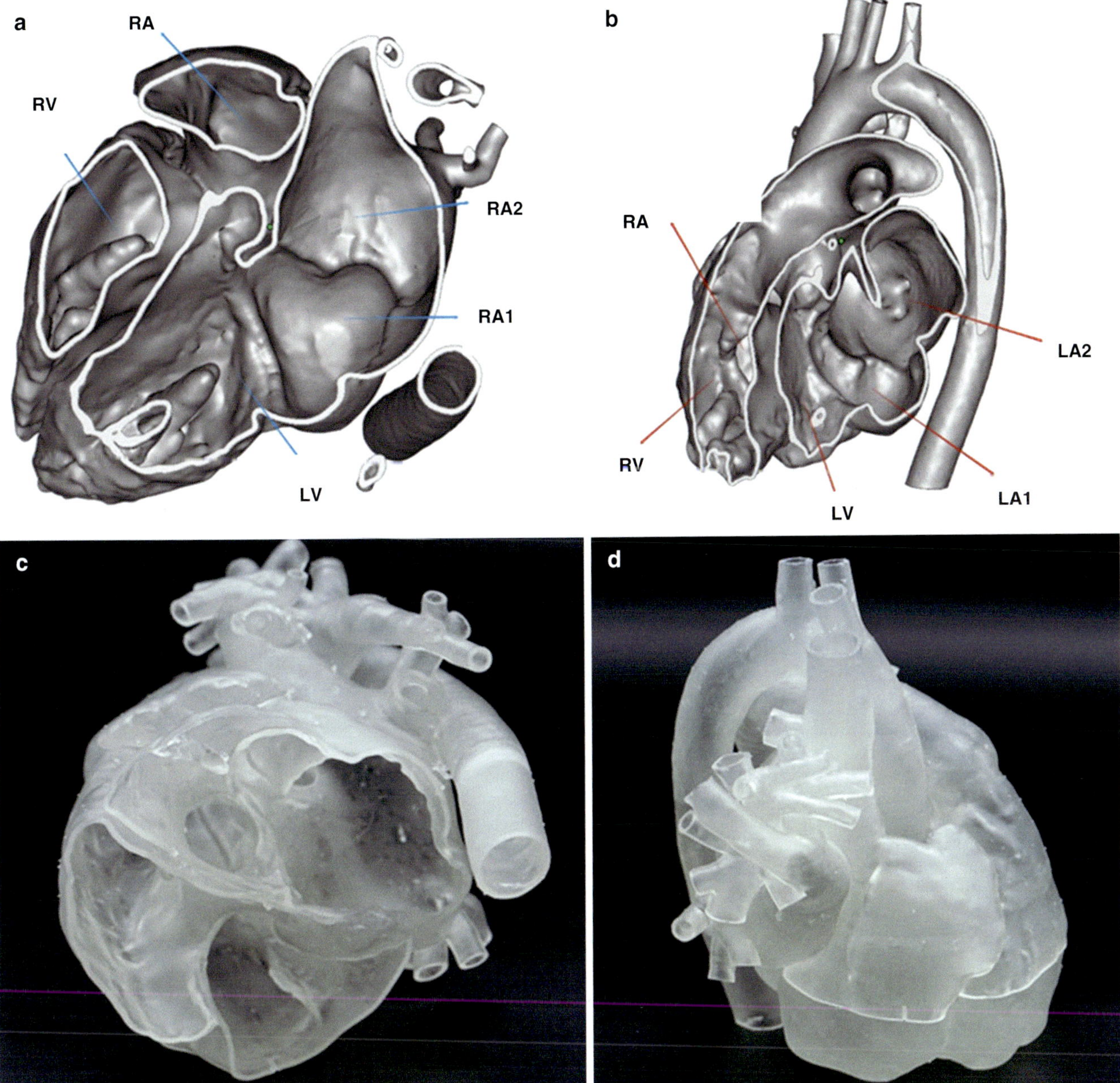

Fig. 5.6 Building the three-dimensional-printed model of the cor triatrium. (**a**) Computer modeling shows the internal structure of the cor triatriatum through a four-chamber view; (**b**) Computer modeling shows the internal structure of the cor triatriatum through the left view; (**c**) The 3D-printed model shows the internal structure of the cor triatriatum; (**d**) The 3D-printed model shows the external structure of the cor triatriatum. The image data, the computer three-dimensional reconstruction, and the 3D-printed model are from Bayi Children's Hospital affiliated with Beijing Military Region General Hospital

three-dimensional reconstruction by a computer can substantiate the anatomical structure and more clearly and intuitively show the abnormal anatomical structure and the spatial position between them (Fig. 5.8). Through a solid model, doctors can more directly discuss the patient's condition and design the treatment plan. If necessary, they can also use the model to simulate the operation, which greatly improves the work efficiency.

5.1.2 Application of 3D Printing Technology in Interventional Treatment of CHDs

In addition to being widely used in the diagnosis and treatment of complex CHDs, a 3D-printed cardiac model can also display the patient's cardiac anatomical information and guide the simulated implantation of an occluder and/or a vascular stent for common CHDs, such as atrial septal defect

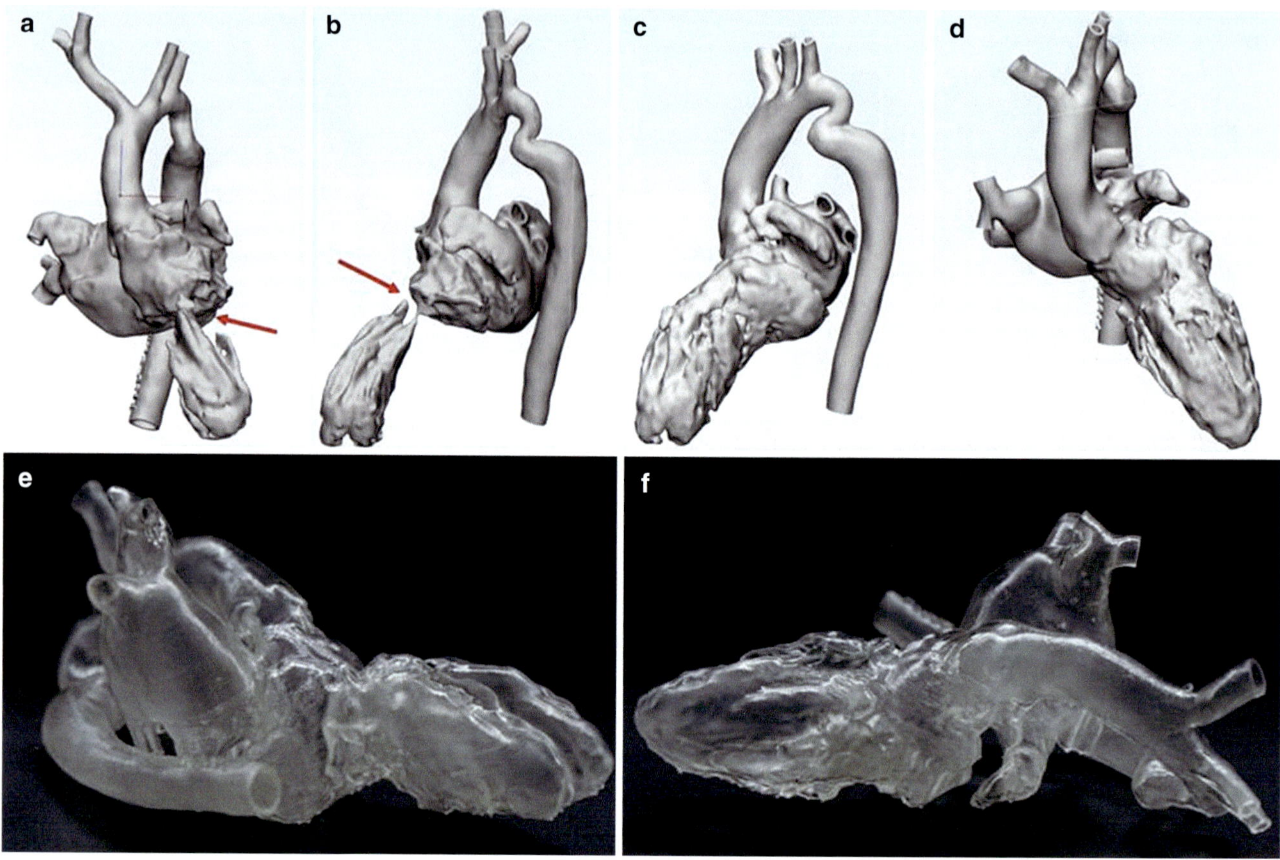

Fig. 5.7 A 3D-printed model of the left ventricular dual-chamber heart was constructed. (**a**) Computer-modeled orthogonal view showing the structure of a systolic left ventricular dual-chamber heart; the red arrow shows the severely narrow part; (**b**) Computer-modeled lateral view showing the structure of a systolic left ventricular dual-chamber heart; the red arrow shows the severely narrow part; (**c**) Computer-modeled lateral view showing the structure of a diastolic left ventricular dual-chamber heart; (**d**) Computer-modeled orthogonal view showing the structure of a diastolic left ventricular dual-chamber heart; (**e**) The 3D-printed model showed the structure of the diastolic left ventricular dual-chamber heart; (**f**) The 3D-printed model showed the structure of the diastolic left ventricular dual-chamber heart. The image data, the three-dimensional computer reconstruction, and the three-dimensional printing model are from the Cardiovascular Surgery Department of Xijing Hospital

and ventricular septal defect, which can increase the success rate of operations and reduce complications.

Atrial septal defect (ASD) refers to an abnormal pathway between the left and right atria formed during development, absorption, and fusion of the original atrial septum during the embryonic period. There are two main types of ASD: primary and secondary ASD. Primary ASD occurs due to septal dysplasia or endocardial cushion dysplasia during embryogenesis. Secondary ASD is caused by secondary atrial septal dysplasia or excessive absorption of primary atrial septal tissue, and the second atrial foramen cannot be closed. Secondary atrial septal defect is usually divided into four types according to its location: (1) Central type defects, located in the middle of the atrial septum, equivalent to the oval fossa, are the most common type, accounting for approximately 70% of the secondary foramen atrial septal defects. (2) Superior cava type, also known as venous sinus type, defects are located above and behind the atrial septum, and there is no obvious boundary between the defect and the entrance of superior vena cava. (3) Inferior cava type defects are located behind the atrial septum; there is no complete atrial septal margin below the defect, but it continues with the entrance of inferior vena cava. The posterior wall of the left atrium constitutes the posterior and inferior margin of the defect. (4) Mixed type defects, i.e., reflect two or more types of large atrial septal defects at the same time. Central type atrial septal defects are more suitable for interventional occlusion. It has been reported that three-dimensional printing technology can be used to guide interventional closure of atrial septal defects. Bennett et al. of Cork University Hospital, Ireland, used three-dimensional echocardiographic data to produce an atrial septal defect model, which clearly showed the location, size, and margin of the atrial septal defect and the spatial structure of other tissues. A three-dimensional heart model has been used in cardiac surgery and interventional cardiac surgery and has important guiding value. Kim [13] and others believe that 3D-printed models can truly and accurately display the cardiac anatomical

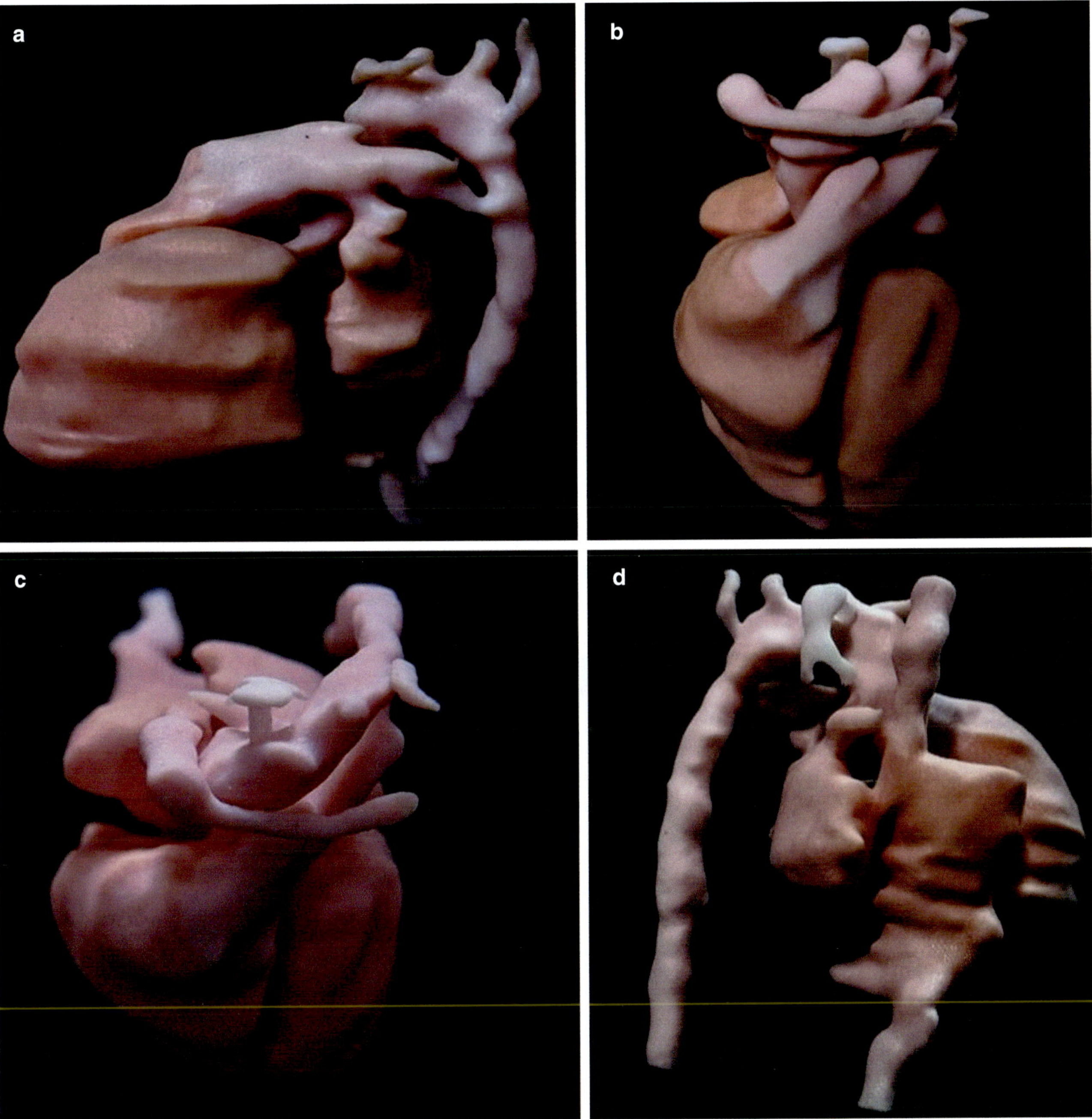

Fig. 5.8 Echocardiographic data were obtained from three-dimensional printed images of the fetal vascular ring heart model. (**a**) left view; (**b**) posterior-anterior view; (**c**) anterior-posterior view; (**d**) right view. The image data and the 3D-printed model are from Tangdu Hospital of Air Force Military Medical University

structure and help surgeons fully understand the location and shape of the defect and its relationship with surrounding tissues. By using different types of catheters and occluders in the models to simulate interventional therapy, appropriate surgical procedures can be formulated to improve the success rate of surgery and reduce radiation exposure and surgical complications. Qiu Xu et al. of Fuwai Hospital created three-dimensional reconstructions from imaging data obtained by three-dimensional echocardiography and CTA by postprocessing software. Twenty-one patients with multiple atrial septal defects were modeled by three-dimensional printing technology. The heart models were simulated by silicone gel printing. The type and location of the occluder were confirmed during the operation. Their model helped solve the difficult problems of occluder placement and high residual shunt rate in interventional closure of multiple atrial septal defects and has important clinical application value. Under the guidance of 3D printing technology, Wang

Zhongmin et al. of Henan People's Hospital found that occluder selection could be simulated in vitro to shorten the operation time and X-ray exposure time and to reduce the failure rate of occluder selection [14].

For complex structural heart disease, the application of 3D printing technology to guide surgery is even more meaningful. The Cardiovascular Surgery Department of the First Affiliated Hospital of Zhengzhou University partnered with the Cardiovascular Surgery Department of Xijing Hospital to treat a patient with giant pseudoaneurysm after mitral valve replacement. They used CTA data modeling to print a heart model to simulate occlusion, simulate the establishment of access through an apical small incision, select the appropriate type of occluder, and determine the occlusion location to avoid interference with the aorta. A 28 mm patent ductus arteriosus occluder was selected and well positioned, without a residual shunt, which proved to have good prognosis, shorten the operation time and X-ray exposure time, and reduce the failure rate associated with occluder selection (Fig. 5.9).

With the development and popularization of 3D printing technology, interventional occlusion can be attempted under 3D model guidance in some patients who were previously contraindicated for the procedure. The inferior vena cava type ASDs are located at the lower part of the atrial septum and continue to the entrance of the inferior vena cava. These defects lack complete margins and clear demarcation. Because there is no effective interval between the posterior and inferior margins to support the ASD occluder, it is easy to cause the occluder to drop off; therefore, interventional treatment is contraindicated, and the treatment mainly depends on surgery. Zhang Yushun et al. from the First Affiliated Hospital of Xi'an Jiaotong University found that the lower edge of inferior cavity ASDs was composed of the inferior vena cava and the inferior wall of the left atrium. As a result, the shape of the inferior cavity ASD was similar to a "T" or "funnel" structure. During the simulated occlusion experiment, it was found that a PDA occluder could adapt well to the special structure of the inferior cavity ASD. The PDA occluder has a shorter umbrella disk and a longer

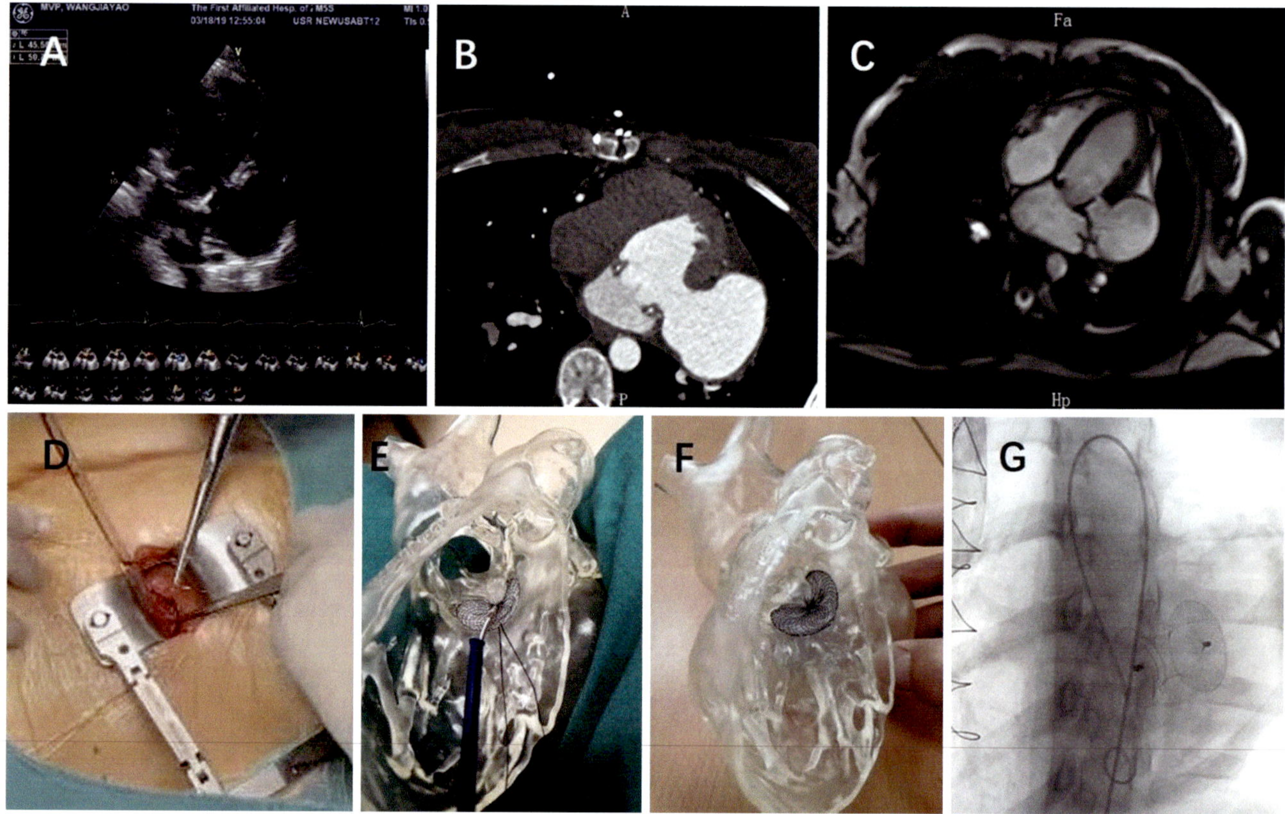

Fig. 5.9 3D printing technique used to guide interventional occlusion of a giant pseudoaneurysm after mitral valve replacement. (**a**) Doppler showing a giant pseudoaneurysm; (**b**) CTA showing a giant pseudoaneurysm; (**c**) magnetic resonance imaging showing a giant pseudoaneurysm; (**d**) small incision through the apex; (**e**) the 3D-printed model was used to simulate occlusion; (**f**) the 3D-printed model was used to select the appropriate occluder to simulate occlusion; (**g**) a 28 mm patent ductus arteriosus occluder was used to completely occlude the giant pseudoaneurysm. The image data and the 3D printing models were obtained from the Cardiovascular Surgery Department of the First Affiliated Hospital of Zhengzhou University and Xijing Hospital

umbrella waist. The shorter skirt edge of the umbrella disk will not have a great impact on the left atrium or cause any occluder displacement. The umbrella waist of the occluder can be well attached to the plane of the inferior vena cava and to the inferior wall of the left atrium, making the occluder very stable. The waist of the PDA occluder will be depressed by compression of the atrial septum above the ASD, providing sufficient extrusion force to fix the occluder. The team also used advanced 3D printing technology to successfully occlude patients with inferior atrial septal defects using a ventricular septal occluder, breaking the long-standing notion that this portion of inferior atrial septal defects could not be treated by interventional therapy.

Ventricular septal defects (VSD) are one of the most common congenital heart diseases, accounting for 20% of all congenital heart diseases. The interventricular septum consists of four parts: membranous septum, inflow septum, trabecular septum, outflow septum, or funnel septum. Ventricular septal defects may occur at various parts of the ventricular septum and can be divided into four types: membranous or perimembranous ventricular septal defect, atrioventricular tubular ventricular septal defect, funnel or subtrunk septal defect, and muscular septal defect. Perimembranous ventricular septal defect is more suitable for interventional occlusion. The authors first confirmed the safety and effectiveness of transcatheter minimally invasive interventional therapy for perimembranous ventricular septal defects (VSD) in 2010. The results were published in Eur Heart J 2010, 31 (18): 2238–45 [15]. In 2014, through a multicenter randomized controlled study, the authors first confirmed that transcatheter minimally invasive interventional techniques, and surgical operations are safe and effective methods for the treatment of perimembranous ventricular septal defects. Interventional therapy has many advantages, such as short operation time, less bleeding during operation, low medical cost, and quick recovery after operation, and has become a "inclusion/exclusion" standard for perimembranous ventricular septal defect. These results were published in JACC. 2014; 63:1159–68 [16].

3D printing technology has achieved good results in the diagnosis and treatment of ventricular septal defects. There are currently many applications of 3D printing technology in the treatment of patients with ventricular septal defect worldwide. In 2008, Kim et al [17]. studied a 30-year-old congenital ventricular septal defect patient. After confirming the existence of a bidirectional-shunt ventricular septal defect heart disease by Doppler echocardiography, CT data were used to print a heart model, and successful occlusion of ventricular septal defect was completed according to the printed model, which showed the relationship between anatomical structure and spatial structure. The study proved that a 3D cardiac physical model is helpful for understanding the pathophysiology of ventricular septal defect anatomy. The model allowed the anatomical structure of the defect to be more accurately displayed, distinguishing the advantages and disadvantages of different operations and interventional treatment and allowing more detailed and accurate surgical plans to be made before operation. In China, Sun Jian and others of Nanjing Children's Hospital successfully completed the surgical closure of children with ventricular septal defects and atrial septal defects using 3D printing technology. Heart models of children were printed by 3D printing technology, the relationship between ventricular septal defect and surrounding tissues was clarified, and the occlusion operation was successfully completed. The study proved that 3D printing technology could overcome the shortcomings of traditional imaging examinations that could not specify the degree of anatomy. Yang Yankun [18] et al. at Fuwai Hospital used CTA to obtain imaging data. A heart model of a patient with ruptured aortic sinus aneurysm was made by using 3D printing technology. The interventional occlusion was simulated on the heart model, and the percutaneous-mediated aortic sinus aneurysm occlusion operation was successfully completed.

Stent implantation is a new method for the treatment of rare vascular diseases such as pulmonary vein stenosis. The operation is difficult and has many complications. Stent implantation is prone to displacement, and stents may cause obstruction of vessels. The effect of previous operations has mainly depended on the surgeon's experience. Olivieri et al [19]. of Washington National Children's Medical Center successfully performed pulmonary vein stent placement in a patient with pulmonary vein stenosis after a CHD operation with the help of 3D printing technology. Echocardiography showed pulmonary vein stenosis and pulmonary venous reflux disturbance in the patient. Images were obtained by CTA angiography, and a 1:1 heart model was created. According to the patient's heart model, the models of pulmonary vein stent and sheath were selected, and a simulated operation of pulmonary vein stent implantation was performed. The Spanish scholar Israel Valverde et al. used MRI data to create heart models with different materials. The heart models were compared with the MR data and angiographic data. The experience of stent implantation was summarized by simulating stent implantation on a 3D-printed model. The most suitable balloon, catheter, and vascular stent were selected to place the stent in the best position in the operation of aortic arch dysplasia.

In short, the continuous progress and development of cardiovascular 3D printing technology not only has important guiding significance for the diagnosis of complex congenital heart diseases and the planning and establishment of surgical procedures, but it can also assist in simulating surgeries, thus playing an increasingly important role in the interventional treatment of congenital heart diseases [20].

5.2 3D Printing of Prenatal Heart Disease

Meng Yang, Jincheng Liu, Jiayou Tang

Congenital heart diseases (CHDs) are a complex specter of malformations difficult to detect, to teach, and to correct. Malformations of the heart and vessels are generally very diverse and heterogeneous so their interpretation is not always simple1. Moreover, it s the most frequent congenital malformation in newborn [1, 21–25], with an estimated incidence about 8–10: 1000 in full-term births, but it could be ten times higher in preterm infants (8.3%) [26, 27]. Furthermore, in early gestation, this incidence is even higher as certain CHDs are complex and not compatible with life and as such have been shown to result in fetal demise. In fact, 50%–60% of the CHDs will eventually require surgical correction, and 25% of these, because of their criticality, can lead to infant mortality [28].

In this setting, the survival or development of disability is crucially dependent on the timing of the diagnosis. For this reason, correct identification in the prenatal period can certainly make the difference between a good or a bad prognosis. Therefore, early prenatal diagnosis of a treatable CHD has been shown to reduce the risk of perinatal morbidity and mortality [29]. It is well known that prenatal diagnosis of CHDs greatly improved the perinatal outcome of these babies, but it is also important insofar as it allows proper counseling of expecting parents, which in turn makes them better aware and able to make a more conscious and serene choice in case of termination of pregnancy or to better prepare them for the management and outcome of their unborn babies.

Conventional two-dimensional (2D) ultrasonography is the gold standard for diagnosis of fetal CHDs, and various methods of antenatal ultrasound assessment of fetal heart are currently available. The "four-chamber view scan" method for screening of the fetal heart proved itself to be less reliable than expected; in fact, several studies [29–31] have shown that the performance of this scan alone is very poor, with a detection rate (DR) of only 48% for CHDs [32]. The additional assessment of the ventricular outflow tracts, which, together with the aforementioned four-chamber view, composes an extended basic fetal scan, increases the DR to 75%, but this is still well under an acceptable rate [33]. The fetal echocardiogram is a more detailed sonographic evaluation of cardiac structures and function, and it is performed by specialist in the prenatal diagnosis of CHD. During a fetal echocardiogram, several imaging modalities can be used, ranging from Color Flow Doppler and M mode to 4D ultrasonography; this is necessary because 2D imaging methods can lack precious spatial information [34]. Fetal echocardiography is a diagnostic method used to identify CHDs in high-risk groups, and in those patients the sensitivity ranges from 60 to 100% [35]; however, in unselected and low-risk pregnancies the DR range can be much lower, going from 35 to 86% [35].

In the modern era, it is now expected that ultrasound must be able to diagnose structural heart disease with precise detail, and so any new diagnostic modalities or tools that improve antenatal detection or counseling comprehension of CHDs are highly welcomed. Despite technological advances in ultrasound machines, increasing experience in fetal medicine, and introduction of study protocols to heart examination, prenatal diagnosis of CHDs remains a challenge. The fetal heart is difficult to examine for many reasons, and it requires extensive training and expertise [29, 36]. The biggest challenges are that the heart is obviously small and changes with gestational age; that it is a dynamic organ (normal fetal heart beat is about 140 bpm); and that it is located in a moving patient (the fetus changes position very often during the ultrasound examination, and this sometimes allows an adequate ultrasound window and sometimes does not). Moreover, there are many fetal and maternal factors that can limit the view (gestational age, fetal position, increased BMI, scarred abdomen, or oligohydramnios).

The cardiac examination of the fetus requires an adequate examiner experience and a continuous feedback-based training of healthcare diagnosis of CHDs. Furthermore, only firsthand experience and adequate training allow the total comprehension of even very complex cardiac pathologies, thus allowing adequate counseling. Indeed, counseling must be as clear and realistic as possible. 3D-printed models of CHDs represent an innovative and useful possibility to improve medical education and training as well as doctor–patient communication. CHD is characterized by complex morphological anomalies in which it is crucial to have a comprehensive understanding of the dimensional and spatial relationship of the intracardiac anatomical structures to understand the disease's physiopathology, embryological origin, and surgical correction procedure [1, 6, 37–56]. 3D-printed CHD models thus allow a unique 3D view of the cardiac anatomy; several studies showed that 3D-printed models are useful in medical education for healthcare professionals, medical students, and doctor–patient communication, both with young patients themselves or their parents [1].

5.3 3D Printing Protocol in Prenatal Diagnosis

5.3.1 Image Acquisition, Segmentation, and Model Design

In order to achieve a better understanding of CHDs, 3D physical models of the heart and vessels can be based on volumetric scans. These scans can be obtained with mainly three methods: computed tomography (CT), magnetic resonance imaging (MRI), and echocardiography imaging data (US). These methods allow a total exploration of all three spatial planes, providing more information than conventional visualization. However, it must be considered that MRI and CT are not very easy methods in prenatal life because they subject the patient (in prenatal diagnosis both the mother and the fetus simultaneously) to either contrast media, anesthesia, or radiation, which can be harmful. The developments in ultrasound scans, both in 3D and 4D, have allowed an adaptation of this tool, extending its capabilities to a complete evaluation of the fetal heart, opening the possibility to the creation of excellent 3D models starting from the raw ultrasound scan [1–3, 29, 57, 58].

The models obtained by echocardiography using 3D/4D-based spatiotemporal imaging collection (STIC) are no different or of inferior quality with respect to CT or MRI-derived models. In fact, the 3D-printed models derived from 3D echocardiography show high accuracy in replicating congenital heart disease, with excellent correlation between standard 2D and 3D model measurements [3, 42, 43, 51, 55, 56]. A very important thing, however, is to obtain a good initial data acquisition, with high-quality imagines, through the ultrasound method of STIC (follow the indications provided in the literature for an optimal STIC). In fact, obtaining an optimal ultrasound volume allows a decrease in segmentation time and the presence of limited noise, thus having a lower possibility of creating artifacts. As general rule, it is important to have a high contrast between the object we ought to reconstruct (in our case the fetal heart) and the surrounding tissues. STIC allows us to improve the visualization of the anatomy and the internal cardiac structures, thus helping the accuracy of the diagnosis of congenital heart defects. This method is also very fast and allows the acquisition of the volume in a few seconds, and so it can be repeated many times until the optimal volume has been acquired. The volume can then be viewed under an infinite number of different views, even without the direct presence of the patient or without the echographic machine, on a PC. This allows us to obtain a lot of information in a very short time (information that is not typically available from conventional 2D images), and to collect and review complex fetal hearts at a later stage and completely offline. STIC is an automatic tool included into the ultrasound probe; it allows the operator to perform a slow scan that generates a single three-dimensional (3D) volume. The acquired volume is composed of a great number of two-dimensional (2D) frames. This volume is recorded by the ultrasound machine, and it is possible to carry out a subsequent analysis of the heart under all the different views and/or planes deemed useful, by presenting an image in the multiplanar and rendering mode showing the positioning of vessels.

After acquiring the ideal volume, there are different ways in which to investigate the fetal heart, depending on the need in the specific case. The multiplanar mode shows the image in three orthogonal planes (axial, sagittal, and coronal), which can be subsequently oriented in all three axes (x, y, z) as well. The rendering mode, by the determination of virtual planes, allows for better morphological assessment of critical internal cardiac structures such as the septum and the atrioventricular valves.

To create a 3D-printed model of the fetal heart, 3D fetal ultrasound scan was obtained with Voluson E8/E10 machine (GE Healthcare, Chicago, IL, USA) using the abovementioned spatiotemporal imagine correlation (STIC). The data were exported directly from the Voluson machine and imported into a specific software called Mimics InPrint (Materialise, Leuven, Belgium) for segmentation (Fig. 5.10). Usually, the time taken to complete the segmentation ranged from 0.5 to 12 h, with an average of 3.5 h. Segmentation is the process that allows the creation of a region of interest (ROI) by specifically selecting a series of voxels (volume units) corresponding to the anatomical structure to be reproduced. There are software that manage the selection of voxels automatically or semi-automatically, but this is not adequate in complex cases of malformations, so manual selection is usually recommended to adequately select the area of interest.

Having the possibility to select the window of interest, we can modulate the 3D reproduction based on the defect you want to highlight. So, the production of a 3D object is not a static mechanism, but a dynamic, modifiable, and modellable one, according to specific needs and specific patient. During this phase, the boundaries of the imagine were verified by a sonographer, changed as needed, and then subsequently precisely defined to obtain an absolutely optimal quality. At the end, a virtual 3D object is generated, leveled, and finally exported as STL files. These files can be further optimized using computer-aided design software in order to eliminate artifacts and noise. Last, the virtual model is transferred to a 3D printer for production. There are numerous options to represent the anatomy of CHD in 3D-printed models such as data preparation and printing materials and also create specific artificial holes to hollowed intracardiac representation to highlight complex relationships between the structures.

There are many materials either rigid or flexible as well as transparent ones to be used as a basis for 3D printing. A very important parameter to factor in is the cost that can be sustained, because different materials and different levels of quality have different costs. Some studies show that the price can indeed radically change, going from USD 1 to USD 200. If the use of model is only to visualize the anatomy, as in the case of medical education and counseling, rigid material would be more than adequate. Usually, it is recommended, if

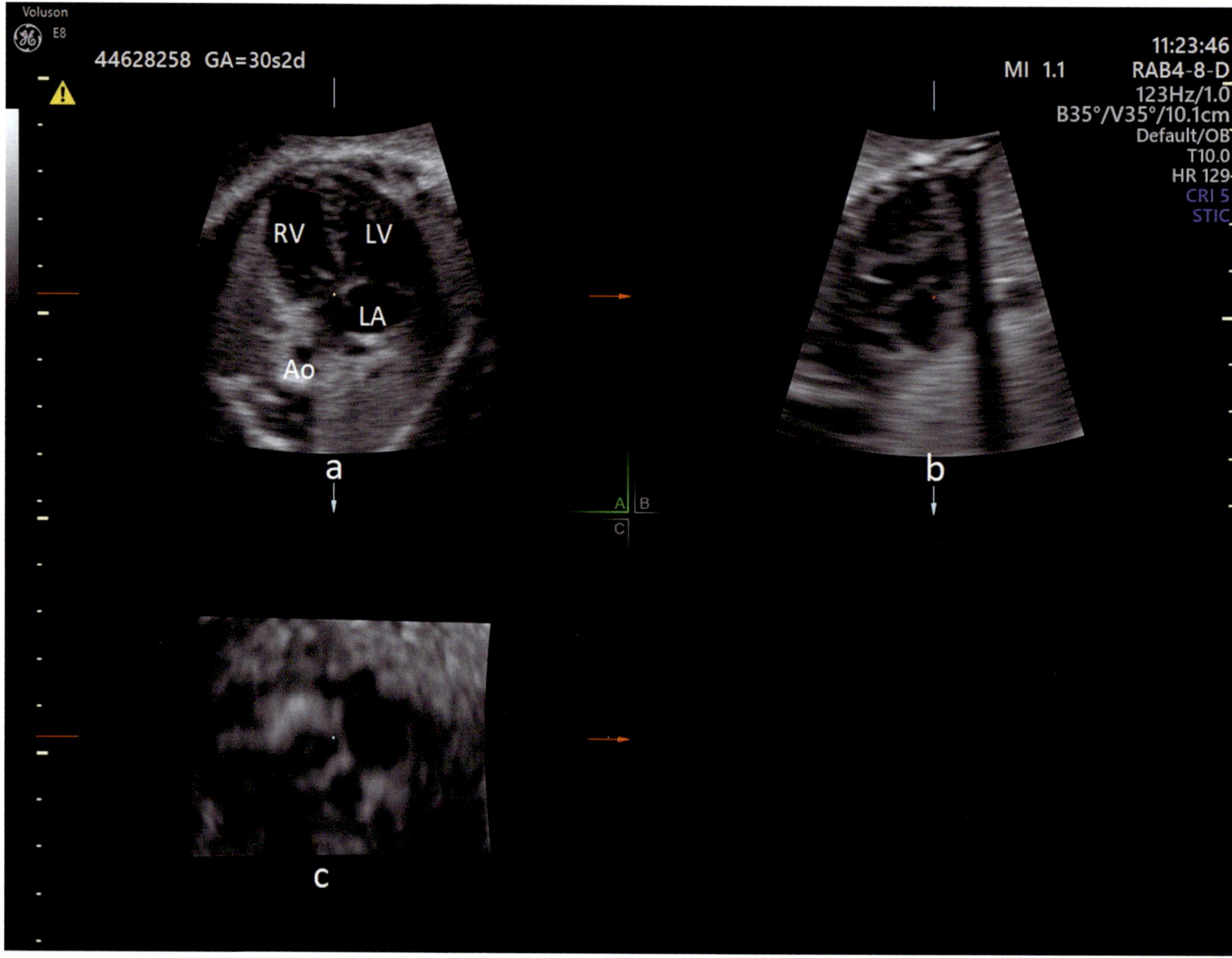

Fig. 5.10 The three-dimensional STIC voucher acquired with the Voluson machine. The volume can be thoroughly examined slice by slice along the three orthogonal planes (**a**, **b**, and **c**). *Ao* Aorta, *RV* right ventricle, *LV* left ventricle, *LA* left atrium

possible, to print the anatomical structures in their real-life dimensions to keep the maximum fidelity, but in prenatal diagnosis, in which the heart is often very small, it is necessary to magnifiy. In our cases, we have amplified the structure five times in all directions, in order to make the final print more comprehensible and allow a macroscopical appreciation of the defects (Figs. 5.11, 5.12, 5.13, and 5.14).

5.3.2 Applications of 3D-Printed Models of CHD in Prenatal Diagnosis [1, 29, 57, 58]

Due to the heterogeneity and complexity of fetal cardiac malformations that may occur, it is essential to have a comprehensive understanding of the dimensional and spatial relationship of the cardiac structures [35]. Until now, the methods for studying and deepening the heart anatomy were pretty much only based on drawn images, diagrams, 2D ultrasound images, or at most through anatomical pieces, which are often not easy to find or otherwise subject to decay [1, 20, 42, 59]. However, a lot of these methods require a 3D mental reconstruction that is not always simple and immediate, especially for those who are not very familiar with these issues, such as other physicians without any CHDs' expertise or the patient itself. This difficult passage is avoided by the presence of the 3D model. Many studies have shown how 3D-printed models are useful to understand anatomic and spatial complexity in CHDs; they represent a valid tool for medical training of all medical personnel, including senior doctor, resident, medical student, and nurses as well [1, 6, 37–56]. In fact, the accuracy obtained with these prints can allow the surgeon to better understand the various cardiac anatomical relationships, and it can also offer the possibility to discuss it clearly in multidisciplinary groups [46, 56]. It can allow maternal–fetal obstetrician to better understand complex cardiac pathologies, also helping him consequently in counseling. The couple, having no medical training, often

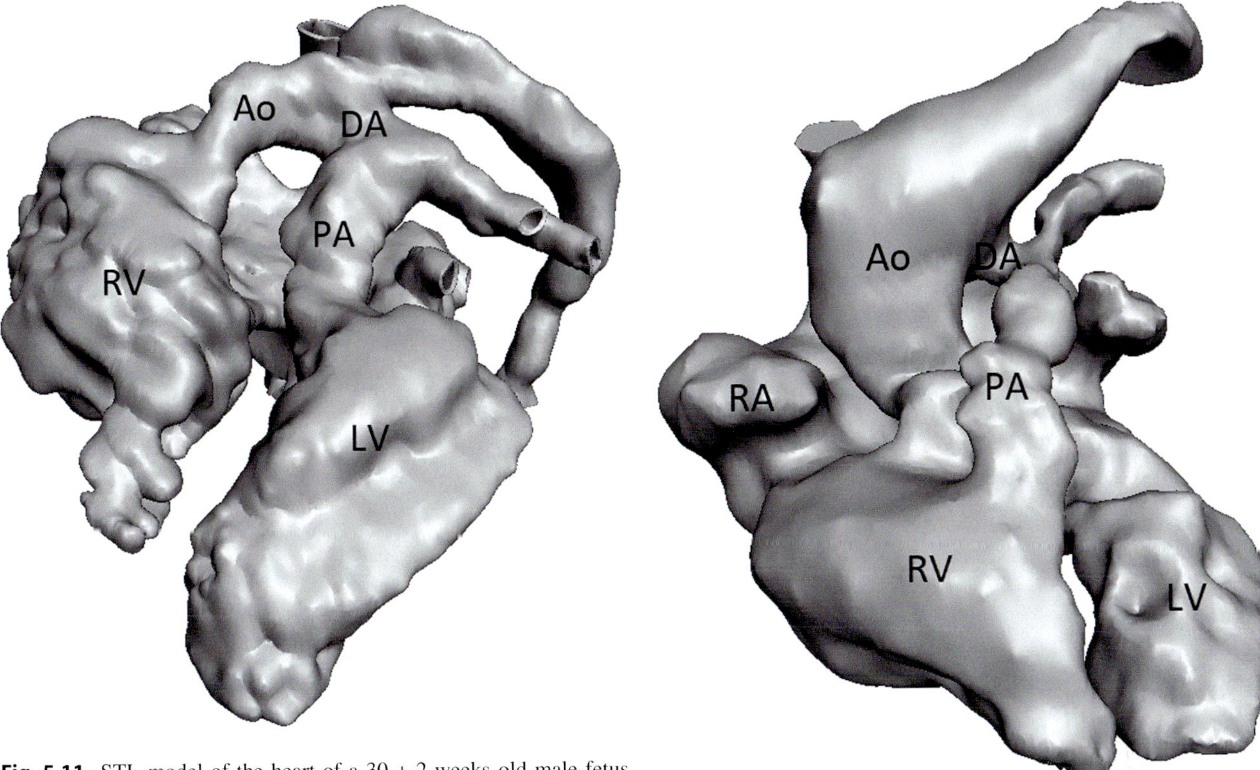

Fig. 5.11 STL model of the heart of a 30 + 2 weeks old male fetus diagnosed with a D-transposition of the great arteries (D-TGA). *Ao* aorta, *PA* pulmonary artery, *RV* right ventricle, *LV* left ventricle, *DA* ductus arteriosus

Fig. 5.12 STL model of the heart of a 25 + 5 weeks old male fetus diagnosed with tetralogy of Fallot. *Ao* aorta, *PA* pulmonary artery, *RV* right ventricle, *LV* left ventricle, *DA* ductus arteriosus, *RA* right atrium

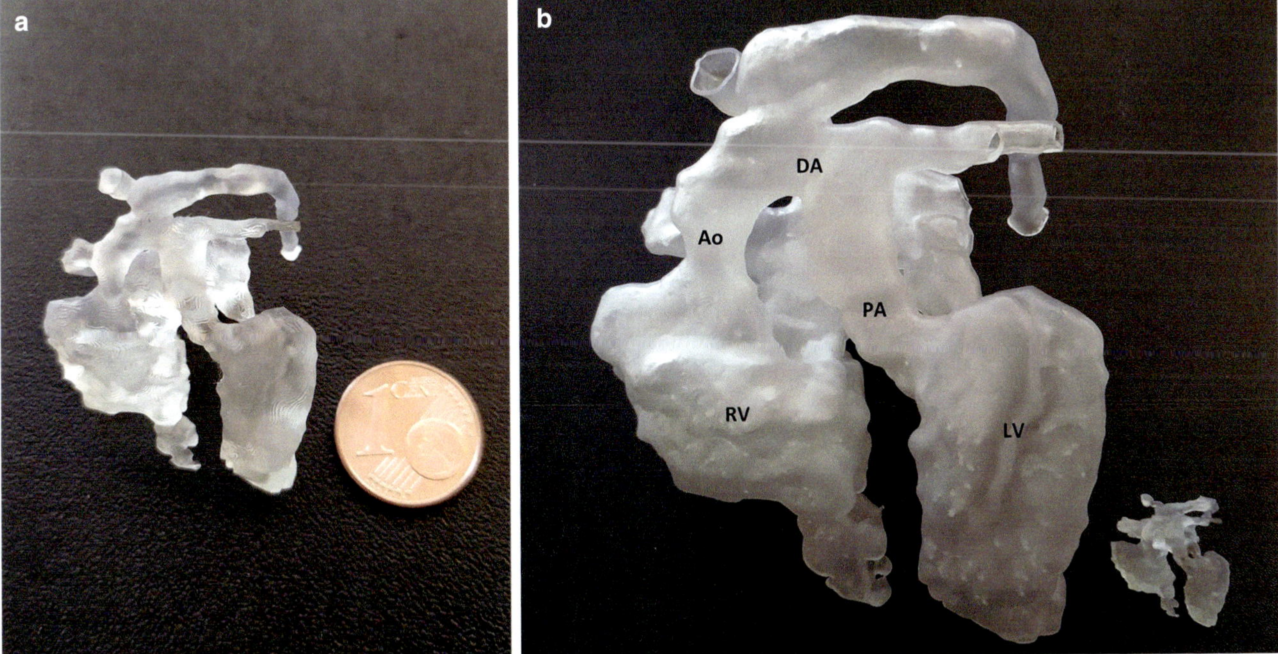

Fig. 5.13 (same model of Fig. 5.11) 3D-printed fetal heart with clear resin both in real dimensions (**a**) and magnified five times (**b**). *Ao* Aorta, *PA* pulmonary artery, *RV* right ventricle, *LV* left ventricle, *DA* ductus arteriosus. The coin is for scale

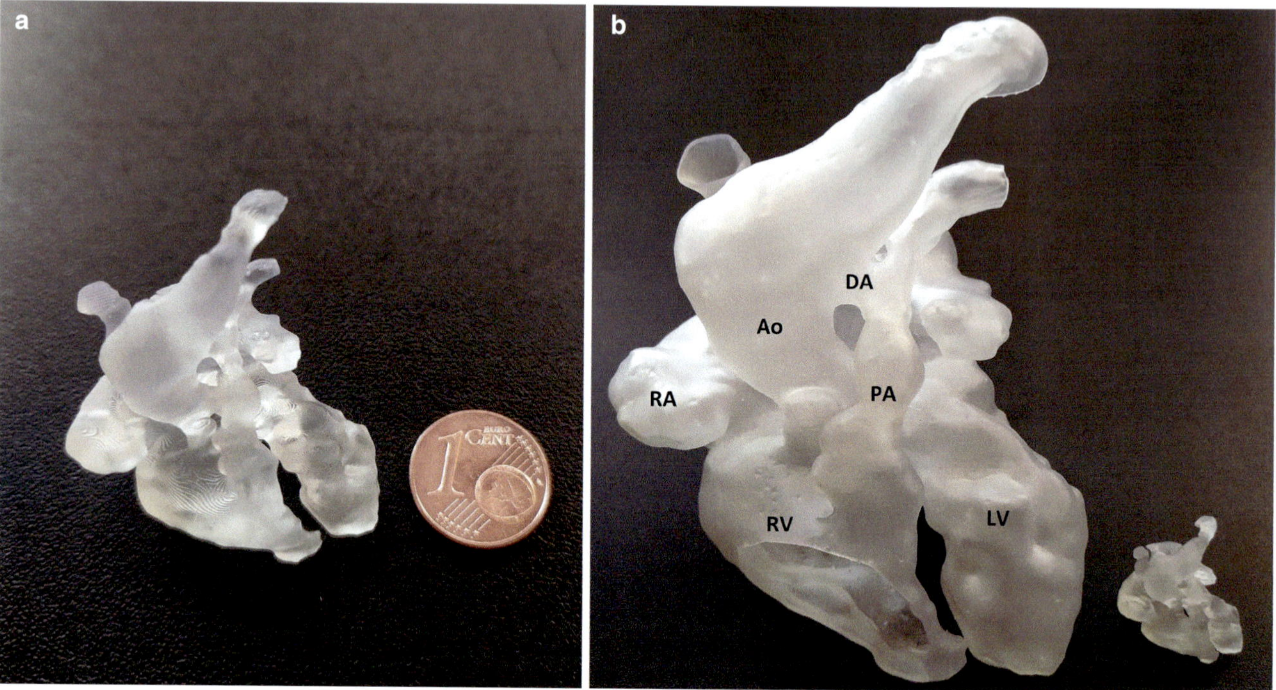

Fig. 5.14 (same model of Fig. 5.12) 3D-printed fetal heart model with clear resin both in real dimensions (**a**) and magnified five times (**b**). *Ao* Aorta, *PA* pulmonary artery, *RV* right ventricle, *LV* left ventricle, *DA* ductus arteriosus, *RA* Right Atrium. The coin is again for scale

hears but does not understand what they are told. Having the opportunity to finally see and touch the fetal pathology definitely helps in understanding and therefore also in the choice of final management. It is also a great help on a psychological level, considering that they are almost always patients with many questions and doubts and they are not fully able to understand the problem.

In conclusion, the production of 3D objects starting from an ultrasound volume is an effective, economic, and easily accessible method. A method that does not require patient sedation has no potentially negative effects on the mother or on the fetus (therefore much safer than CT and MRI) and for which acquisition programs are very fast (STIC), without however worsening the quality of the final 3D object. This method allows adequate training for doctors operating in the field of maternal–fetal medicine, allows a greater possibility of understanding by non-expert medical staff (residents, nurses, etc.), and provides a solid and valid help for counseling.

Finally, a brief mention of the possibility of having a reproduction of a customized heart [60] is needed. The 3D-printed hearts discussed so far are used mainly for counseling and/or for medical operator training (both for physiology and for pathology) and they are generic printed models, which represent a set of fetuses with that particular condition. However, there is also the possibility of having a "personalized 3D heart," with the exact three-dimensional reproduction of the heart of that fetus, in order to be able to reason and visualize the fetal condition specifically, without generalizations. Some couples in this way can perceive a greater empathy, a greater involvement, and understanding to what their real condition is. It is also important to remember how each heart, independently from the underlying pathology it has been labeled with, will always have small anatomical variations that make it unique. For this reason, having a customized heart (for example of a very particular and complex case) can provide useful information, also educational, to all medical staff. If you make an STIC voucher (where therefore the ultrasound volume is optimal), the final resolution will be excellent. Furthermore, the high-quality conditions allow us to cut the production times because the number of artifacts and imperfections decreases (which otherwise must be eliminated later). The segmentation times in this case are always around 2 h, and the printing time is 1 h for the life-sized version and 10 h for the magnified one, therefore an absolutely acceptable timing.

References

Section 5.1

1. Lau I, Sun Z. Three-dimensional printing in congenital heart disease: a systematic review. J Med Radiat Sci. 2018;65:226–36.
2. Samuel BP, Pinto C, Pietila T, Vettukattil JJ. Ultrasound-derived three-dimensional printing in congenital heart disease. J Digit Imaging. 2015;28:459–61.

3. Olivieri LJ, Krieger A, Loke Y-H, Nath DS, Kim PCW, Sable CA. Three-dimensional printing of intracardiac defects from three-dimensional echocardiographic images: feasibility and relative accuracy. J Am Soc Echocardiogr. 2015;28:392–7.
4. Yoo SJ, Spray T, Austin EH III, Yun TJ, van Arsdell GS. Hands-on surgical training of congenital heart surgery using 3-dimensional print models. J Thorac Cardiovasc Surg. 2017;153:1530–40.
5. Anwar S, Singh GK, Varughese J, Nguyen H, Billadello JJ, Sheybani EF, Woodard PK, Manning P, Eghtesady P. 3D printing in complex congenital heart disease across a spectrum of age, pathology, and imaging techniques. JACC Cardiovasc Imaging. 2017;10:953–6.
6. Hadeed K, Dulac Y, Acar P. Three-dimensional printing of a complex CHD to plan surgical repair. Cardiol Young. 2016;26:1432–4.
7. Yoo SJ, Thabit O, Kim EK, Ide H, Yim D, Dragulescu A, Seed M, Grosse-Wortmann L, van Arsdell G. 3D printing in medicine of congenital heart diseases. 3D Print Med. 2015;2:3.
8. Hua Z, Yang X, Liu K. Improving surgical outcomes of double outlet far from right ventricle using 3D printing technology. Chin J Thorac Cardiovasc Surg Clin. 2016;5:532–6.
9. Zhao L, Fan T, Bin L. Application value of 3-D printed cardiac model in preoperative evaluation and surgical planning of double outlet right ventricle. J Zhengzhou Univer (Med Ed). 2018;53:351–4.
10. Kurup HK, Samuel BP, Vettukattil JJ. Hybrid 3D printing: a game-changer in personalized cardiac medicine? Expert Rev Cardiovasc Ther. 2015;13:1281–4.
11. Valverde I, Gomez G, Coserria J, Suarez-Mejias C, Uribe S, Sotelo J, Velasco M, De Soto J, Hosseinpour A, Gomez-Cia T. 3D printed models for planning endovascular stenting in transverse aortic arch hypoplasia. Catheter Cardiovasc Interv. 2015;85:1006–12.
12. Shiraishi I, Yamagishi M, Hamaoka K, Fukuzawa M, Yagihara T. Simulative operation on congenital heart disease using rubber-like urethane stereolithographic biomodels based on 3D datasets of multislice computed tomography. Eur J Cardiothorac Surg. 2010;37:302–6.
13. Kim MS, Hansgen AR, Wink O, Quaife RA, Carroll JD. Rapid prototyping: a new tool in understanding and treating structural heart disease. Circulation. 2008;117:2388–94.
14. Wang Z, Liu Y, Xu Y, Gao C, Chen Y, Luo H. Three-dimensional printing-guided percutaneous transcatheter closure of secundum atrial septal defect with rim deficiency: first-in-human series. Cardiol J. 2016;23:599–603.
15. Yang J, Yang L, Wan Y, Zuo J, Zhang J, Chen W, Li J, Sun L, Yu S, Liu J, Chen T, Duan W, Xiong L, Yi D. Transcatheter device closure of perimembranous ventricular septal defects: mid-term outcomes. Eur Heart J. 2010;31:2238–45.
16. Yang J, Yang L, Yu S, Liu J, Zuo J, Chen W, Duan W, Zheng Q, Xu X, Li J, Zhang J, Xu J, Sun L, Yang X, Xiong L, Yi D, Wang L, Liu Q, Ge S, Ren J. Transcatheter versus surgical closure of perimembranous ventricular septal defects in children: a randomized controlled trial. J Am Coll Cardiol. 2014;63:1159–68.
17. Kim MS, Hansgen AR, Carroll JD. Use of rapid prototyping in the care of patients with structural heart disease. Trends Cardiovasc Med. 2008;18:210–6.
18. Yang Y, Hong Z, Xu Z. A case of rupture of aortic sinus aneurysm occluded by catheter with the assistance of 3D printing technology. Chin J Inter Cardiol. 2014:135–6.
19. Olivieri L, Krieger A, Chen MY, Kim P, Kanter JP. 3D heart model guides complex stent angioplasty of pulmonary venous baffle obstruction in a mustard repair of d-TGA. Int J Cardiol. 2014;172:E297–8.
20. Vukicevic M, Mosadegh B, Min JK, Little SH. Cardiac 3D printing and its future directions. JACC Cardiovasc Imaging. 2017;10:171–84.

Section 5.2

21. Australian Institute of Health and Welfare. Cardiovascular disease Australian facts 2011. Canberra: Australian Institute of Health and Welfare; 2011. p. 220.
22. Mitchell SC, Korones SB, Berendes HW. Congenital heart disease in 56,109 Births: incidence and natural history. Circulation. 1971;43:323–32.
23. Van der Linde D, Konings EE, Slager MA, et al. Birth prevalence of congenital heart disease worldwide: a systematic review and meta-analysis. J Am Coll Cardiol. 2011;58:2241–7.
24. Wren C, Birrell G, Hawthorne G. Cardiovascular malformations in infants of diabetic mothers. Heart. 2003;89:1217–20.
25. Tuo G, Pini Prato A, Derchi M, Mosconi M, Mattioli G, Marasini M. Hirschsprung's disease and associated congenital heart defects: a prospective observational study from a single institution. Front Pediatr. 2014;2:99–102.
26. Hoffman JL, Kaplan S. The incidence of congenital heart disease. J Am Coll Cardiol. 2002;39:1890–900.
27. Moons P, Sluysmans T, De Wolf D, et al. Congenital heart disease in 111 225 births in Belgium: birth prevalence, treatment and survival in the 21st century. Acta Paediatr. 2009;98:472–7.
28. Bravo-valenzuela NJ, Borges Peixoto A, Araujo Junior E. Prenatal diagnosis of congenital heart disease: a review of current knowledge. Indian Heart J. 2018;70:150–64.
29. Badreldeen IA. The new 3D/4D based spatio-temporal imaging correlation (STIC) in fetal echocardiography: a promising tool for the future. J Matern Fetal Neonatal Med. 2014;27(11):1163–8.
30. Crane JP, LeFevre ML, Winborn RC, et al. Randomized trial of prenatal ultrasonographic screening: impact on the detection, management, and outcome of anomalous fetuses. The RADIUS Study Group. Am J Obstet Gynecol. 1994;171:392–9.
31. Stoll C, Alembic Y, Dott B, et al. Evaluation of prenatal diagnosis of congenital heart disease. Prenat Diagn. 1998;18:801–7.
32. Achiron R, Glaser J, Gelernter I, Hegesh J, Yagel S. Extended fetal echocardiographic examination for detecting cardiac malformations in low risk pregnancies. BMJ. 1992;304:671–4.
33. Carvalho JS, Mavrides E, Shinebourne EA, Campbell S, Thilaganathan B. Improving the effectiveness of routine prenatal screening for major congenital heart defects. Heart. 2002;88:387–91.
34. Carvalho JS, Allan LD, Chaoui R, Copel JA, De VOre GR, Hecher K, Lee W, Munoz H, Paladini D, Tutschek B, Yagel S. ISUOG practice guidelines (updated): sonographic screening examination of the fetal heart. Ultrasound Obstet Gyecol. 2013;41:348–59.
35. Randall P, Brealey S, Hahn S, et al. Accuracy of fetal echocardiography in the routine detection of congenital heart disease among unselected and low risk populations: a systemic review. BJOG. 2005;112:24–30.
36. Devore GR, Falkensammer P, Sklansky MS, Platts LD. Spatio-temporal image correlation (STIC): new technology for evaluation of the fetal heart. Ultrasound Obstet Gynecol. 2003;22:380–7.
37. Valverde I, Gomez G, Gonzales A, et al. Three- dimensional patient-specific cardiac model for surgical planning in Nikaidoh procedure. Cardiol Young. 2015;25:698–704.
38. Bhalta P, Tretter JT, Chikkabyrappa S, Chakravarti S, Mosca RS. Surgical planning for a complex double-outlet right ventricle using 3D printing. Echocardiography. 2017;34:802–4.
39. Biglino G, Capelli C, Wray J, et al. 3D-manufactured patient-specific models of congenital heart defects for communication in clinical practice: feasibility and acceptability. BMJ Open. 2015;5:1–8.
40. Biglino G, Capelli C, Leaver LK, Shievano S, Taylor AM, Wray J. Involving patients, families and medical staff in the evaluation

of 3D printing models of congenital heart disease. Commun Med. 2015;12:157–69.

41. Biglino G, Capelli C, Koniordou D, et al. Use of 3D models of congenital heart disease as an education tool for cardiac nurses. Congenit Heart Dis. 2017;12:113–8.
42. Costello J, Olivieri L, Krieger A, et al. Utilizing three- dimensional printing technology to assess the feasibility of high-fidelity synthetic ventricular septal defect models for simulation in medical education. World J Pediatr Congenit Heart Surg. 2014;5:421–6.
43. Costello JP, Olivieri LJ, Su L, et al. Incorporating three- dimensional printing into a simulation-based congenital heart disease and critical care training curriculum for resident physicians. Congenit Heart Dis. 2015;10:185–90.
44. Farooqi KM, Lengua CG, Weinberg AD, Nielsen JC, Sanz J. Blood pool segmentation results in superior virtual cardiac models than myocardial segmentation for 3D printing. Pediatr Cardiol. 2016;37:1028–36.
45. Farooqi KM, Gonzalez-Lengua C, Shenoy R, Sanz J, Nguyen K. Use of a three dimensional printed cardiac model to assess suitability for biventricular repair. World J Pediatr Congenit Heart Surg. 2016;7:414–6.
46. Garekar S, Bharati A, Chokhandre M, et al. Clinical application and multidisciplinary assessment of three dimensional printing in double outlet right ventricle with remote ventricular septal defect. World J Pediatr Congenit Heart Surg. 2016;7:344–50.
47. Greil GF, Wolf I, Kuettner A, et al. Stereolithographic reproduction of complex cardiac morphology based on high spatial resolution imaging. Clin Res Cardiol. 2007;96:176–85.
48. Jones TW, Seckeler MD. Use of 3D models of vascular rings and slings to improve resident education. Congenit Heart Dis. 2017;12:578–82.
49. Kappanayil M, Koneti NR, Kannan RR, Kottayil BP, Kumar K. Three-dimensional-printed cardiac prototypes aid surgical decision-making and preoperative planning in selected cases of complex congenital heart diseases: early experience and proof of concept in a resource-limited environment. Ann Paediatr Cardiol. 2017;10:117–25.
50. Kiraly L, Tofeig M, Jha NK, Talo H. Three-dimensional printed prototypes refine the anatomy of post-modified Norwood-1 complex aortic arch obstruction and allow presurgical simulation of the repair. Interact Cardiovasc Thorac Surg. 2016;22:238–40.
51. Loke Y, Harahsheh AS, Krieger A, Olivieri LJ. Usage of 3D models of tetralogy of Fallot for medical education: impact on learning congenital heart disease. BMC Med Educ. 2017;17:54–61.
52. Ma XJ, Tao L, Chen X, et al. Clinical application of three- dimensional reconstruction and rapid prototyping technology of multislice spiral computed tomography angiography for the repair of ventricular septal defect of tetralogy of Fallot. Genet Mol Res. 2015;14:1301–9.
53. Mottl-Link S, Hubler M, Kuhne T, et al. Physical models aiding in complex congenital heart surgery. Ann Thorac Surg. 2008;86:273–7.
54. Olejnik P, Nosal M, Havran T, et al. Utilisation of three- dimensional printed heart models for operative planning of complex congenital heart defects. Kardiol Pol. 2017;75:495–501.
55. Olivieri LJ, Krieger A, Loke YH, et al. Three-dimensional printing of intracardiac defects from three-dimensional echocardiographic images: feasibility and relative accuracy. J Am Sco Echocardiogr. 2015;28:392–7.
56. Olivieri LJ, Su L, Hynes CF, et al. "Just-In-Time" simulation training using 3-D printed cardiac models after congenital cardiac surgery. World J Pediatr Congenit Heart Surg. 2016;7:164–8.
57. Townsend K, Pietila T. 3D printing and modeling of congenital heart defects: a technical review. Birth Defects Research. 2018;110(13):1091–7. https://doi.org/10.1002/bdr2.1342.
58. Chen SA, Ong CS, Hibino N, Baschat AA, Garcia JR, Miller JL. 3D printing of the fetal heart using 3D ultrasound imaging data. Ultrasound Obstet Gynecol. 2018;52(6):808–9. https://doi.org/10.1002/uog.19166.
59. Lim KH, Loo ZY, Goldie S, Adams J, McMenamin P. Use of 3D printed models in medical education: a randomized control trial comparing 3D prints versus cadaveric materials for learning external cardiac anatomy. Anat Sci Educ. 2016;9:213–21.
60. Sun Z, Lau I, Wong YH, Yeong CH. Personalized three-dimensional printed models in congenital heart disease. J Clin Med. 2019;8(4):522.

6 Valvular Disease and Three-Dimensional Printing

Jiayou Tang, Yang Liu, Da Zhu, Yanyan Ma, Fanglin Lu, Fang Fang, Xiaoke Shang, Jian Yang, Yongjian Wu, Xin Pan, and Haibo Zhang

6.1 Transcatheter Aortic Valve Replacement and Three-Dimensional Printing

Jiayou Tang, Yang Liu, Da Zhu

Aortic valve disease is a common heart valve disease. The epidemiological data suggest that the incidence of aortic valve disease is as high as 3%–7% in people over 65 years of age and that it tends to increase with age [1, 2]. The causes of aortic valve disease include degenerative diseases, mucoid degeneration, congenital bicuspid aortic valve, and rheumatic heart disease. As the population in China ages, people with degenerative valvular diseases will exhibit major pathological changes. Severe aortic valve disease can lead to increased cardiac load, which leads to chest tightness, shortness of breath, angina pectoris, dizziness, syncope, and other typical symptoms, resulting in left heart failure and even sudden death. According to the 2017 American Heart Association/American College of Cardiology and the 2017 European Society of Cardiology guidelines for valvular disease [3, 4], once patients are clinically diagnosed with severe valvular stenosis or insufficiency and have obvious symptoms and progressive decline in cardiac function, surgical repair or replacement of the diseased aortic valve should be performed in a timely manner. In reality, some patients with advanced age, severely impaired left ventricular function, or multiple comorbidities are considered to be contraindicated or high risk for traditional open-heart surgery. Transcatheter aortic valve replacement (TAVR) is an emerging minimally invasive valve replacement operation that uses interventional catheter technology to compress the stent and artificial biological valve in vitro and deliver them to the position of the aortic valve to complete the implantation of the prosthetic valve and restore valve function. This type of intervention is less invasive, does not require cardiopulmonary bypass, and results in rapid postoperative recovery [5]. It is increasingly being promoted in clinical practice. Based on strong evidence-based medical studies, the 2017 American College of Cardiology and American Heart Association guidelines also consider TAVR as the preferred/primary treatment for elderly patients with high-risk aortic stenosis. More recently, results of the Partner 3 (Safety and Effectiveness of the SAPIEN 3 Transcatheter Heart Valve in Low Risk Patients With Aortic Stenosis) study showed that in low-risk patients with aortic stenosis, the composite endpoints of death and major adverse events after TAVR were significantly lower than that after surgical aortic valve replacement, and the death, stroke, and rehospitalization rates at 1 year were significantly reduced [6, 7].

TAVR was first introduced in China in 2010 and officially commercialized in China in 2017. However, potentially serious complications, such as aortic annulus rupture, coronary artery occlusion, electrical conduction block, peripheral vascular injury, and prosthetic valve thrombosis, displacement, and paravalvular leakage still hinder the more widespread application of this technique. Among these complications, rupture of the aortic annulus and obstruction of the coronary ostia are the more dangerous and urgent complications that often lead to rapid deterioration and even death of the patients. On the other hand, paravalvular leakage, valve

J. Tang · Y. Liu · Y. Ma · J. Yang (✉)
Xijing Hospital, Xi'an, China

D. Zhu
West China Hospital of Sichuan University, Chengdu, China

F. Lu
Changhai Hospital, Naval Medical University, Shanghai, China

F. Fang · H. Zhang
Beijing Anzhen Hospital, Affiliated with Capital Medical University, Beijing, China

X. Shang
Union Medical College Affiliated with Tongji Medical College, Wuhan, China

Y. Wu
Fuwai Hospital, Chinese Academy of Medical Sciences, Beijing, China

X. Pan
Chest Hospital Affiliated with Shanghai Jiaotong University, Shanghai, China

J. Yang et al. (eds.), *Cardiovascular 3D Printing*, https://doi.org/10.1007/978-981-15-6957-9_6

displacement, conduction block, thrombosis, and other complications often lead to a poor prognosis, increasing the risk of surgery and the possibility of rehospitalization. Therefore, accurate preoperative evaluation to guide the selection of the appropriate types and size of prosthetic valve and the development of an intraoperative strategy to lessen the procedural risk are crucial when planning the TAVR procedure.

TAVR is different from the conventional thoracotomy heart operation. The operators cannot directly see the entire aortic root during the operation, nor can they open the heart to examine its internal anatomical structures. Therefore, evaluation of preoperative imaging and intraoperative navigation are very important. Computed tomography, magnetic resonance imaging, transthoracic or transesophageal echocardiography, and other imaging modalities typically display tomographic images on two-dimensional (2D) screens. Before TAVR, the chief surgeon/interventionist needs to mentally reconstruct the 2D images into three-dimensional (3D) structure. 3D printing technology can transform the 2D image data of the aortic root and valve of patients into 1:1 life-size 3D physical models, providing information that is difficult to display by traditional imaging methods. The goal is to greatly simplify and standardize the complicated process and make TAVR surgery more accurate and safer. 3D printing technology, which is being used more and more extensively in the medical field, not only improves patient education but also assists in developing the operation strategy. The use of 3D-printed model-based in vitro simulations of the TAVR procedure can also lead to improvements and innovation of the design of TAVR prosthesis and equipment [8].

6.1.1 Pathophysiology of Aortic Stenosis

Aortic valve stenosis is mainly caused by congenital abnormalities of the valve, degeneration/calcification of the valve associated with aging, and/or fusion/calcification of the aortic cusp/leaflets as sequelae of the rheumatic process (Fig. 6.1). The cross-sectional area of aortic valve opening in the normal adults is typically ≥ 3.0 cm^2. When the area of an aortic valve opening is narrowed to one-third of the normal size or less, obstruction of blood flow typically occurs. When the area is less than 1.5 cm^2, pressure gradient and blood flow velocity across the aortic valve start to increase. Hemodynamically significant aortic stenosis causes insufficient blood supply to systemic organs of the body and increases the afterload of left ventricle, which typically remodels as concentric hypertrophy. As the coronary arteries originate from the aortic cusps, aortic stenosis also reduces coronary blood flow, which, in association with left ventricular hypertrophy, may lead to cardiac arrhythmia and sudden death. In general, during the compensatory period, patients may not have symptoms. In the decompensated phase, symptoms such as fatigue, laborious dyspnea, angina, dizziness or syncope, and even sudden cardiac death occur in 10–20% of cases.

6.1.2 Pathophysiology of Aortic Insufficiency

Aortic insufficiency can also be caused by degenerative calcification of the aortic valve, rheumatic valve disease,

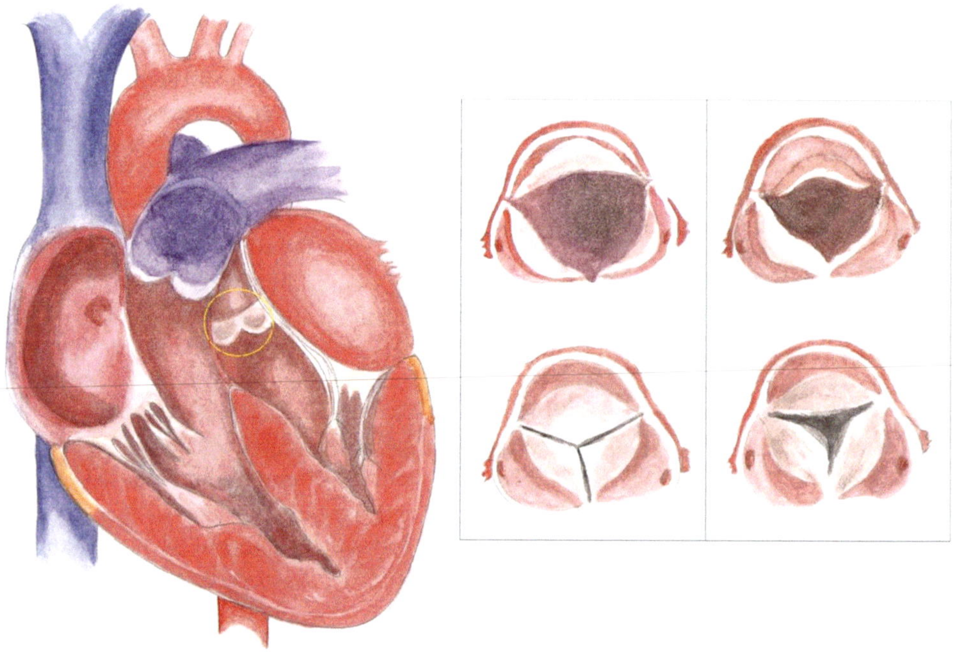

Fig. 6.1 Diagram showing normal and stenosed aortic valves

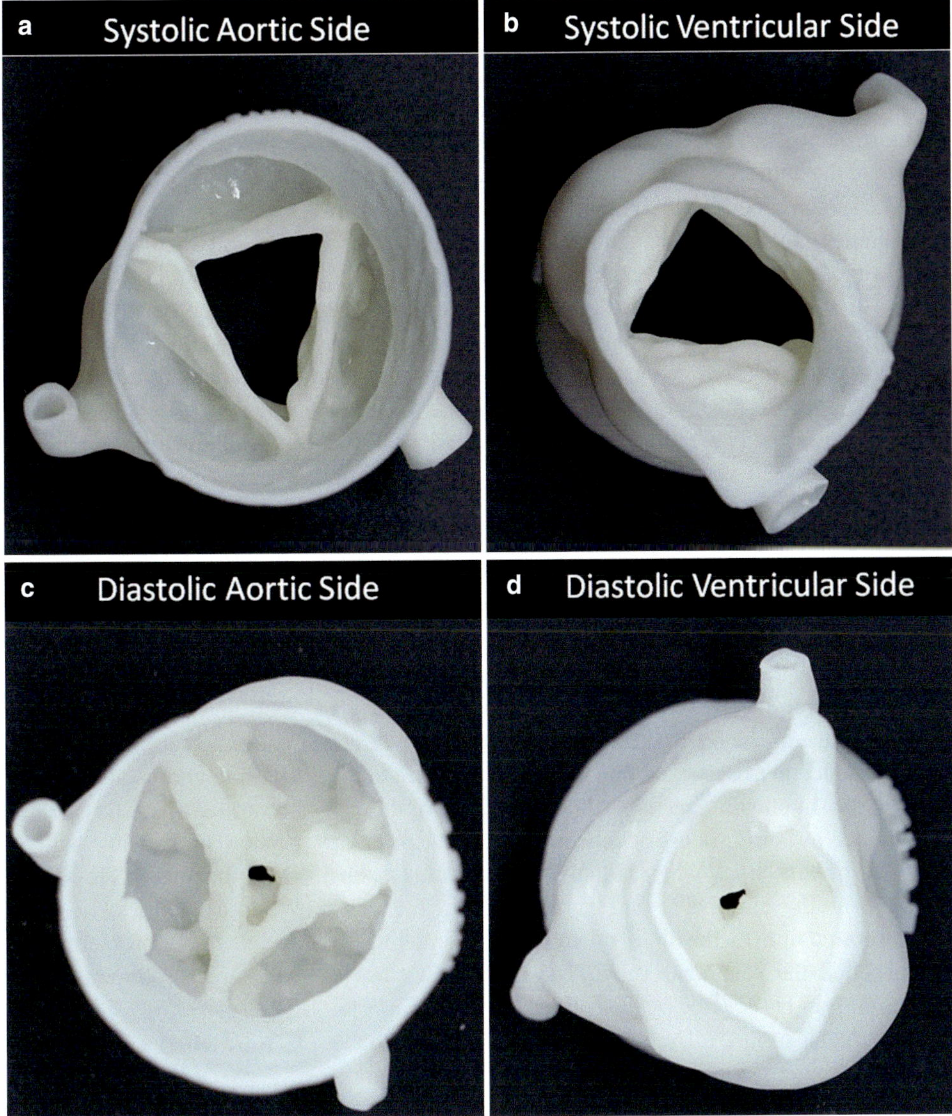

Fig. 6.2 3D-printed model of aortic insufficiency. (**a**, **b**) Systolic phase observed from the aorta (**a**) and the ventricular (**b**) side. (**c**, **d**) Diastolic phase observed from the aorta (**c**) and the ventricular (**d**) side of the valve insufficiency gap

and congenital valve malformation (Fig. 6.2). Hypertension is associated with dilatation of the sinotubular junction, which in turn may cause malcoaptation of the aortic valve leaflets, leading to aortic insufficiency. In addition, degeneration of the elastic fibers is caused by medial cystic necrosis of the annulus, and the expansion of the annulus may also cause incomplete closure of the aortic valve. Furthermore, any dilation of the ascending aorta, aneurysm, or aortic dissection may result in incomplete closure of the aortic valve.

Aortic valve insufficiency allows some of the blood ejected forward from the left ventricle to the ascending aorta during systole to regurgitate backward into the ventricle during diastole, which increases the ventricular preload. The left ventricle in turn has to work harder to pump the excess regurgitant blood volume into the ascending aorta in the next systole, which increases the ventricular afterload. In the early stages, the left ventricle compensates by increasing the intensity of the myocardial contractions, which gradually leads to left ventricular myocardial hypertrophy, and progressive left ventricular expansion leads to a decrease in the left ventricular systolic function and ejection fraction. When this occurs, the left ventricle is unable to maintain the necessary cardiac output, at which point left ventricular congestive heart failure occurs. Sometimes left ventricular failure, even in the initial period, can be irreversible, depriving patients of the opportunity for further treatment. A large amount of aortic regurgitation also causes a decrease in diastolic blood pressure and causes the reduced perfusion of the coronary arteries. Patients may suffer from angina pectoris symptoms and even sudden death. Increased diastolic pressure in the left ventricle causes increased pressure in the left atrium, leading to the enlargement of the left atrium and the occurrence of atrial fibrillation.

6.1.3 Anatomy of the Aortic Root and Aortic Valve

In contrast to direct observation of the overall anatomical structure during surgery, the focus during TAVR is to obtain images of the aortic root and aortic valve under dynamic status. The surgeon focuses not only on the aortic annulus (virtual annulus), leaflet, and the sinotubular junction, but also needs a more comprehensive evaluation of the height of the ostium of the coronary artery, the size and volume of the coronary sinus, the left ventricular outflow situation, and the condition of the ascending aorta. At the same time, the surgeon also needs to take into consideration cardiac contraction and diastole. The following is a brief review of the anatomy of the left ventricular outflow tract and the aortic root:

6.1.3.1 Aortic Root

The aortic root is continuous with the left ventricular outflow tract, located at the right rear of the funnel of the right ventricular outflow tract; the posterior margin is located between the mitral orifice and the ventricular septal muscle. It extends from the plane of the left ventricular muscular outflow tract from the attachment of the semilunar valve of the aorta to the plane of the sinotubular junction. About two-thirds of the circumference of aortic root is attached to the left ventricular muscular outflow tract, whereas the other one-third is continuous with the aortic valve and the mitral valve fiber. The aortic root comprises the sinus of Valsalva, the interleaflet triangle, and the semilunar valve. The aortic valve has a fibrous core and is covered by the endothelium on its arterial and ventricular surfaces. The aortic root forms a ring with the left ventricular component that supports the wall of the aorta and continues upward to form the elastic fibrous wall of the sinus of Valsalva. This ring is called the anatomical ventriculoarterial junction. The lowest points of aortic valve attachment are below the anatomical ventriculoarterial junction.

6.1.3.2 Aortic Valve Leaflet and Sinus

The aortic valve normally consists of three semilunar valves with the aortic valvular attachment margin arching over the anatomical ventriculoarterial junction. Behind each valve, the walls of the aorta bulge outward to form the sinuses of Valsalva. When closed, the leaflets converge toward the center along the margin of the junction (the midpoint of the free margin forms thickened nodules, known as the nodules of Arantius). When the ventricle contracts, blood rushes upward, pushing the aortic valve away from the center. During ventricular diastole, the valve leaflet passively descends into the center of the arterial cavity. When the valve is morphologically normal, the three leaflets meet along the margin of the junction and support the flow of blood from the aorta to prevent backflow into the ventricle. Two of the three aortic sinuses give rise to coronary arteries, hence the names left, right, and non-coronary sinus.

If the aortic valve is formed with only two leaflets instead of three, it is called a bicuspid aortic valve (BAV). If three leaflets are fused by calcification to form two leaflets, it is also classified as a bicuspid valve. The bicuspid valve is the most common congenital aortic stenosis deformity, with a prevalence of about 2% in the population. It has a special anatomical structure, asymmetrical valve leaflet shape, large oval raphe of sinus, obstructed blood flow at the mouth of the valve, increased flow velocity, and an eddy current, resulting in valve thickening and asymmetrical calcification. Meanwhile, due to its own genetic mechanism and the abnormal blood flow impinging on the aortic wall, it is more prone to aortic wall lesions such as ascending aorta dilatation and aortic aneurysm. Patients often have an enlarged ascending aorta. During TAVR operations, complications such as valve displacement and paravalvular leakage are prone to occur, leading to a significantly increased risk of death both in the short and long term. For these reasons, a number of large-scale clinical studies of TAVR in Western countries listed bicuspid aortic valve as an exclusion criterion [9]. In China, according to existing evidence-based medical data, the proportion of patients with various types of bicuspid aortic valves having TAVR (40%–50%) is much higher than that in Western countries (1.6%–9.3%), so a bicuspid aortic valve is an inevitable problem for TAVR in China. Common BAV types are as follows (Fig. 6.3):

6.1.3.3 Aortic Annulus and Transcatheter Aortic Valve Replacement of a Virtual Annulus in the Aortic Root

The aortic annulus is not shaped like a simple ring. In fact, the actual aortic annulus consists of at least three rings and one crown-shaped ring. The three-dimensional shape of the aortic valve is like that of the tripod of a crown, and the attachment point of the leaflet forms the base of the crown. A "virtual annulus" exists at the bottom of the crown and is determined by the plane of the three lowest attachment points. This plane marks the entrance of the left ventricular outflow tract into the aortic root; it is also the area where the TAVR valve is anchored. This ring has no real anatomical boundaries and can only be measured from images, which explains why it is defined as a "virtual" ring. The ring at the top of the crown is a real ring—the sinotubular junction, which consists of the aortic sinus crest and the valve junction points. The connection plane of the sinus is the outlet of the aortic root, extending upward into the ascending aorta. The attachment of the meniscus of the aortic leaflets crosses

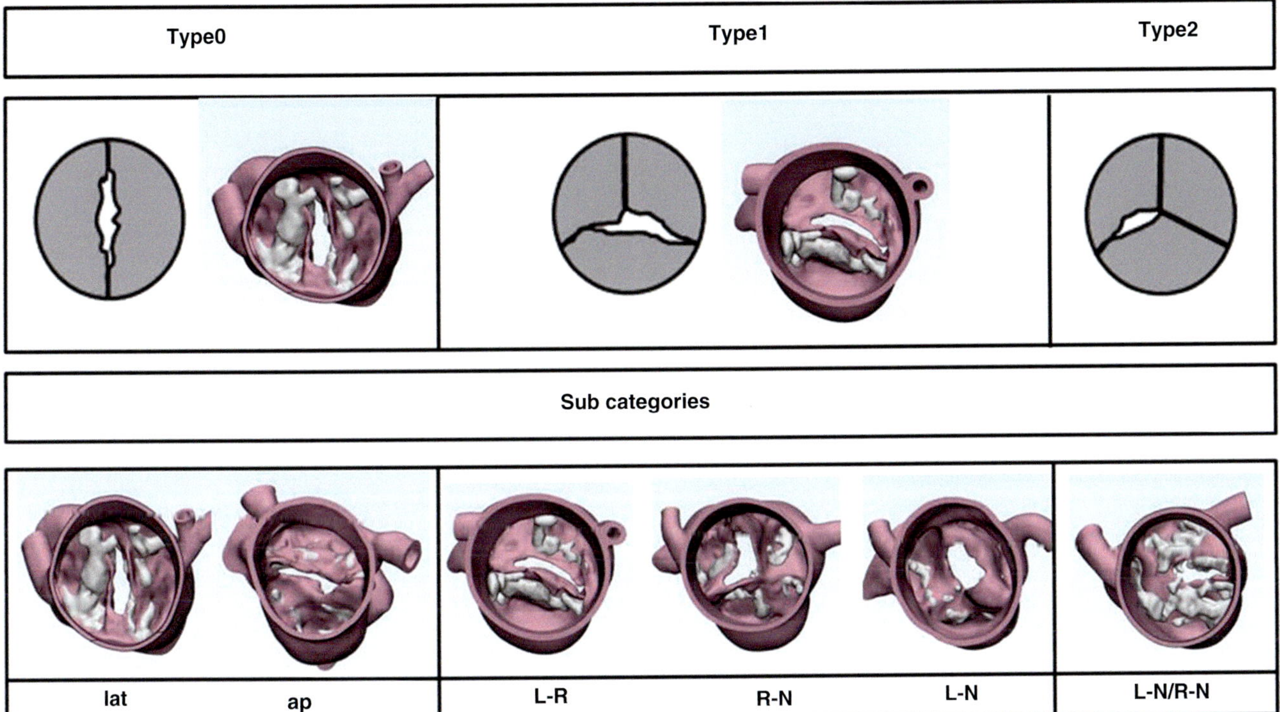

Fig. 6.3 Bilobular aortic valve classification

another real ring, the dissected ventriculoarterial connection. Only part of the aortic valve attaches to the ventricular muscle. Most of the non-coronary leaflet and part of the left coronary leaflet are continuous fibers of the anterior mitral valve or aortic valve. The thickened end of the valve forms a "fibrous triangle," which enables the aortic valve to adhere with stability to the top of the left ventricle.

At present, preoperative evaluation of both the surgical aortic valve replacement and the transcatheter aortic valve replacement depends mainly on transthoracic/transesophageal echocardiography and cardiac computed tomography angiography (CTA). Echocardiography, in particular, can provide an accurate assessment of aortic stenosis, of the type and severity of aortic insufficiency, and a useful evaluation of postprocedure hemodynamic parameters [10] (Fig. 6.4).

However, both techniques can only show the aortic root as a two-dimensional/three-dimensional image. For the cardiologist, it takes time to understand and mentally visualize a static three-dimensional concept. 3D printing technology can present the entire aortic root structure to the cardiologist as a dynamic model based on the imaging data and computer modeling. The model not only shows the three-dimensional multifaceted picture of the ascending aorta, coronary ostia, aortic annulus, leaflets, sinus, and the morphological and pathological changes in the left ventricular outflow tract but also provides a good opportunity for simulating the operation in vitro [11] (Fig. 6.5).

6.1.4 Transcatheter Aortic Valve

At present, numerous transcatheter valves for TAVR are available worldwide, and clinical research on these products has gone hand in hand with their development. Of the dozens of transcatheter valve products on the market, some early examples, including the SAPIEN Transcatheter Heart Valve System (Edwards Lifesciences Corporation, Irvine, CA USA), the CoreValve (Medtronic, Minneapolis, MN USA), and the Evolut R (Medtronic), show good outcomes when used in high-risk patients. In general, the transcatheter valve is composed of a nickolinum alloy metal stent (some of the transapical valves have positioning keys). The valve leaflets, which are made of pig heart valve, pig pericardium, or cow pericardium, are sutured into the stent, which is then compressed and placed in the conveyor. The valve release mode is divided into self-expanding valves and balloon-dilated valves. The approach can be transvascular or transapical (Fig. 6.6).

In-depth studies of the transcatheter valve resulted in the development of a new generation of transcatheter valves represented by the SAPIEN 3, the Evolut R, the Lotus (Boston Scientific, Marlborough, MA USA), and others. This new generation comprised transcatheter valves with fewer defects; a significant decrease in the incidence of paravalvular leakage, conduction block, and other complications; and the characteristics of recyclability, small-size delivery systems, and automatic positioning. Compared with events in

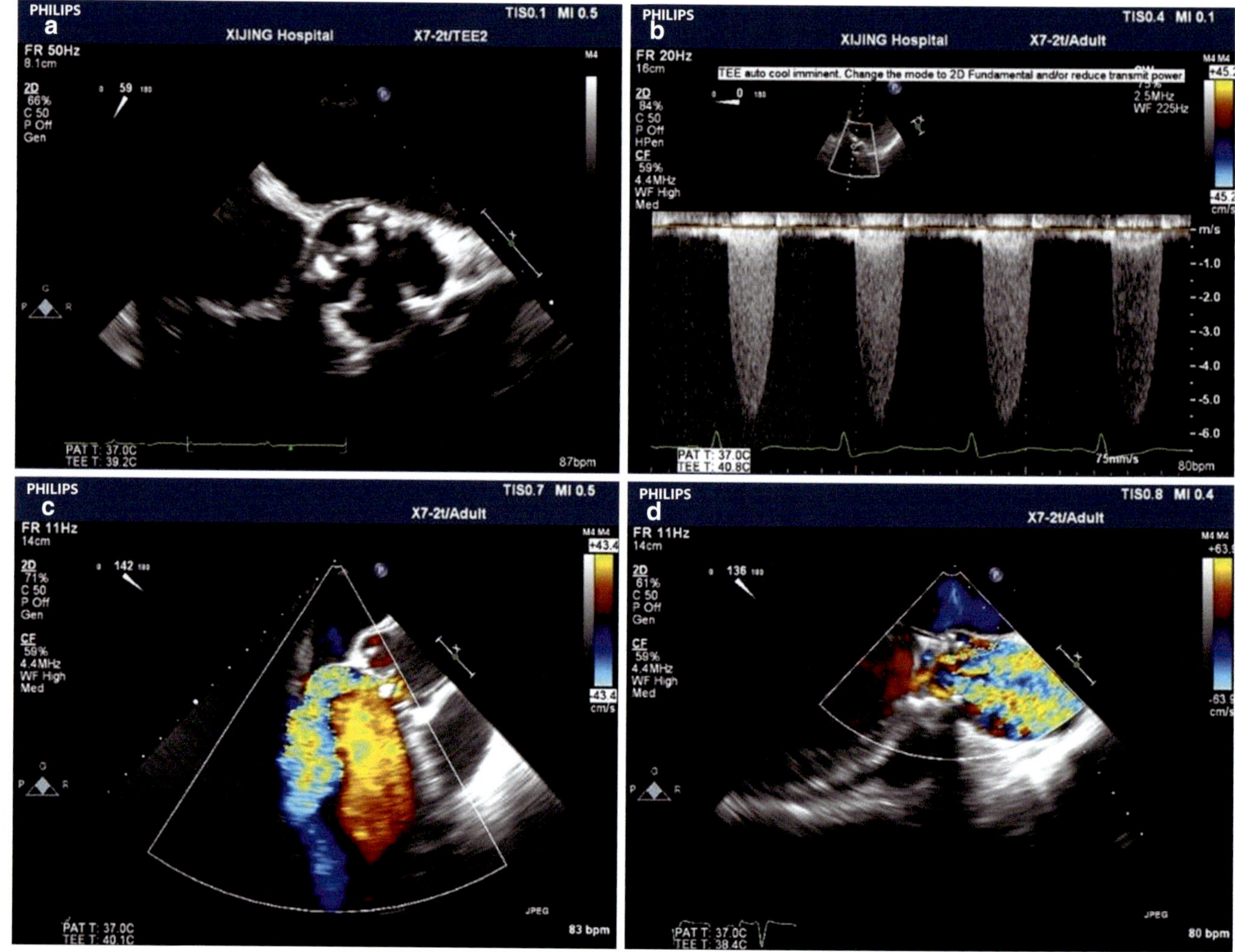

Fig. 6.4 Echocardiography in the diagnosis of aortic valve disease. (**a**) Anatomical view of the short-axis view of the aortic valve. (**b**) Doppler measurement of transvalvular blood flow velocity and pressure gradient. (**c**) Color Doppler assessment of aortic valve regurgitation. (**d**) Color Doppler assessment of aortic valve blood flow, regurgitation, and paravalvular leakage after TAVR. Images were obtained from the Department of Cardiovascular Surgery of Xijing Hospital

other countries, China's TAVR technology and instrument research and development started relatively late. Since Prof. Dr. Ge Junbo et al. successfully completed the first TAVR operation in China on October 3, 2010, more than 1000 operations have been completed in mainland China. Seven different aortic valve products have been introduced. In 2017, breakthroughs were made in domestic valves. The Venus A valve (Qiming Co., Hangzhou, Zhejiang Province, China), inserted by a transvascular approach, and the J-Valve (Suzhou Jiecheng Co., Wujiang, Jiangsu Province, China), inserted via a transapical approach, were approved by the China Food and Drug Administration (CFDA), laying a foundation for the rapid development of TAVR in China [12–14]. The world's first preinstalled valve, the Venibri (Hangzhou Qiming Co.), was used in the first-in-man study in 2018 and has been shown at several international conferences in surgical demonstrations. The second-generation retrievable Venus A Plus (Hangzhou Qiming Co.) was successfully implanted in patients in the Second Affiliated Hospital of Zhejiang University Medical College. Follow-up studies on the Shanghai minimally invasive VitaFlow (MicroPort Medical, Shanghai, China) valve have been completed, and the valve has entered the China Food and Drug Administration approval process. Meanwhile, the SAPIEN XT valve (Edwards) and the Taurus One valve (PeiJia Medical, Suzhou, Jiangsu Province, China) are also being studied in clinical trials. Until now, the Venus A valve and the J-Valve, both made in China, have been used in heart centers of as many as 100 hospitals. In 2018 alone, the number of implants in China exceeded 1000, benefiting large numbers of critically ill elderly patients (Fig. 6.7).

At present, TAVR is done mainly via two approaches: the transfemoral approach and the apical approach. TAVR via the femoral artery is the mainstream treatment, mainly for

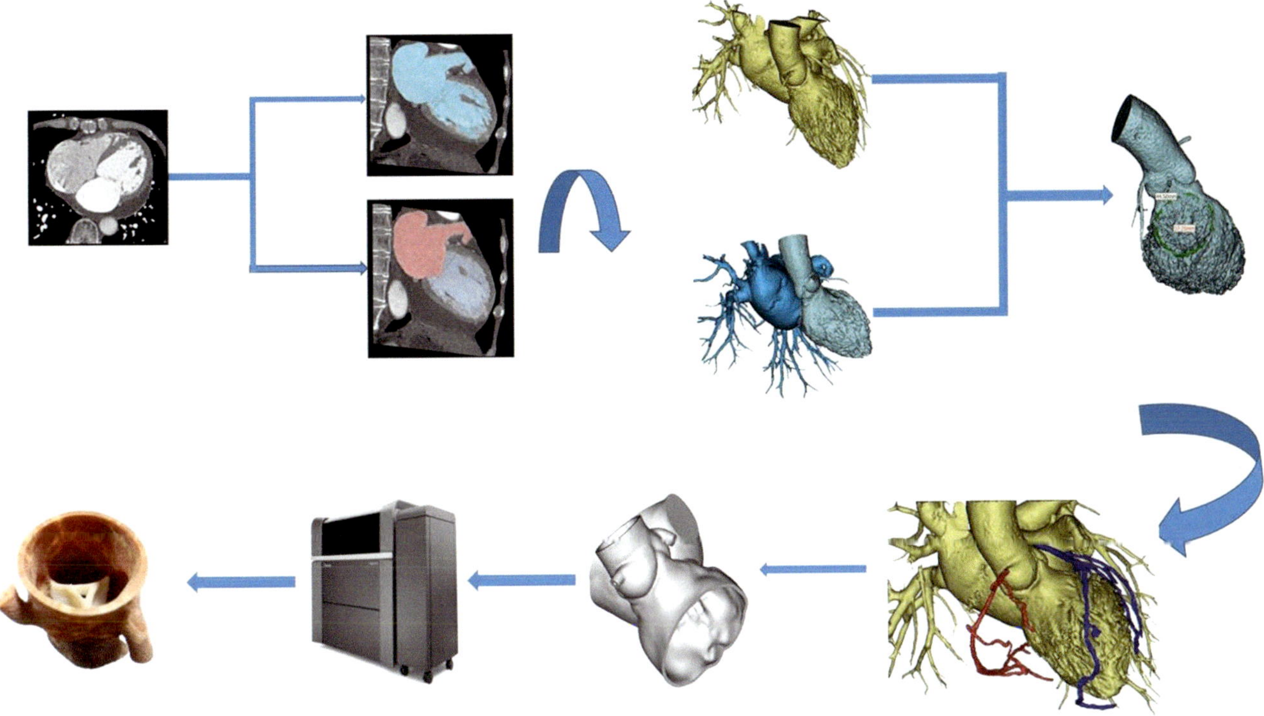

Fig. 6.5 Preoperative computed tomography angiography data were obtained to display aortic valves and adjacent structures in a 3D-printed model

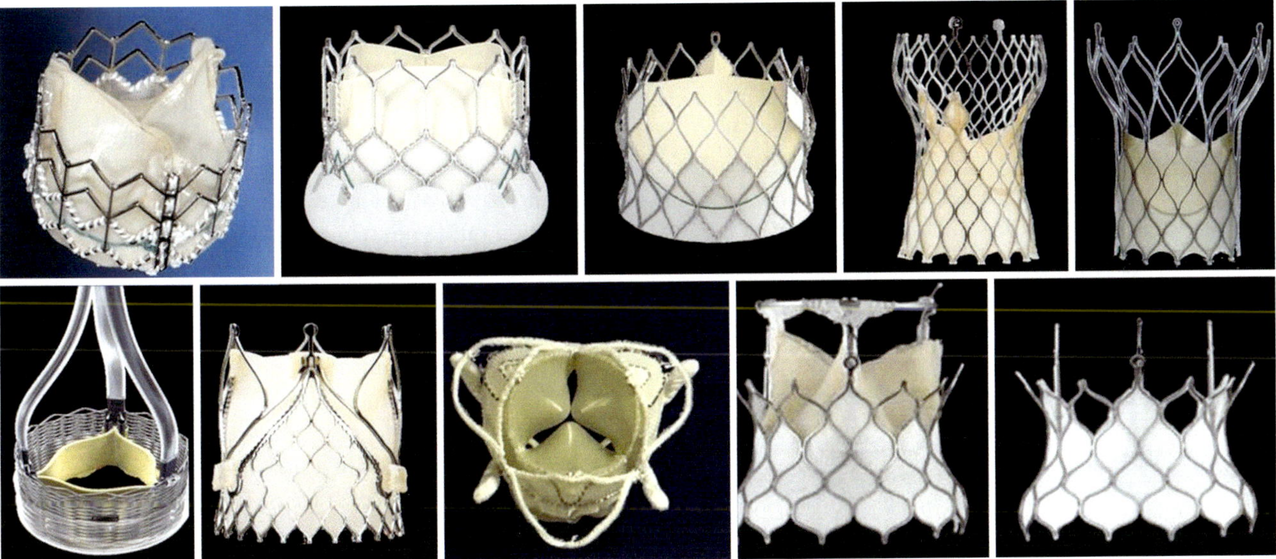

Fig. 6.6 Representational transcatheter aortic valve types. Including Venus A-valve, VitaFlow MicroPort Valve, Taurus One valve, J-Valve, CoreValve, Lotus valve, and SAPIEN XT valve

aortic valve stenosis. This procedure usually requires predilation with a balloon and simultaneous aortic root angiography to visualize the coronary artery and the annulus. Then, the compressed transcatheter valve in the conveyance system is delivered to the stenotic area and released. Afterward, angiography and transesophageal echocardiography are performed to evaluate the position and morphological characteristics of the prosthetic valve and the paravalvular leakage (Fig. 6.8).

Currently, transapical TAVR is designated primarily for patients with no or difficult peripheral vascular access or those with aortic valve insufficiency. The operative steps usually require an apical incision and purse-string sutures (Fig. 6.9). The catheter and guide wire are used to establish

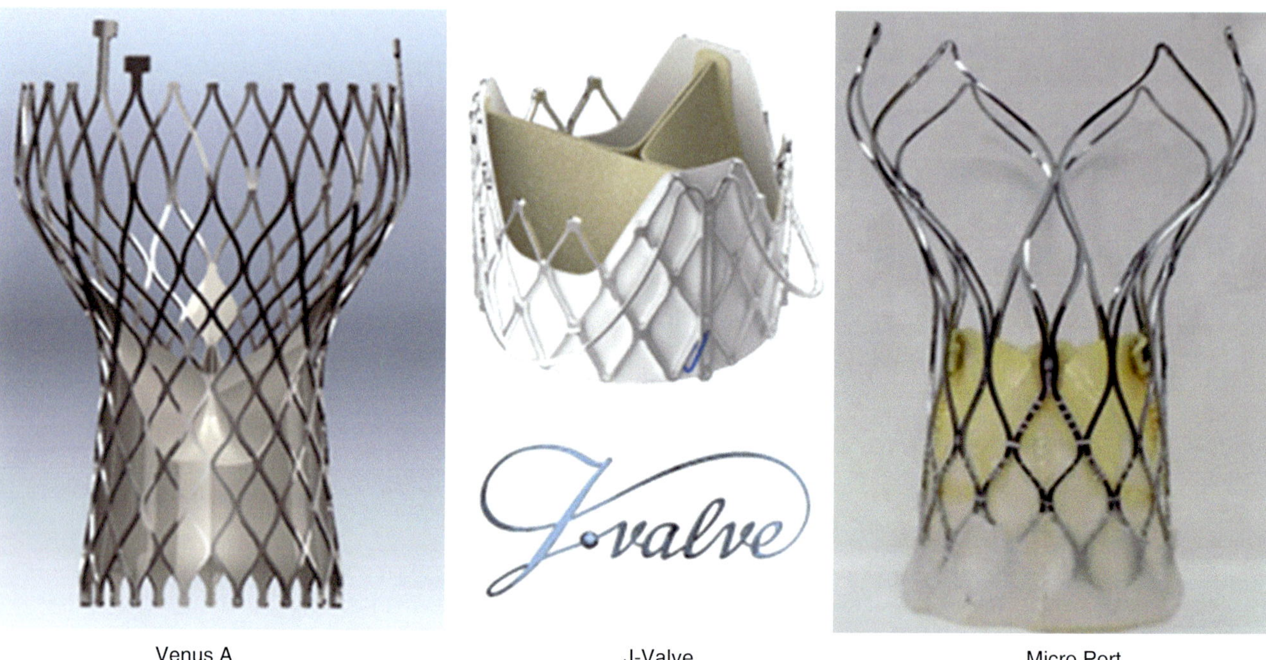

Fig. 6.7 Schematic diagrams of transcatheter aortic valves made in China

access to the transaortic valve via the incision. The compressed stent valve is transported through the apical approach through the guide wire pathway across the autologous aortic valve. The stent valve is positioned in the aortic sinus. After the valve is released, the morphological characteristics, the position of the valve, and the degree of paravalvular leakage are observed by angiography.

With the development of TAVR technology and the increase in material science research, innovations in transcatheter valves can provide solutions to avoid many intraoperative and postoperative complications. However, aortic valve diseases are complicated, with great individual differences, and the many complications that can occur in elderly patients increase the intraoperative risks and uncertainties associated with TAVR surgery. Therefore, applying interdisciplinary 3D printing technology to perioperative evaluation is worthwhile [15].

6.1.5 Advantages of Three-Dimensional Printing in Transcatheter Aortic Valve Replacement

Compared with the benefits of traditional imaging technology, the advantages of 3D printing in TAVR surgery are as follows: (1) identification of anatomical details and prediction/prevention of complications preoperatively; (2) ongoing enhancement of surgical teaching techniques; and (3) optimization of TAVR device development and design [16–18]. At present, the TAVR industry in China is still in its infancy. In addition to further research and the development of a new generation of devices, the prevention and treatment of common clinical TAVR complications are also of particular importance. Common postoperative complications of TAVR include valve displacement, paravalvular leakage, stroke, vascular complications, arrhythmia, and acute kidney injury. Based on current experience, preoperative transesophageal echocardiography and CTA assessment alone cannot meet the requirements of accurate preoperative assessment. The introduction of 3D printing technology has added new concepts, methods, and means for perioperative assessment. 3D printing was first used in the medical field in orthopedics and stomatology. Because the printing materials were mainly hard materials, its application in cardiology was limited. With the continuous improvements in printing technology and progress of printing material research and development, 3D printing has been applied more and more widely in the cardiovascular field in recent years. For TAVR surgery, using composite materials of different levels of hardness and flexibility and images based on real anatomical information, the individualized leaflet shape was printed from 3D static information. This process can help simulate the implantation of valves, prevent complications, and serve as a reliable clinical platform for testing, optimizing, and validating new instruments and TAVR devices [19].

6.1.5.1 Evaluation of Paravalvular Leakage

Paravalvular leakage, which is the most common complication after TAVR, refers to the phenomenon of blood flow returning to the left ventricle along the gap outside the pros-

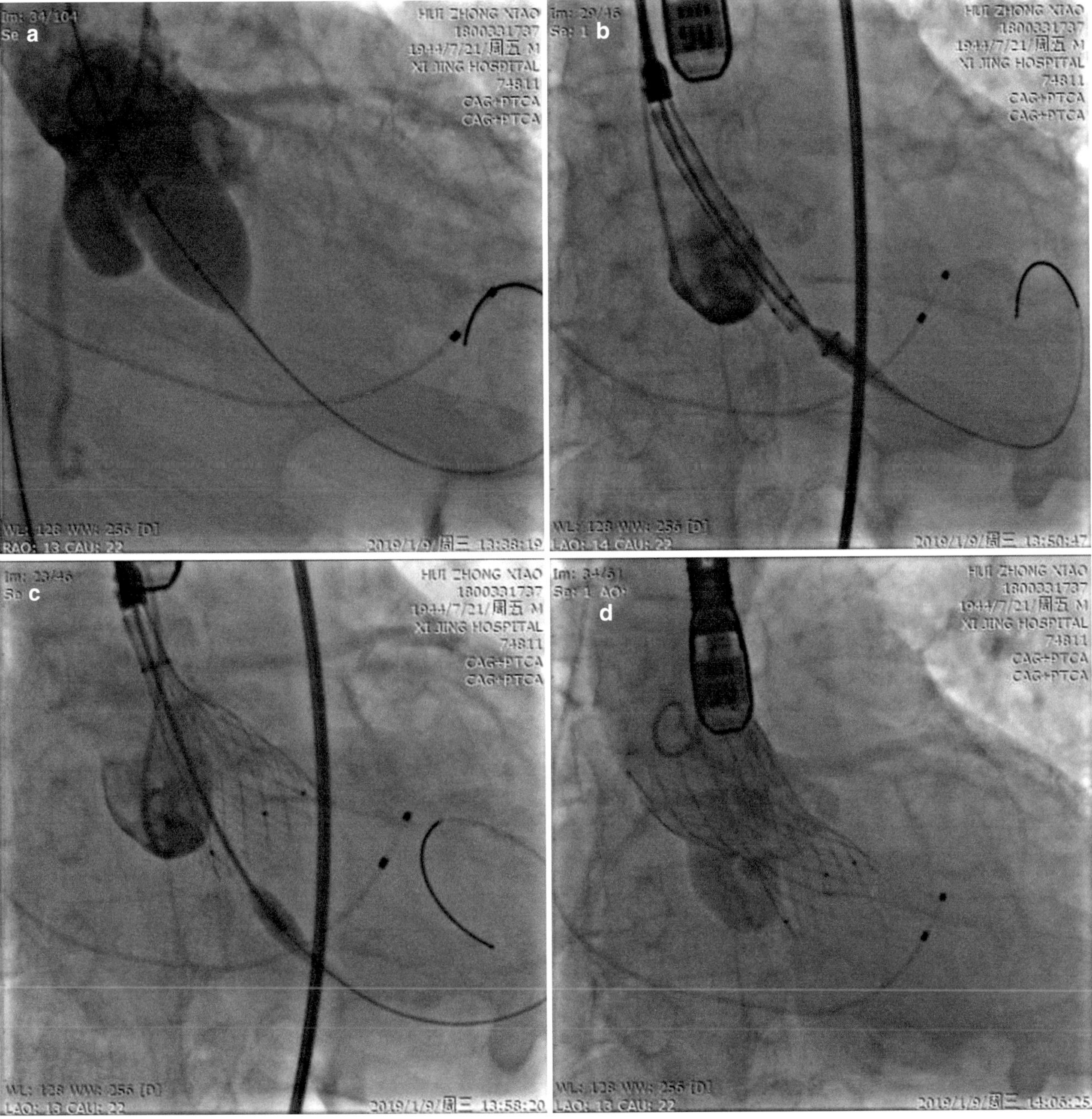

Fig. 6.8 The procedure of transcatheter aortic valve replacement via the femoral artery. (**a**) Balloon dilation of a stenosed aortic valve and simultaneous aortic root angiography. (**b**) Compressed bracket valve crossing the stenosed aortic valve via the transfemoral delivery system. (**c**) Angiography at the same time after partial release of the stent valve to observe the shape and location of the valve. (**d**) Stent valve angiography after complete release was performed to observe the shape, location, and paravalvular leakage of the valve. Images were obtained from the Department of Cardiovascular Surgery of Xijing Hospital

thetic valve during ventricular diastole after replacement of the stent valve. In the Placement of Aortic Transcatheter Valves I (PARTNER I) trial, the incidence of moderate and severe paravalvular leakage was as high as 7.8% and 11.8%, respectively, and it directly affected the prognosis of the patients [20, 21]. The incidence of paravalvular leakage has decreased significantly with the use of the new-generation valves and a better understanding of optimal valve size, suture line design, and implantation techniques. In the Placement of Aortic Transcatheter Valves II (Partner II) study, moderate and severe disk leakage rates were reduced to 5.4% and 3.7%, respectively [22]. In a study of the new generation of SAPIEN 3 valves, the results of a 1-year follow-up examination showed no severe paravalvular leakage.

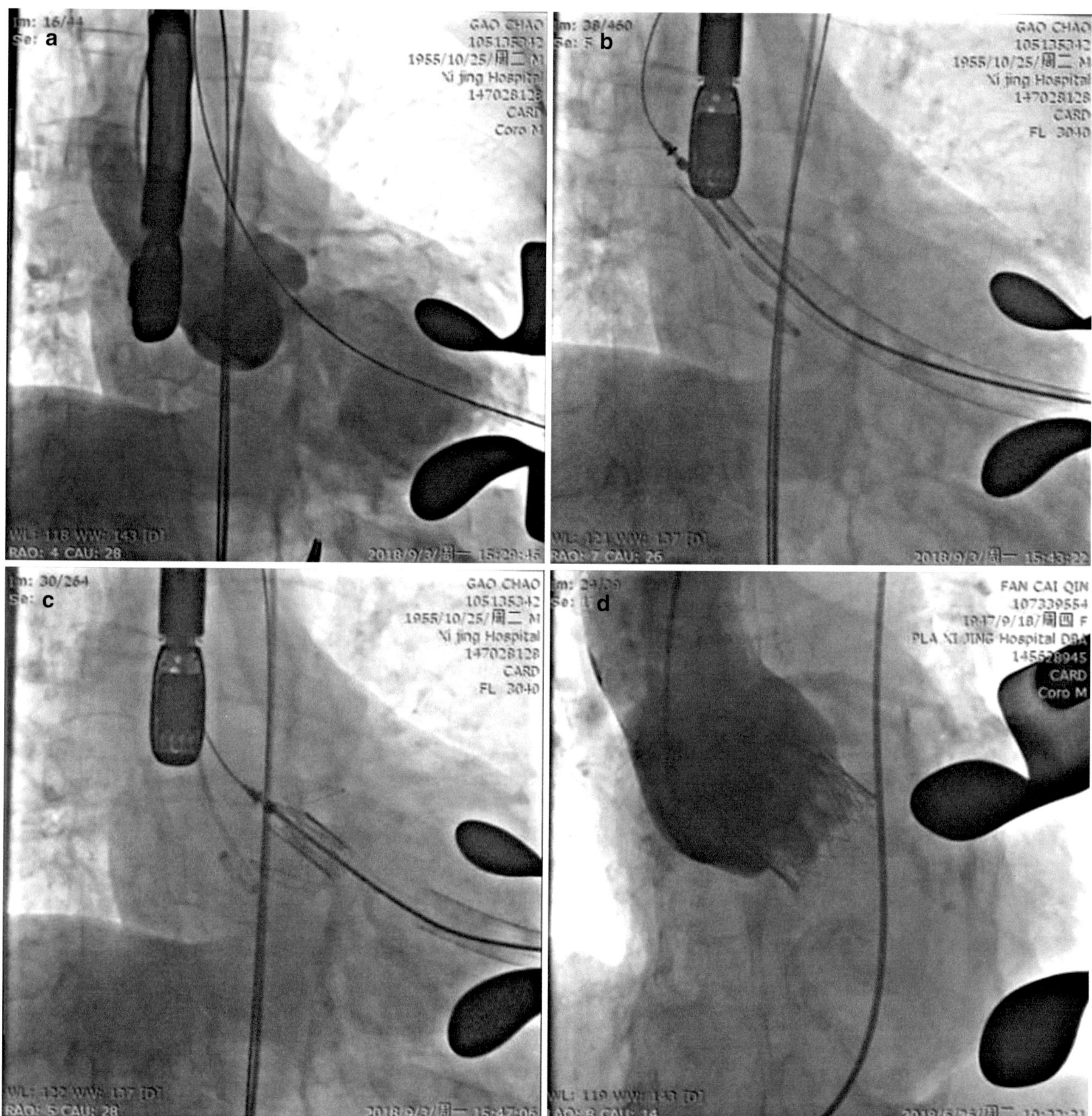

Fig. 6.9 Operational procedure of transapical transcatheter aortic valve replacement. (**a**) Establishment of a transaortic valve approach through an apical incision; concurrent angiography shows aortic valve insufficiency. (**b**) Compressed bracket valves across autologous aortic valves through the apical delivery system; (**c**) Stent valve partial positioner for intra-aortic sinus, to observe the shape and position of the valves. (**d**) Stent angiography after complete release of the valves to observe the shape and position of the valves and paravalvular leakage. Images were obtained from the Department of Cardiovascular Surgery of Xijing Hospital

The results also showed that mild paravalvular leakage had no significant effect on the 1-year mortality rate, which is a definite advantage over the previous generation of valves.

Nevertheless, being able to predict paravalvular leakage before TAVR is of great significance when developing a surgical strategy and selecting a valve. In preoperative mainstream CTA assessment, no matter what kind of software is used, such as Mimics or 3 Mensio, one can identify only calcification of valve leaflets and the valve ring, thereby indicating the risk of paravalvular leakage (qualitative), but the degree of paravalvular leakage cannot be accurately determined (quantitative). To overcome this problem, researchers from the Georgia Institute of Technology (Atlanta, GA, USA) and the Piedmont Heart Institute (Atlanta, GA, USA) used a multimaterial 3D printer to print a model of the aortic root [11]. By controlling the "diameter and bending wavelength" of the printed material, the model was able to better simulate the physiological characteristics of the aortic tissue. This model could even show the special conditions of the valve leaflets, such as calcification deposits and valve leaflet thickening, and accurately and completely depict the anatomical information. The results suggest that the 3D model can show exactly which patients are likely to develop paravalvular leakage and can even show the location and severity of the complication. Even though TAVR surgery has become more mature internationally, this method can still help to formulate more accurate surgical strategies, including selection of valve type, implantation strategy, and prevention of complications [16]. At present, in China, for cases with complicated anatomical conditions, being able to simulate the implantation strategy before surgery using a 3D-printed model is an indispensable way to effectively and accurately guide the operative procedure and to avoid and reduce complications.

6.1.5.2 Prediction of the Possibility of Conduction Block

TAVR, like a traditional thoracotomy with surgical aortic valve replacement, frequently causes heart block. The overall incidence of conduction abnormalities requiring permanent pacemaker implantation after TAVR is still higher than that after surgical aortic valve replacement. With the continuous relaxation of indications and the younger age of the population requiring surgery, this complication has attracted more attention from researchers. Postoperative conduction block may be due to calcified plaque displacement, which causes sustained pressure or permanent damage to the atrioventricular conduction system at the junction of the right coronary valve and the non-coronary valve, and the ventricular end of the prosthetic valve may also damage the conduction system located at the ventricular septum. Other risk factors include oversizing of the prosthetic valve, left ventricular outflow tract stenosis, aortic calcification near the root of the valve, preoperative partial atrioventricular block (right bundle branch block is the most common), and a too-low valve release position. Studies have shown that the expansion of prosthetic valve stents below the aortic annulus increases the incidence of conduction abnormalities, especially left bundle branch block. Conduction block usually occurs immediately after the release of the valve or 24 to 48 h after the operation, and the patients often need permanent pacemakers. TAVR may cause left and right bundle branch block and atrioventricular block. Fifty percent of cases of atrioventricular block occur within 1 week after TAVR and 80% within 1 month, but some cases occur 1–6 months after surgery [23, 24].

Researchers from the Georgia Institute of Technology and the Piedmont Heart Institute printed a model of aortic stenosis with calcification, used measurements to select a balloon of the right size for predilation, and further selected different stent valves to simulate the valve replacement procedure [11]. By using a carefully simulated 3D model, the researchers were able to more easily detect the direction of the deviation of the balloon during dilation and to clearly observe how the orientation of the stent valve would be affected by severe calcification after further release, thus determining the probability of conduction block. The results suggested that calcification of valve leaflets generally does not affect conduction when the volume of the aortic sinus is sufficient. Severe calcification of the root and annulus can easily cause lateral displacement of the stent valve, thereby causing conduction block. Through in vitro simulation and comparing the effects of implanting different valves, combined with the actual clinical effect, the researchers also found that the shorter transcatheter valve frame may be the cause of less conduction block. This result is consistent with the results of a meta-analysis of 11,210 patients published by Windecker et al., suggesting that the rate of permanent pacemaker implantation when using the SAPIEN valve was 6%, whereas that with the CoreValve was 28% [25].

Therefore, analysis of in vitro simulation of 3D-printed models can further improve the accuracy of preoperative evaluation and provide effective preoperative guidance for TAVR operations. In the future, as new valves become available, evaluation with 3D printing can, to a certain extent, provide reliable information about what kind of balloon and valve to choose, where to release the stent, how to avoid placing the stent too deep, how to avoid choosing large-diameter valves, and how to choose valves with short frames for patients with right bundle branch block, thereby greatly reducing the incidence of these complications.

6.1.5.3 Acute and Delayed Coronary Artery Occlusion

Acute or delayed coronary artery occlusion refers to the phenomenon whereby the stent valve pushes the self-leaflet or calcified tissue to the coronary artery ostium immediately after TAVR or during the long-term follow-up period, resulting in coronary artery occlusion and myocardial infarction. Common risk factors include (1) a large calcification at the edge of the left and right coronary sinuses; (2) a coronary ostium that was too close to the annular plane of the aortic valve, especially when the distance was <10 mm; (3) a sinus diameter < 30 mm or aortic root calcification with a ratio close to 1.0 of the diameter of valvular sinus; and (4) long aortic valve leaflets [26]. However, the risk factors for late-onset coronary occlusion have not yet been determined. Some high-risk patients have good postoperative coronary blood flow but could still have a late-onset coronary occlusion postoperatively. With these patients, one needs to pay special attention to any abnormal symptoms that occur in the week following the procedure. Whether this late-onset coronary occlusion is associated with placement of the valve is unknown. During TAVR, the valve should not be placed too high, and aortography should be performed to confirm that the valve does not block the entrance to the coronary artery. The degree of calcification of the aortic valve should be carefully assessed before surgery; the distance from the coronary sinus to the aortic valve sinus should be accurately measured; and the ratio of the diameter of the sinus to that of the valve should be calculated. Currently, there is no clear standard that would prohibit patients from receiving TAVR in order to avoid coronary sinus obstruction. Therefore, it is very important to accurately evaluate the dynamic changes in the anatomical structure before the operation.

3D printing technology in the field of medicine is becoming more sophisticated. One can not only print models using materials of different hardnesses and colors but one can also print a transparent model, which greatly facilitates clinical observation and simulation. Researchers used soft materials to print the aortic root, the sinus, and the coronary arteries and could measure on the solid model the height of the coronary ostia and the ratio of the diameter of sinus to that of the annulus, which could further be used to evaluate the risk to the coronary artery compared with information obtained using CTA.

For patients with severe calcification of the valve leaflet and the annulus or with high-risk coronary artery occlusion of the bicuspid aortic valve, their CTA data can be dumped out of Digital Imaging and Communications in Medicine files for further 3D modeling. Calcified tissues and valve annulus and valve leaflet tissues can be processed with different colors and layered, and 3D models can be printed by combining flexible and rigid materials. In the Department of Cardiovascular Surgery of the Xijing Hospital, cardiologists used the 3D-printed TAVR model to simulate balloon dilation in vitro and the release of the valve to evaluate whether a patient is likely to have a coronary artery occlusion during TAVR and the possibility of a delayed coronary artery occlusion after the operation. If the patient is really at high risk of coronary artery obstruction, the results obtained from the in vitro simulation can be used to guide the preparation of the intraoperative plan (Fig. 6.10). A coronary artery guide wire can be used as a preventive measure when it is anticipated that occlusion will occur during valve implantation, and the coronary "chimney" technique or the long stent implantation technique can be used to solve the problem intraoperatively [27]. So et al. have shown 3D printing can stratify the risk of coronary artery obstruction in patients with high-risk aortic root anatomy undergoing TAVR [28].

Although the incidences of acute coronary obstruction and delayed coronary obstruction are low, the consequences are often serious. Moreover, these patients are difficult to deal with, and the long-term prognosis of coronary "chimney" technology and other associated technologies still needs to be studied. The variety of different transcatheter valves on the market, such as the J-Valve with positioning keys, reflects a certain role in coronary protection. Researchers in the Department of Cardiovascular Surgery of Xijing hospital found that, by recreating the clinical situation using an in vitro 3D-printed model and by using the three U-shaped positioning keys of the J-Valve that could grasp the leaflets, they could not only firmly locate the bracket valve in the aortic rings but could also limit the ability of the thickened leaflets to move to the coronary ostia, thereby avoiding coronary blocking (Fig. 6.11).

6.1.5.4 Treatment of a Bicuspid Aortic Valve

With the development of TAVR instrumentation and the increasing number of operations performed, more and more patients with BAV are being identified. TAVR is increasingly used in the treatment of bicuspid aortic stenosis, and more and more researchers are concerned about the clinical outcomes. Because of the special anatomical structure and mechanical performance of the BAV, especially a type 0 bicuspid valve, treatment with TAVR is prone to complications such as paravalvular leakage, valve displacement, and aortic dissection, which make the operation more difficult and riskier than that performed on a tricuspid aortic valve. One study compared the imaging data of 400 patients, showing that the circumferential areas of their bicuspid aortic valves, the sinus, and the inner diameter of the ascending aorta were significantly larger than those of the normal tricuspid aortic valve and that the bicuspid aortic valve had more severe eccentric calcification [29]. In a study published in 2017, in which 1427 patients with characteristic Asian and European bicuspid aortic valve structures were compared, more European patients had moderately severe insufficiency, whereas the diameters of the annulus, sinus, and the ascending aorta of the Asian patients were significantly greater than those of the European patients [30].

Recent studies have shown that the surgical success rate and mortality rate using TAVR to treat a bicuspid aortic valve were not significantly different from those using TAVR to treat the tricuspid aortic valve, but it did increase the incidence of paravalvular leakage and of valve-in-valve implantation. At the same time, other major problems with bicuspid valves during TAVR are that the valve is prone to displacement: too high a position caused the valve to migrate into the ascending aorta, and too low a position led to conduction block and the increased probability of valve-in-valve implantation. Therefore, using TAVR to treat bicuspid aortic stenosis remains a challenge. 3D printing technology has spe-

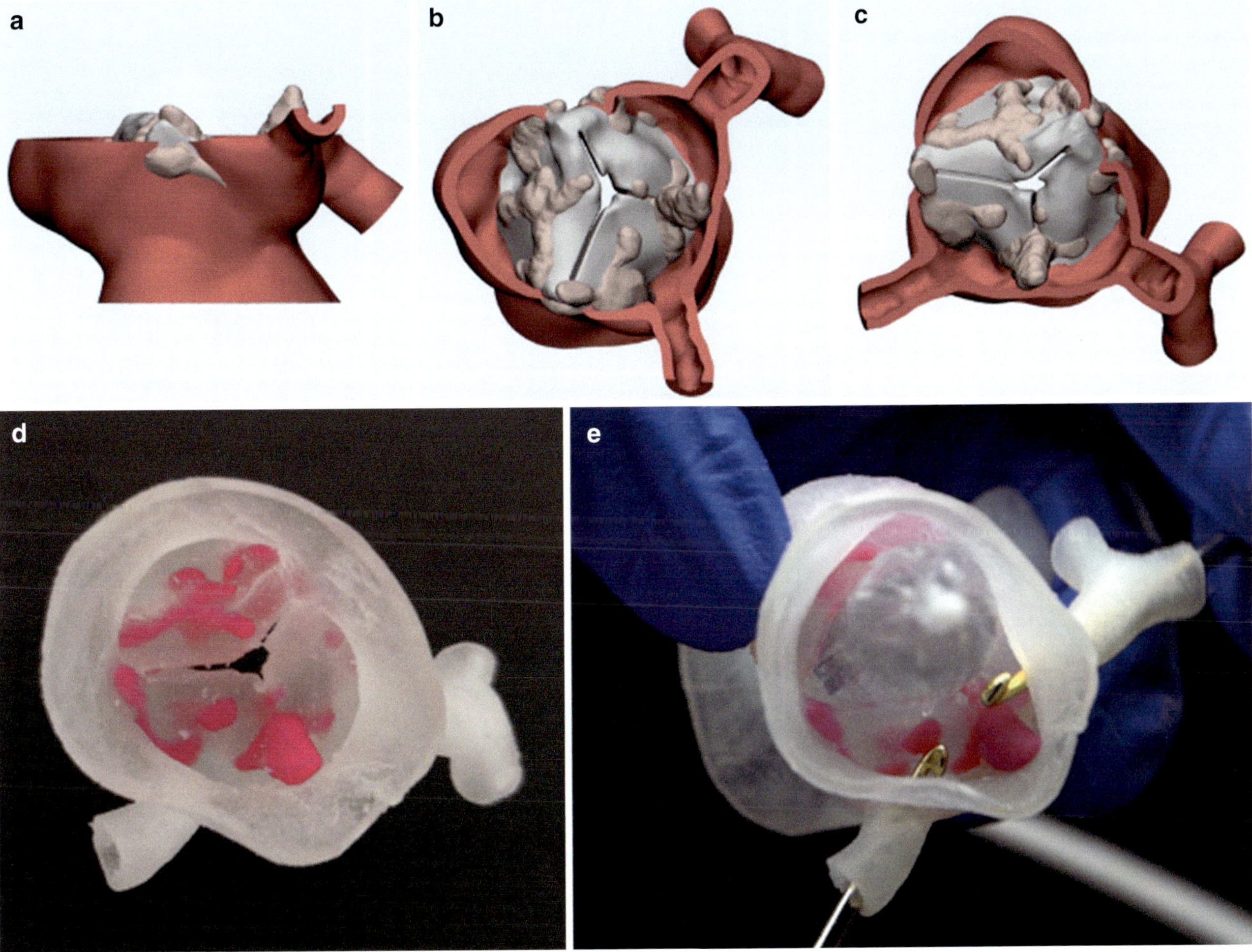

Fig. 6.10 The Department of Cardiovascular Surgery of Xijing Hospital used a three-dimensional (3D) aortic valve model to evaluate the risk of coronary artery occlusion using balloon dilation in vitro. (**a–c**) A computer-generated 3D model shows the calcification of the valve lobe and the height of the coronary artery in patients at risk of coronary artery occlusion. (**d, e**) 3D-printed model and balloon dilation simulation in vitro. Image data, 3D computer reconstruction, and 3D-printed model are from the Department of Cardiovascular Surgery of Xijing Hospital

cific advantages for treating the bicuspid aortic valve with TAVR. First, the 3D model can clearly show the root structure of the aortic valve, the spatial position of the bicuspid valve, the distribution of the calcifications, and the sizes of the aortic sinus and the coronary ostia. Second, a 3D-printed model can be used preoperatively to determine a good projection angle for the surgeons. After all, the annulus is visible as a plane under the X line in patients with BAV, so it is not possible to determine whether the implanted valve is in the right position. In addition, the surgeon can use in vitro simulation to practice the cross-valvular technique and the feel of releasing the valve. Finally, with in vitro simulation, a new generation of instruments with a retrievable, high-radial-support force and an antileakage device can be used during the operation, such as the SAPIEN 3, the Lotus, and the Venus-A Plus, to compare the fitness of each valve for different patients horizontally, to select the best transcatheter valve (Fig. 6.12).

6.1.5.5 Prevention of Vascular Complications

The TAVR approach is divided into a vascular approach and an apical approach, of which the femoral artery approach accounts for more than 90% with less trauma, a more convenient operative procedure, and fewer complications. Elderly patients usually present with a poor overall condition: Some have vessels with severe atherosclerosis, calcification, aortic arch plaques, ulcers, or large calcified plaques and even porcelain aorta. Such patients are prone to vascular injury and other serious consequences when they undergo TAVR via a vascular approach. Preoperative assessment of vascular CTA images can help identify most vascular lesions, thus prompting the surgeon to choose another approach if necessary. However, for various reasons, with some patients there is no alternative but to perform TAVR through a conventional approach. In this situation, 3D printing technology offers great advantages

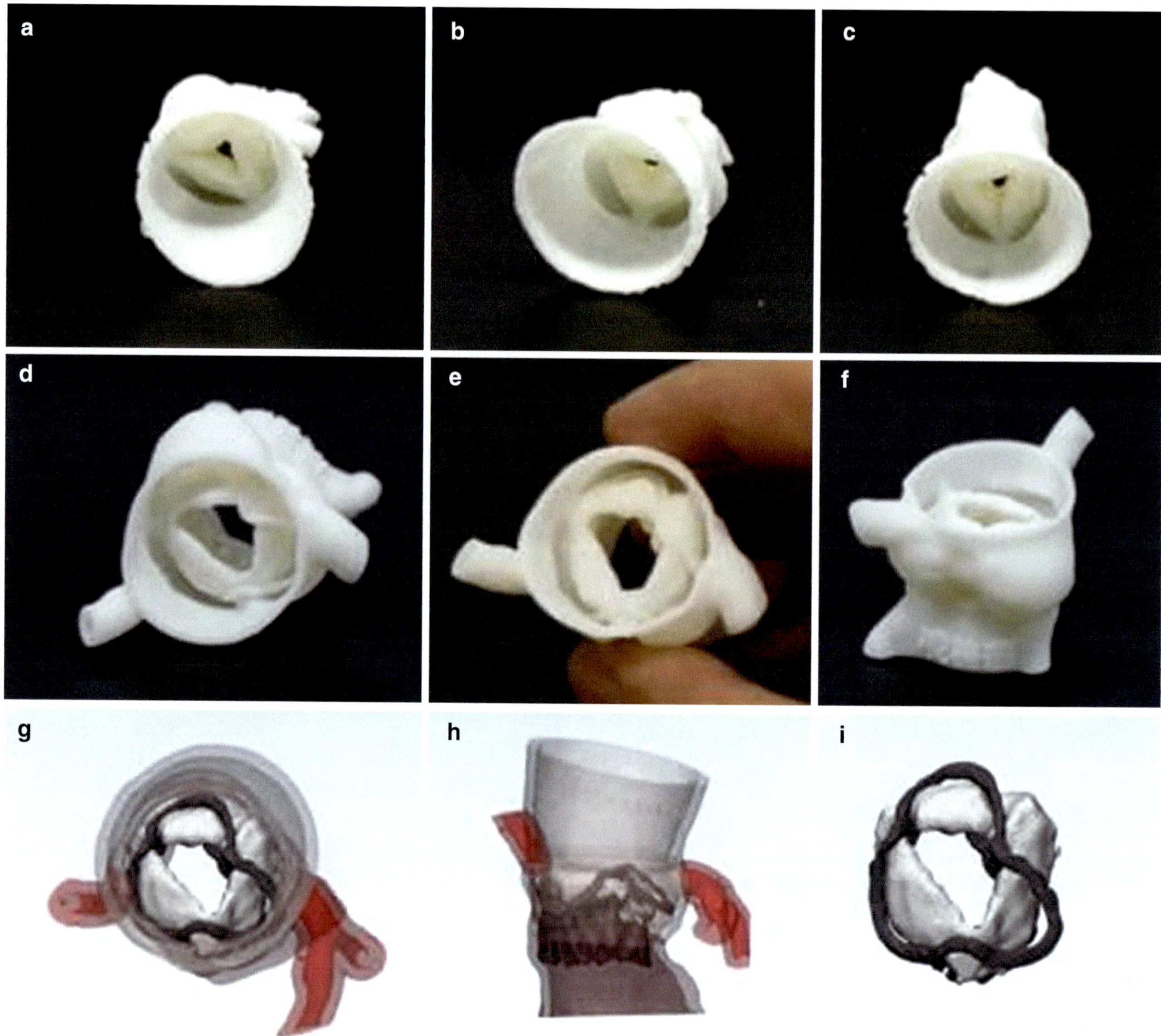

Fig. 6.11 Assessment of a three-dimensional (3D)-printed model for patients with high coronary risk in the Department of Cardiovascular Surgery of Xijing Hospital before and after transcatheter aortic valve replacement. (**a-c**) Aortic valve lengthening, thickening, and stenosis from different angles. (**d–f**) Multi-angle view of a 3D model after placement of a J-Valve; G–I 3D modeling and segmentation processing, respectively, can illustrate stent valves and their effect on the coronary artery. Image data, 3D computer reconstruction, and 3D-printed model were obtained from the Department of Cardiovascular Surgery of West China Hospital and Xijing Hospital

by allowing the creation of 3D vascular models to analyze the vulnerable parts of the blood vessels. These models can be used to help the surgeon carefully manipulate the catheter guide wire during the operation or to guide the implantation of a valve transporter with capture technology, thereby reducing the risk of vascular complications (Fig. 6.13). Preoperative simulation with a 3D-printed model can also encourage surgeons to consider endovascular stent repair before TAVR in some patients with thoracic and abdominal aortic aneurysms.

6.1.6 Optimization of the Platform of a Three-Dimensional In Vitro Simulation Model Before Transcatheter Aortic Valve Replacement Surgery

A high-precision composite 3D-printed model not only depicts the patient-specific anatomical structure statically but also identifies potential surgical problems and risks through dynamic in vitro simulation of balloon dilation and valve release, which helps the surgical team formulate surgi-

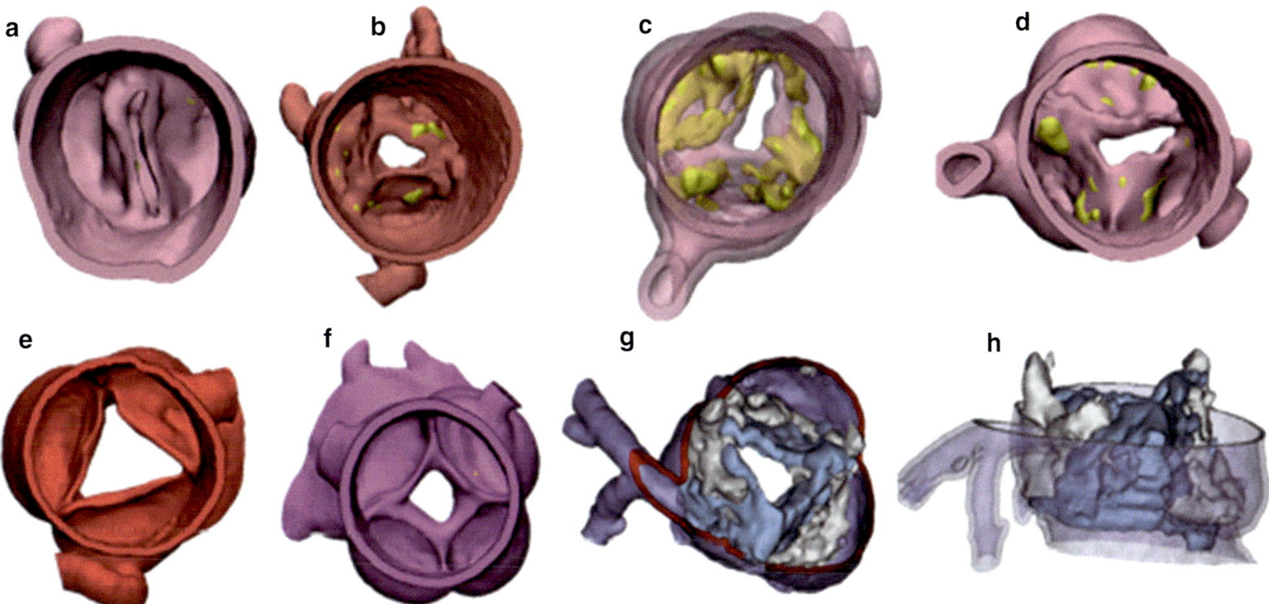

Fig. 6.12 Three-dimensional reconstruction of bicuspid aortic valve, tricuspid aortic valve, and quadricuspid aortic valve. (**a–d**) Different types of bicuspid aortic valve models. (**e**) Tricuspid aortic valve model. (**f**) Quadricuspid aortic valve model. (**g, h**) Tricuspid aortic valve three-dimensional reconstructed section and side display. Image data and 3D reconstruction model were obtained from the Department of Cardiovascular Surgery of Xiangya Second Hospital and Xijing Hospital

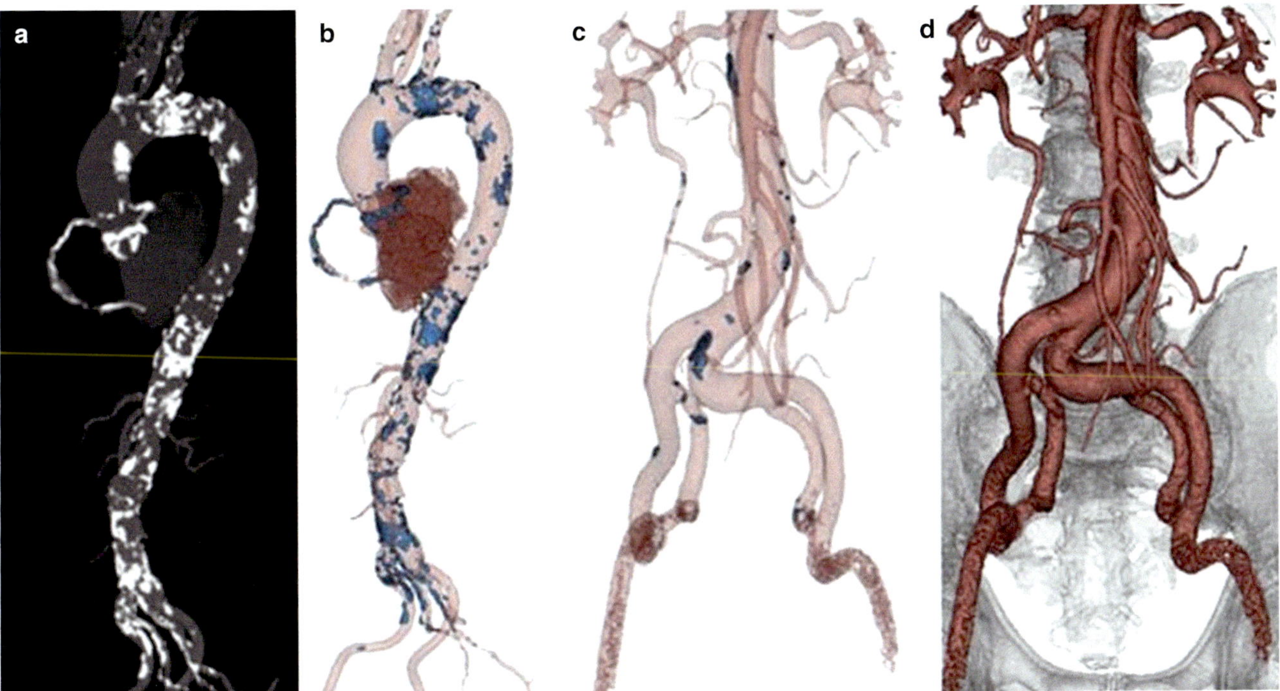

Fig. 6.13 Three-Dimensional models were used to analyze the vascular lesions along the pathway. (**a, b**) Three-dimensional (3D) images were used to process calcified plaques. (**c, d**) 3D images were used to analyze the distortion of the vascular access. Image data and computer 3D reconstruction models are from the Department of Cardiovascular Surgery of Xijing Hospital

cal strategies and avoid complications. On this basis, a variety of flexible materials with characteristics similar to those of human heart tissue can be used to print a 3D model of the aortic valve and surrounding structures. By creating a pulsating fluid platform, one can accurately construct a model that includes the motion of the beating heart, thereby simulating a dynamic version of a diseased heart valve. At the same time, with the aid of high-speed cameras, X-ray imaging equipment, and an ultrasound probe, researchers can simulate the real intervention therapy of human disease, measure the blood flow velocity before and after valve replacement, and obtain similar clinical pathological data from X-ray contrast imaging and ultrasound Doppler imaging (Fig. 6.14). With this kind of platform, one can achieve the following: (1) complete preoperative simulation of TAVR, which speeds up the learning curve and reduces the operative risk, and (2) a way to test, optimize, improve, and verify the instruments used for TAVR.

With the development of technological resources and the accumulation of clinical experience, TAVR is considered safe and is usually the first choice for high-risk patients with a faulty aortic valve. The indications and the range of applications for this minimally invasive surgical technique are expanding. The key improvements in TAVR include better

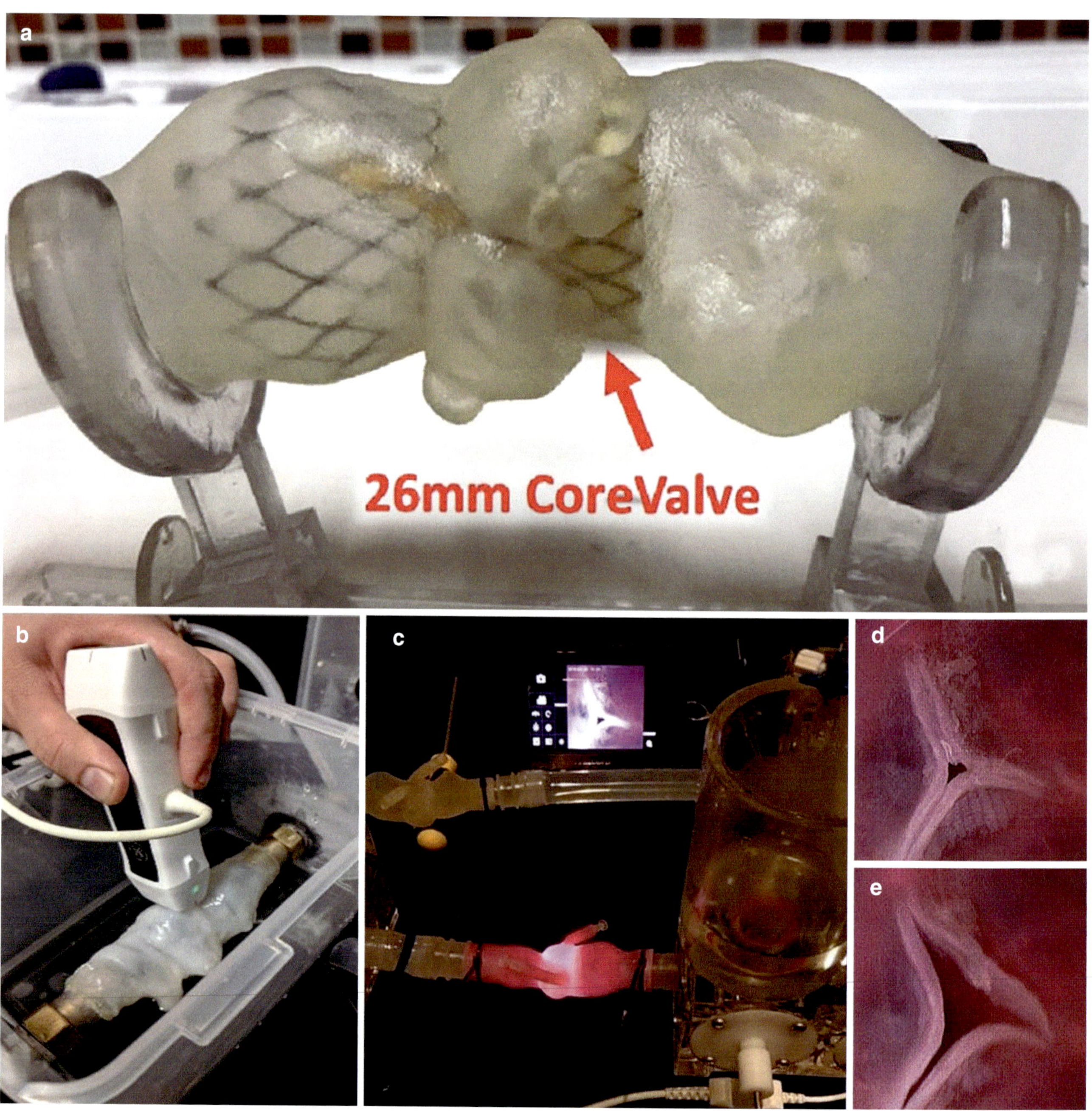

Fig. 6.14 An in vitro simulator for a 3D-printed model. (**a**) In vitro simulator with a 26 mm CoreValve mounted inside; (**b**) Ultrasound Doppler Pulse flow detection using a 3D-printed model. Valve closure during the diastolic phase. (**c**) In vitro simulator with a camera mounted inside; (**d**) Valve close during the diastolic phase; (**e**) Valve open during the systolic phase. Testing system and 3D-printed model from the Prince of Wales Hospital, Hong Kong, and Department of Cardiovascular Surgery, Xijing Hospital

patient selection, selection of tailored biological prostheses, and innovative valve design. Using 3D-printed models can help identify potential complications in complex cases before intervention. The 3D model of the whole heart provides training opportunities for transvascular and transapical TAVR. 3D-printed models for planning and simulating valve surgery can help identify risks and select the best parameters. In addition, the flexible material can display and simulate the functional characteristics of severe degenerative aortic stenosis. The pathological hemodynamic environment of severely calcified aortic stenosis can be fully reproduced in these 3D-printed models to improve surgical planning for patient-specific TAVR [31].

With the continuous development of TAVR procedures, an increasing number of operations, accumulated experience, and continuous progress in the development of instruments, minimalist TAVR operations are being carried out at more and more centers outside China. Minimalist TAVR can be performed in the general catheter laboratory, using local anesthesia, transthoracic cardiac ultrasound, the peripheral arterial approach, subcutaneous puncture, and a vascular suture device. TAVR is becoming greatly simplified, even without the presence of a surgeon standby table. Although more and more centers in China can perform TAVR procedures, most of them are still moving along the learning curve. Centers that have performed less than 100 operations total need to be approached with caution, because their ability to perform successful operations is still far behind that performed in countries outside China. However, minimalist TAVR is not an easy procedure; strict, rigorous preoperative evaluation is still needed. The good news is that working with a 3D-printed model can speed up the operator's learning curve, reduce intraoperative complications, and play a helpful role in promoting minimalist TAVR.

6.2 Transcatheter Mitral Valve Therapy and Three-Dimensional Printing

Jiayou Tang, Yang Liu, Yanyan Ma

Mitral stenosis (MS) is one of the most common valvular diseases threatening people's health. Most cases of MS are sequelae of rheumatic fever; the remaining cases are due to congenital stenosis, senile mitral annulus, and subannular calcification. Mitral insufficiency (MI) is caused mainly by valvular degeneration and rheumatic fever or is secondary to myocardial infarction or left atrial or ventricular remodeling or dysfunction, which may be associated with atrial fibrillation. According to the latest epidemiological survey data from developed countries, MI is the type of valvular disease with the highest incidence in people over 65 years old. Studies have shown that the long-term effect of the surgical treatment of mitral valve disease is significantly better than that of drug treatment. However, some patients with MS secondary to rheumatic fever are younger, and replacement of the valve significantly affects their quality of life. Meanwhile, for many senior high-risk patients with multisystemic disease, valve replacement may cause higher surgical risk and lower survival benefit. European experiences demonstrate that the surgical success rate for these patients is only 50%; for patients with severe functional regurgitation, this rate drops to 16% [32]. Therefore, clinicians have focused on minimally invasive treatment of mitral valve diseases. In 1984, Inoue and his colleagues first reported percutaneous balloon mitral valvuloplasty (PBMV). Then Lock et al. successfully used a polyethylene balloon catheter to expand MS in 1985. Minimally invasive techniques for MS developed rapidly. After decades of hard work, Prof. Francesco Maisano of the University of Zurich in Switzerland was the first to complete transcatheter MI treatment based on edge-to-edge technology using the MitraClip (Abbott, Chicago, IL, USA) device, which triggered worldwide interest and further attempts to treat high-risk patients with MI. On June 12, 2012, surgeons at the Rigshospitalet in Copenhagen, Denmark, completed the world's first human transcatheter mitral valve replacement (TMVR) procedure, marking the entrance of mitral valve replacement into the minimally invasive era.

Over the past 5 years, an endless stream of mitral valve intervention and replacement devices has emerged, and news of successful clinical trials has been frequently reported. However, the widespread promotion and popularization of this technology are still extremely limited, not only because of the peculiarities of the structure of the mitral valve but also because of the difficulty of preoperative screening and evaluation. At present, expert consensus is that the preoperative evaluation of patients for transcatheter mitral valvuloplasty and replacement depends mainly on the use of imaging including transesophageal echocardiography and computed tomography (CT). The mitral valve is a three-dimensional structure with diversified normal anatomy and pathologies. It has a complex structure that changes dynamically during the cardiac cycle. Therefore, preprocedural planning for mitral valve intervention by imaging modality alone has significant limitations. It is often difficult to appreciate how an interventional device would sit in the mitral annulus or alter the structure of the mitral valve, or to identify preoperatively potential risks and problems that one may encounter during the operation. Therefore, a new type of spatial stereoscopic model for observation and simulation is urgently needed in clinical treatment.

The intersection of three-dimensional (3D) printing technology and medicine is gradually revealing its advantages. Applications are becoming more widespread and intricate, from the early 3D printing for learning and educating about the rigid overall structure to the subsequent printing of artificial bones and joint prostheses to simulate objects to be implanted. Consequently, in vitro simulations using 3D-printed artificial organs and soft models show that it is especially important for clinicians to provide information that is difficult to display with traditional imaging modalities. This chapter focuses on the basic knowledge of mitral valve disease and explores the development of 3D printing technology, its interdisciplinary integration with heart disease, and its impact on mitral valve interventions.

6.2.1 Anatomical Features of the Mitral Valve

When one is studying mitral valve disease, it is not enough to focus only on the valve itself. What is needed is a comprehensive assessment of the so-called mitral valve complex, which comprises the mitral valve and its adjacent structures, including the mitral valve leaflets, annulus, and subvalvular structures (including the chordae and papillary muscles), as well as important adjacent structures including the circumflex coronary artery and the left ventricular outflow tract. Previous understanding of the mitral valve complex relied mainly on the results of anatomical studies. It was found that the mitral valve leaflet consists of a larger anterior leaflet and a smaller posterior leaflet. The anterior leaflet occupies one-third of the entire annulus due to its relationship with the aortic valve and septum, also known as the aortic valve leaflet. The posterior leaflet occupies the remaining two-thirds of the annulus, also known as the mural leaflet. The atrial and ventricular endocardium continues on the surface of the leaflets. The mitral leaflets are naturally asymmetrical. Neither are the junctions of the mitral leaflets, papillary muscles, and chordae.

The mitral annulus is a soft leaflet attachment structure defined as the attachment points of the mitral valve leaflets to the left atrium and ventricle. Different from the aortic annulus, the mitral annulus is a 3D saddle-shaped structure, not D-shaped or circular. The posterior mitral annulus is a noncontinuous fibrofatty structure, so the texture is soft and thus more dilatable than the anterior mitral annulus. It is difficult to accurately evaluate the mitral annulus using traditional two-dimensional (2D) imaging. However, with 3D echocardiography [33–35] or 3D-computed tomography angiography (CTA), 3D modeling of 3D ultrasound Digital Imaging and Communications in Medicine [DICOM] data can reveal the spatial structure of the mitral valve [34, 35]. The spatial structure of the annulus can be measured dynamically (Fig. 6.15).

The papillary muscles and the chordae connect the leaflets and annulus on one side and the ventricle wall on the other side. There are about 24 chordae and their attached papillary muscles in the ventricular chamber under the mitral valve. The individual differences in the distribution of the papillary muscles and the connection area are very complicated, depending on the distribution of the coronary artery and other factors. The inferior papillary muscle is supplied with blood from the posterior descending branch of the left ventricle. The superior papillary muscle is supplied by the diagonal branch, the circumflex artery, or the obtuse marginal branch of the left coronary artery. The lesions vary with different papillary muscles and chordae.

The composition of the mitral valve complex varies from individual to individual, so does the complexity of the lesion.

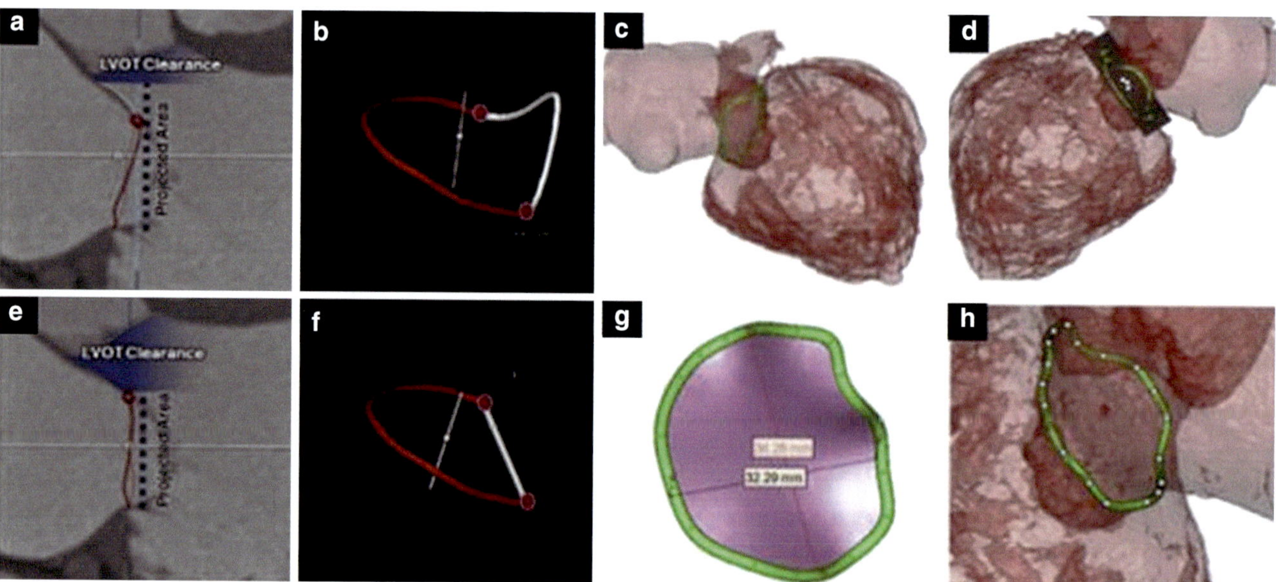

Fig. 6.15 Three-dimensional (3D) imaging of the mitral annulus. (**a–d**) Computed tomography and 3D model images of the saddle-shaped mitral annulus. (**e–h**) Computed tomography and 3D modeling images of the horizon-shaped mitral annulus. Image data and computerized 3D reconstruction model from the Department of Cardiovascular Surgery, Xijing Hospital

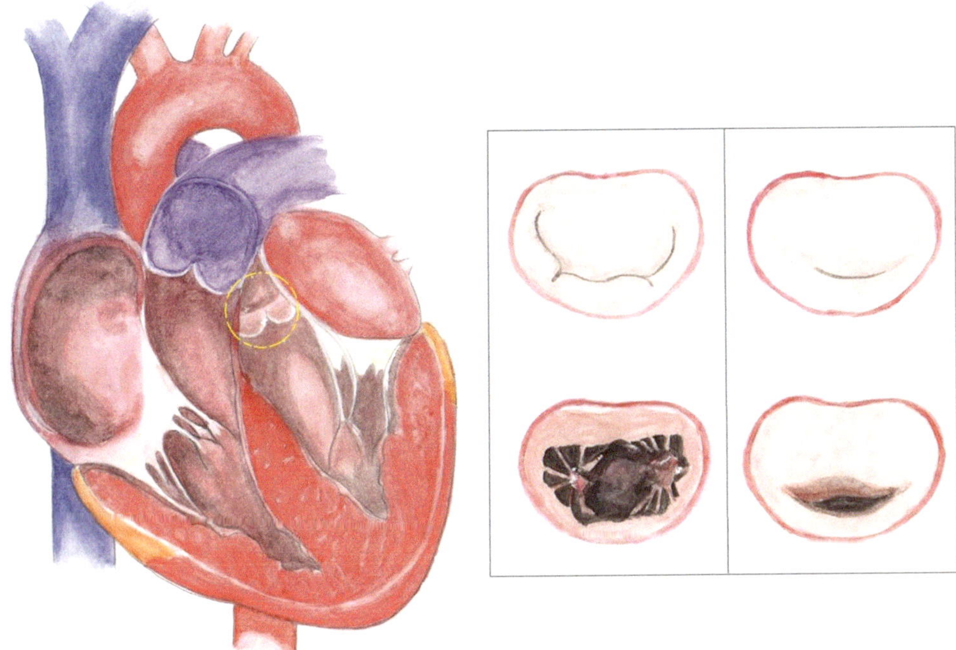

Fig. 6.16 Schematic diagram of mitral stenosis

Clinicians have found that transthoracic echocardiography cannot clearly show the mitral valve complex and that sometimes even the lesions of the mitral valve leaflets cannot be seen clearly. One can obtain a clear view of the mitral valve leaflets and annulus with transesophageal echocardiography, which can provide comprehensive evaluation of the mitral valve complex. CTA assessment can be used to observe the mitral valve leaflet and subvalvular structures in different sections, but the inability to detect differential pressure and regurgitation during mitral valve motion renders this modality unsatisfactory. Therefore, the ability to access a 3D image rather than a 2D image is of great significance for clinical work [32, 36, 37].

6.2.2 Pathophysiology of Mitral Stenosis

The normal adult mitral valve orifice area is 4–6 cm^2. When the valve orifice area is <2.0 cm^2, hemodynamic changes are considered clinically significant. When the area of the valve orifice is reduced to 1.5–2.0 cm^2, the patient has mild stenosis; when the valve area is 1.0–1.5 cm^2, the patient is moderately stenotic; and a patient with a valve area of <1.0 cm^2 has severe stenosis. When the patient is severely stenotic, the left atrial pressure can be as high as 20–25 mmHg (1 mmHg = 0.133 kPa) to allow blood to flow through the narrow mitral valve. Elevated left atrial pressure can lead to increased pulmonary vein and pulmonary capillary pressure, resulting in labored dyspnea. When the left atrial pressure exceeds 30 mmHg, clinical manifestations such as difficulty in breathing, cough, and cyanosis appear. As the disease progresses, the left atrium increases in size and the right heart pressure increases, which can lead to atrial fibrillation and right heart dysfunction. Normally, it can be as long as 10 years from the time symptoms of initial rheumatic carditis appear to the development of significant mitral stenosis; thereafter, symptoms will gradually progress and atrial fibrillation and right heart failure may develop during the next 10–20 years (Fig. 6.16).

6.2.3 Pathophysiology of Mitral Insufficiency

The mitral valve consists of four parts: the leaflets, the annulus, the chordae, and the papillary muscles, any of which can cause structural abnormalities or dysfunction, leading to mitral regurgitation. During systole, the mitral valve, affected by long-term inflammation, exhibits degeneration and shortening such that it cannot close normally. The blood from the left ventricle flows into the left atrium. The early stage can be asymptomatic or the patient can exhibit palpitations and chest tightness; the main sign is a ventricular systolic murmur. In patients who had rheumatic carditis, it can take as long as 20 years for symptoms of significant mitral regurgitation to appear. Progress is rapid after heart failure. Mild mitral regurgitation may have no obvious symptoms or may involve only mild discomfort. Common symptoms of severe mitral regurgitation include labored dyspnea, fatigue, and significantly reduced tolerance for activity. Long-term follow-up data have shown that cardiac function in patients with mitral regurgitation is significantly improved after surgery compared to after drug therapy. Even in patients with heart failure or atrial fibrillation, the result is the same (Fig. 6.17).

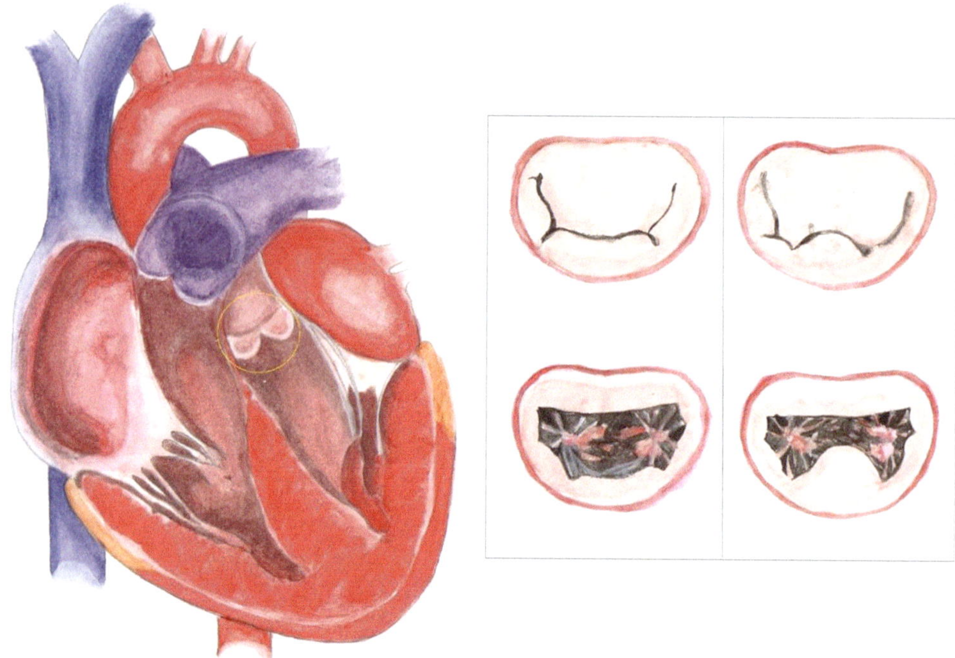

Fig. 6.17 Schematic diagram of mitral insufficiency

At present, the preoperative evaluation of mitral valve disease relies mainly on the results of transthoracic and transesophageal echocardiography. These imaging methods can accurately evaluate the type and severity of mitral stenosis and regurgitation, which also has a positive effect on the evaluation of perioperative hemodynamic parameters [34] (Fig. 6.18).

At present, ultrasound data have been used to perform 3D printing, which can clearly show the anatomical structure of the mitral valve, including the morphology of the anterior and posterior leaflets, the different leaflet openings, and the closing states of the systolic and diastolic phases (Fig. 6.19).

In addition, the application of CTA data, especially four-dimensional dynamic image data, can also be used in vitro for 3D printing to model the mitral anatomy, including the anterior and posterior lobes and the chordae. Papillary muscles and their relationship with the internal structures of the heart can be displayed, and mitral stenosis and insufficiency can be visualized clearly (Fig. 6.20).

6.2.4 Three-Dimensional Printing Technology and Interventional Therapy for Mitral Stenosis

Although medication can alleviate the symptoms of mitral stenosis, it does not cure the obstructed blood flow induced by the stenotic valve. The 2017 American College of Cardiology/American Heart Association guidelines state that if a patient with mitral stenosis requiring intervention does not have a left atrial thrombus or moderate or severe mitral regurgitation, and the leaflets are of good quality, percutaneous balloon mitral valvotomy (PBMV) is preferred to surgery (class/level of recommendation: I, b). For asymptomatic patients, the indication for PBMV is moderate to severe mitral stenosis (mitral valve area ≤ 1.5 cm^2), accompanied by pulmonary hypertension at rest or exercise. If the patient is planning to become pregnant or to undergo non-cardiac surgery, PBMV can also be considered. In addition, patients who are unable to undergo surgery due to advanced age or high surgical risk or patients with severely deformed valve leaflets may choose PBMV as a palliative treatment if there is no thrombus in the left atrium and there is no moderate or severe regurgitation in the mitral valve.

Following is a brief description of PBMV: Using the Seldinger technique, the cannula is inserted through the right femoral vein, and a Brockenbrough needle is delivered through the right femoral vein to puncture the interatrial septum. After a successful puncture, the femoral vein puncture hole and the atrial septum puncture hole are expanded with a 14 Fr dilator, then delivered into the balloon catheter (Inoue balloon catheter system) via a guidewire, and the balloon is inflated under fluoroscopy so that the narrow orifice of the mitral valve is dilated. After the expansion is completed, repeat left and right cardiac catheterization is done to observe the effect of expansion (Fig. 6.21).

Mitral balloon dilatation is a minimally invasive procedure, but complications can still occur: (1) A malignant arrhythmia can be caused by the device entering the left ventricle. (2) Mitral regurgitation can occur after dilation: Most mitral regurgitation is characterized by reflux at the junction of the valve leaflet. The main cause of reflux at the non-

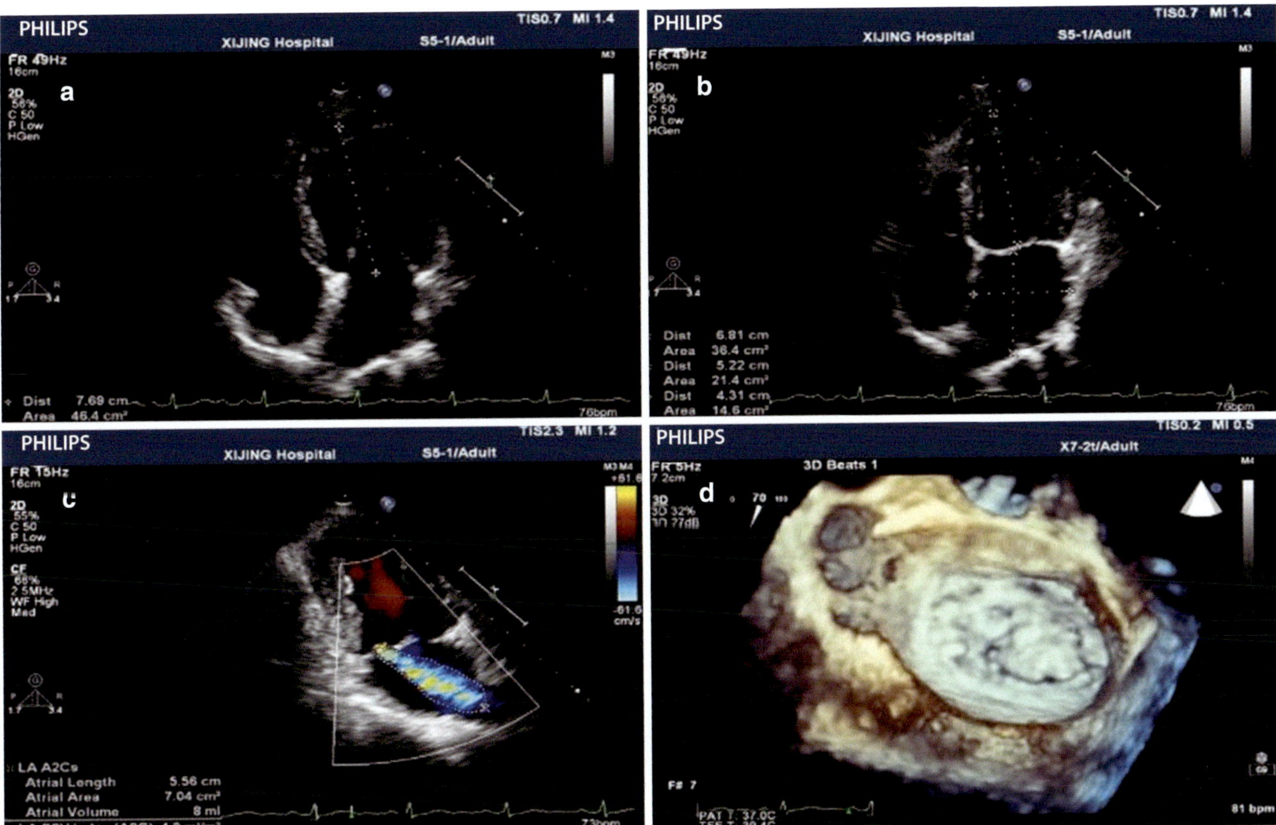

Fig. 6.18 Echocardiographic images of mitral valve disease. (**a**) Four-chamber view of diastolic mitral valve. (**b**) Four-chamber view of systolic mitral valve. (**c**) Color Doppler assessment of the mitral insufficiency. (**d**) Color Doppler three-dimensional assessment of the location, type, and severity of mitral insufficiency. Image data from the Department of Cardiovascular Surgery, Xijing Hospital

junction is a lobular tear or damage to the chordae. Patients with significant mitral regurgitation had a lower 8-year event-free survival rate (no cardiac death, mitral valve replacement, secondary PBMV, heart failure requiring hospitalization, or embolization). (3) Atrial septal defect can be caused by a puncture: The incidence of a left-to-right shunt in the atrial septum after PBMV is 3%–16%, determined by oximetry. Generally, about 60% of patients with defects have defects that self-close, have minimal left-to-right flow (pulmonary circulation blood flow/systemic blood flow [Qp/Qs] < 2.0], and good clinical tolerance. Multiple punctures can lead to an unrecoverable atrial septal defect. (4) Pericardial tamponade, a cardiac complication also caused by puncture, has a reported incidence in the foreign literature of 0.6%–5% and in the domestic literature of 0.5%–1.5%. Patients with a small amount of pericardial effusion do not need any special treatment. Those who are stable can continue to have PBMV. A moderate-to-large quantity of pericardial effusion can cause acute pericardial tamponade, which requires immediate pericardial puncture decompression; severe cases need to be switched to open thoracic surgery.

Because PBMV is a palliative operation and prone to complications, it is performed only rarely in China, so the number of patients having PBMV is small. Many clinicians prefer their patients with mitral stenosis to have open surgery. According to the guidelines, the current recommended preoperative evaluation method, transthoracic echocardiography, can provide information on leaflet lesions, valve area, blood flow rate, and transvalvular pressure, but it is hard to predict the direction and degree of the tear based on valve leaflet adhesions. For some elderly high-risk patients with mitral stenosis accompanied by calcifications, cardiac ultrasound cannot provide further comprehensive assessment. After all, mitral valve leaflet calcification is a relative contraindication for PBMV.

The introduction of 3D printing technology can make up for the deficiency of the 2D echocardiographic images. 3D modeling is performed in the diastolic and systolic phases based on the patient's cardiac CTA images or the 3D transesophageal echocardiography Digital Imaging and Communications in Medicine (DICOM) file, and the leaflet and annulus lesions are layered and printed with materials of different hardness to obtain a patient-specific left heart sys-

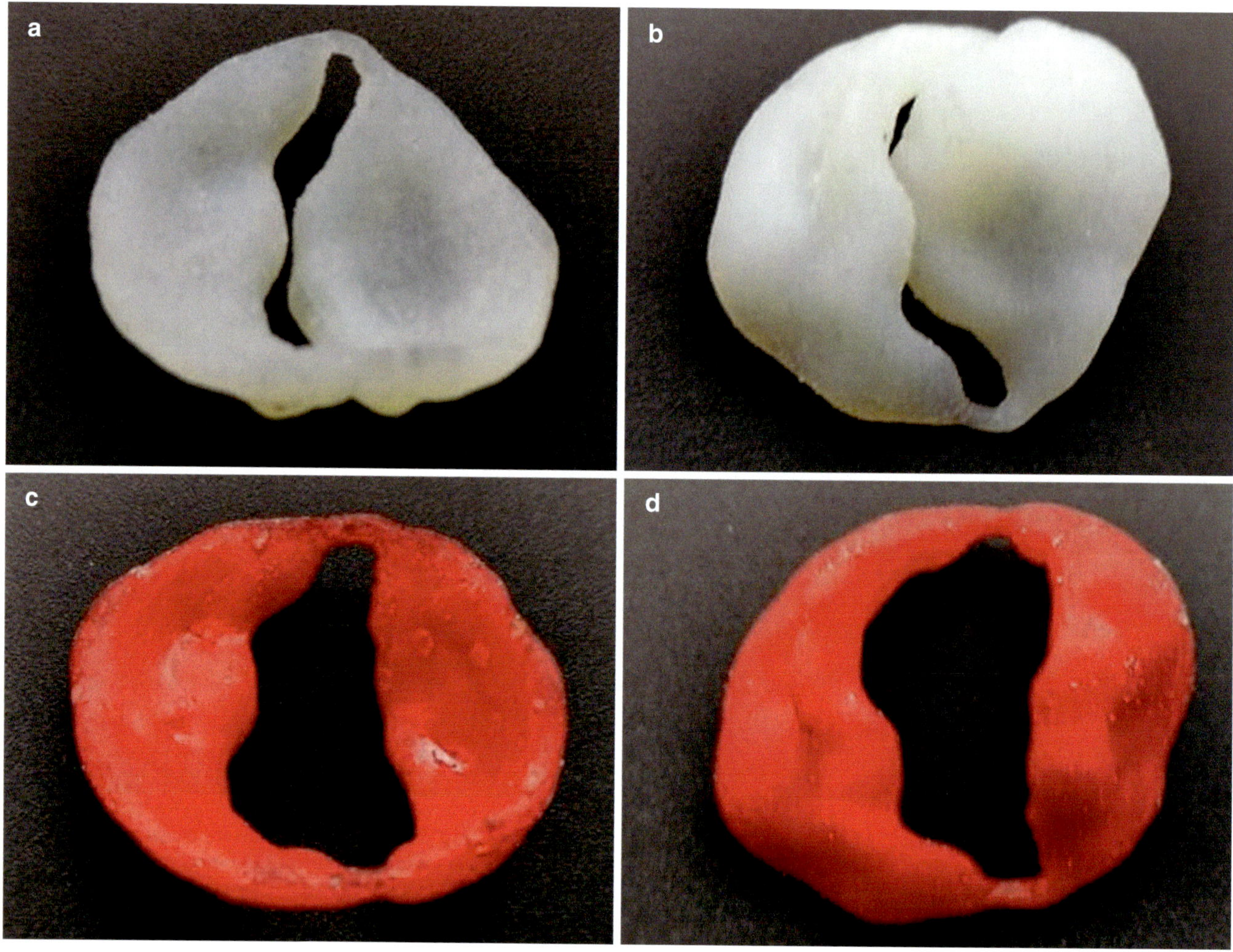

Fig. 6.19 Three-dimensional-printed normal mitral valve model based on echocardiographic data. (**a**) Images of systolic closed mitral valve from the atrial view. (**b**) Systolic closed mitral valve from the ventricular view. (**c**) Diastolic closed mitral valve from the atrial view. (**d**) Diastolic closed mitral valve from the ventricular view. Image data and 3D-printed model from the Department of Cardiovascular Surgery, Xijing Hospital and National Additive Manufacturing Innovation Center

tem model. Using such a model, a better assessment can be made, and the following clinical benefits can be obtained:

1. For patients with a large left atrium, preoperative simulation with a 3D printing model can help the physician select the appropriate angle and position of the atrial septal puncture to avoid pericardial tamponade due to puncture position deviation, poor interventional operations, or an iatrogenic atrial septal defect caused by multiple punctures.
2. The 3D printing model shows the structure of the left atrial appendage and the left ventricle. The preoperative simulation guides clinicians to avoid damaging the left atrial appendage and to prevent ventricular perforation or malignant arrhythmia caused by the balloon.
3. For patients with severe mitral stenosis, practical simulation on the 3D model can help the surgeon find the appropriate angle and direction for pushing the balloon and reducing the actual operation time and the radiation intake.
4. Using a 3D model made of materials of different levels of hardness, combined with biomimetic materials that simulate the mass and mode of adhesion of the patient's valve, and simulating balloon dilation can better predict the degree of tearing of the leaflets, thus judging the postoperative probability and degree of mitral regurgitation. This approach not only benefits patient screening but can also assist the surgeon in selecting the appropriate balloon size during surgery.

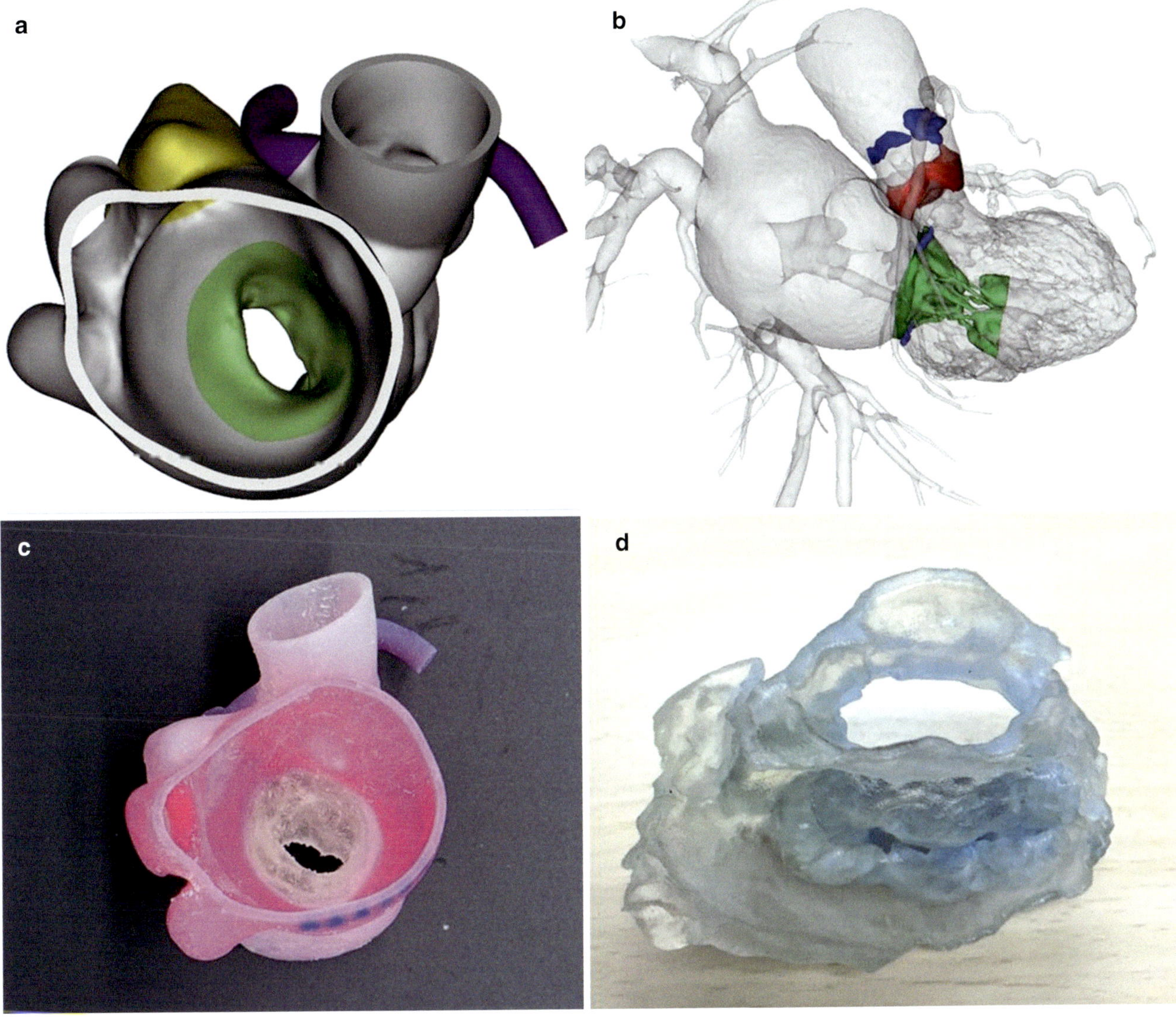

Fig. 6.20 Three-dimensional (3D)-printed mitral valve model based on computed tomography angiography data. (**a**) Computer modeling shows mitral stenosis from the atrial view. (**b**) Computer modeling shows mitral insufficiency, visible chordae, papillary muscles, and their relationship with the internal structures of the heart. (**c**) 3D-printed model shows mitral stenosis from the atrial view. (**d**) 3D-printed model shows mitral insufficiency from an atrial view. Image data, computer 3D reconstruction, and 3D printing model from the Prince of Wales Hospital, Hong Kong, and Department of Cardiovascular Surgery, Xijing Hospital

6.2.5 Three-Dimensional Printing and Interventional Treatment of Mitral Insufficiency

Mitral regurgitation is a common valvular heart disease with a tenfold incidence of aortic stenosis. In China, the prevalence of mitral regurgitation in patients over the age of 60 is 13.4%, and the number of patients with grade 3+ mitral regurgitation or more requiring treatment could reach ten million, but the actual number of patients undergoing mitral valve surgery is only 40,000 per year. According to the pathogenesis, mitral regurgitation can be divided into organic and functional; according to the timing of clinical presentation, mitral regurgitation can be divided into acute and chronic. Patients with mild mitral regurgitation may not have clinical symptoms for a long time, and their prognosis is good; patients with severe mitral regurgitation may be accompanied by symptoms such as palpitations, chest tightness, and shortness of breath. Patients with acute severe mitral regurgitation have poor tolerance for surgery and a high risk of death; the 5-year incidence of cardiovascular death and events in patients with chronic severe asymptomatic mitral regurgitation is 14 ± 3% and 33 ± 3%, respectively. Patients with severe heart failure have an annual mortality rate of 34%. Clinical studies have shown that drug therapy can only improve the symptoms of patients with mitral

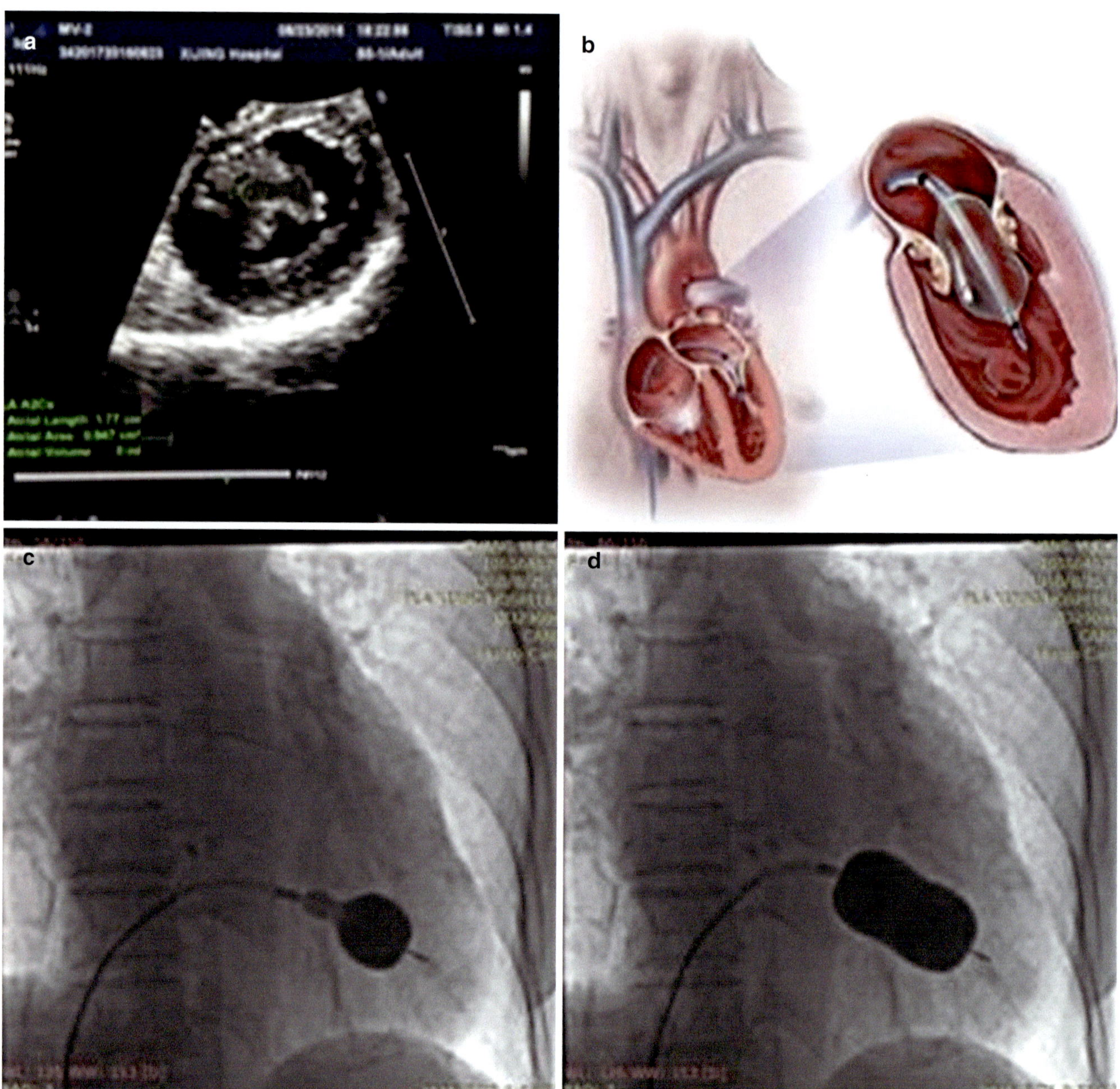

Fig. 6.21 Balloon dilatation of mitral stenosis. (**a**) Transcranial ultrasound assessment of the mitral valve area. (**b**) Percutaneous balloon mitral valvuloplasty approach and schematic diagram. (**c**) The balloon through the stenotic mitral valve under X-ray guidance. (**d**) The balloon is inflated under X-ray guidance. The imaging data are from the Department of Cardiovascular Surgery, Xijing Hospital

regurgitation; it cannot extend their survival time. Surgical valve repair or replacement is considered a standard method of treating mitral regurgitation and has been shown to relieve symptoms and prolong patient survival times. However, about half of the patients with mitral regurgitation are not treated effectively because of high-risk factors such as low heart function, comorbidities, and advanced age. In the past decade, the rapid development of transcatheter mitral interventional therapy has brought new hope to patients with mitral regurgitation.

In general, mitral regurgitation interventional techniques can be divided into two categories: transcatheter mitral valve repair (TMVr) and TMVR. According to different technical principles, TMVr can be divided into (1) percutaneous edge-to-edge mitral valve repair [MitraClip; MitralStitch (Hangzhou DeJin Medtech Co, Hangzhou, China)]; ValveClamp (Hanyu Medical Technology, Shanghai, China); (2) percutaneous mitral annuloplasty (Cardioband, Edwards Lifesciences, Irvine, CA USA), including direct and indirect annuloplasty; and (3) percutaneous mitral artificial chordae implant (NeoChord, NeoChord, St. Louis Park, MN, USA; MitralStitch).

TMVR technology includes interventional autologous mitral valve implantation, valve-in-valve implantation after bioprosthetic replacement, and valve-in-ring implantation after valvuloplasty, among others. The first tests in humans of the first-generation valves, such as the Edwards CardiAQ valve (Edwards Lifesciences, Irvine, CA, USA), the Neovasc Tiara valve (Neovasc, Richmond, BC, Canada), the Abbott Tendyne valve (Abbott Laboratories, Lake Bluff, IL USA), and the Medtronic Intrepid valve (Medtronic, Minneapolis, MN USA), have been completed and showed specific clinical effects. For the midvalvular portion of the bioprosthetic valve and the annular valve after valvuloplasty, the prosthetic valve and annulus can provide radial support. The current interventional aortic valve can be used to complete the TMVR. The orthotopic valve implantation technique for patients with mitral regurgitation with a mitral valve without significant calcification is the true TMVR. Although many products (>50) are available for TMVR, most of them are in the preclinical stage, limited by the anatomical specificity of the mitral valve and adjacent structures, and the difficulty of screening and evaluating preoperative patients. Although some products were tested in clinical trials, the results were poor.

6.2.6 Three-Dimensional Printing and Transcatheter Mitral Valve Repair

In 2003, the world's first transcatheter mitral valvuloplasty was used clinically. The team pushed a MitraClip mitral valve clamp device into the left atrium and left ventricle through the femoral vein of a patient with MI who had been placed under general anesthesia. With the guidance of 3D ultrasound and radiography, they used the device to clamp the middle of the anterior and posterior mitral lobes, so that the mitral valve was transformed from a large single hole to a small double hole during systole, thus reducing the MI. Transcatheter edge-to-edge mitral valve repair has since been performed in more than 60,000 patients worldwide.

The 2017 American Heart Association guidelines and the US Food and Drug Administration both recommended MitraClip for the treatment of primary MI. The Endovascular Valve Edge-to-Edge Repair Study I (EVEREST I) feasibility study and other registries and studies such as the Two-Phase Observational Study of the MitraClip System in Europe (ACCESS-EU), the Percutaneous Mitral Valve Repair in Cardiac Resynchronisation Therapy (PERMIT-CARE) feasibility study, the transcatheter mitral valve intervention (TRAMI) registry, the Getting Reduction of Mitral Insufficiency by Percutaneous Clip Implantation (GRASP) registry, and the Cardiovascular Outcomes Assessment of the MitraClip Percutaneous Therapy for Heart Failure Patients with Functional Mitral Regurgitation (COAPT) trial have proved that the MitraClip is also beneficial for functional MI. However, multicenter experiences found some problems with this device, such as damage to blood vessels and the atrial septum caused by its large size; insufficient alternative sizes; complicated operative procedures; a long learning curve; a long operative time; and the need for multiple clamping. Also, patient screening is strict and patient evaluation is difficult. Therefore, an American team printed a patient-specific 3D mitral valve model based on 3D transesophageal echocardiographic data so that the lesion of the mitral valve leaflet and the structures of the left atrium and ventricle could be seen stereoscopically. As a result, the clinicians could analyze surgical procedures and select the clamping position in vitro.

The simulation of leaflet clamping in vitro can help clinicians understand the working principle of the device, accelerate learning, and master the operative technology, thereby effectively improving the preoperative evaluation efficiency and surgical plan guidance. However, the fly in the ointment is that the simulation does not permit the surgeons to assess the therapeutic effect of MI after valve leaflet clamping. With the development of 3D printing technology, the in vitro simulated surgical device will not only display the surgical procedure but also obtain the hydrodynamic data through the laser or ultrasonic probe, so as to more realistically reflect the effect of the operation.

Mitralign (Edwards Lifesciences, Irvine, CA USA) is a representative product for annuloplasty. It is used to suture the edge of the annulus; it tightens itself to reduce the annulus. It is ineffective for MI due to injury of the valve leaflet or chordae and is suitable only for secondary MI. Cardioband is a type of valvuloplasty ring that can be delivered to the mitral annulus through the venous approach combined with puncturing the atrial septum, the shrinkage ratio of which can reach 25–30%. The principle behind the NeoChord is to send the artificial chordae through the apical approach into the left ventricle with one end connected to the myocardium of the left ventricle and the other end connected to the mitral valve to form artificial chordae, thereby improving MI. Based on current research data, it is very effective and safe in the case of simple posterior lobe P2 prolapse; it is less effective for other kinds of prolapse or MI. MitralStitch is a Chinese-made, patented product produced solely by Hangzhou DeJin Medtech, Hangzhou, China. Compared with the simple edge-to-edge and non-physiological treatment modes of the MitraClip system currently available on the international market, the MitralStitch mitral valve repair system is more diverse, more in line with the patient's natural physiological state, and can achieve the implantation of the artificial chordae (Fig. 6.22). The apical approach of the MitralStitch makes the operating distance shorter and the instrument

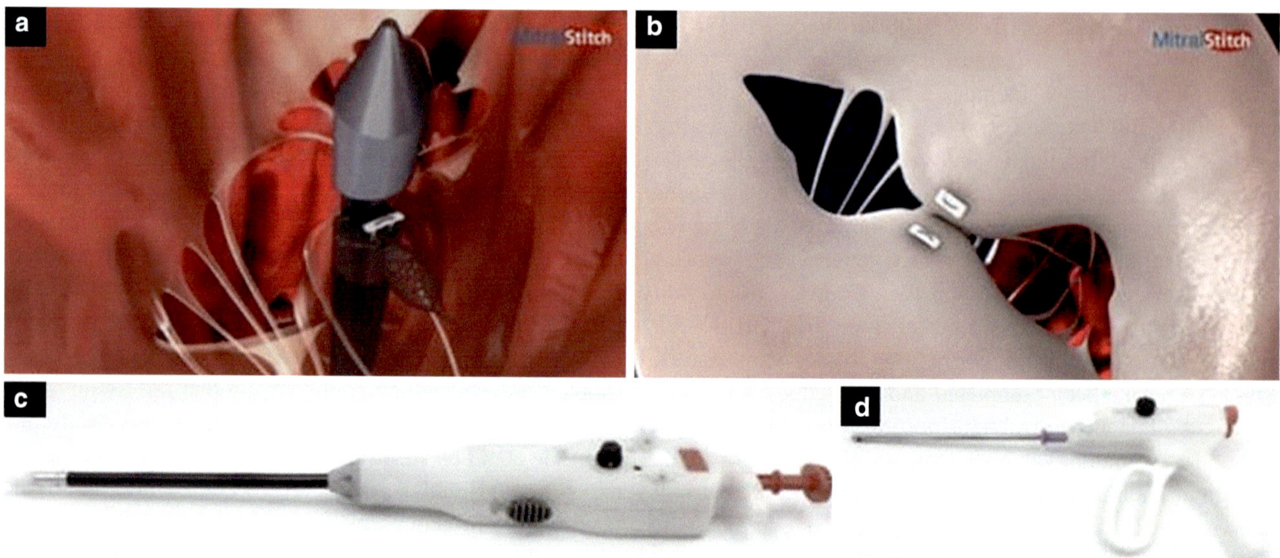

Fig. 6.22 MitralStitch device (Hangzhou DeJin Medtech Co, Hangzhou, China) patented and made in China. (**a**) Working principle of the device. (**b**) Edge-to-edge stitching. (**c**) Delivery device. (**d**) Locking device

more controllable. The significance of the MitralStitch is that patients with MI do not have to choose thoracotomy, and they can be effectively treated with a minimally invasive operation without cardiac arrest, extracorporeal circulation, and angiography. MitralStitch is easier for the surgeon to operate than other instruments, which are cumbersome and time-consuming. In addition, ValveClamp, a device invented at the Zhongshan Hospital, which is affiliated with Fudan University and Shanghai Hanyu Medical, has the advantages of larger valve capture space, easier operation, smaller delivery system (14 Fr), and more sizes. Its operating time is also much shorter than those of other TMVr devices. The catheter operating time is only 10–15 min. Its safety and effectiveness have been verified in hundreds of animal experiments. The preliminary clinical trial results were good.

Current technologies and devices for interventional mitral valve repair have their own strengths and weaknesses. The edge-to-edge suture and mitral annuloplasty are relatively complete procedures that have been used extensively and that have proved in clinical research studies to be beneficial in preventing mitral annulus expansion. The disadvantages are that the edge-to-edge suture and mitral annuloplasty usually do not completely correct the mitral regurgitation; some instruments are too complicated to operate within the small incision through the apex; and the operation takes a long time. Although the artificial chord technique is more attractive in theory, it is difficult to compare its effects with those of other operations because of limited hands-on experience. The benefit of artificial chordae technology is that it replicates proven surgical techniques and is performed without extracorporeal circulation and cardiac arrest; it also retains the possibility of subsequent surgical or transcatheter mitral valve repair or replacement. The shortcomings of this technique include the following: (1) It still requires a thoracotomy incision that, although a smaller incision, is more invasive than a puncture. (2) Experience is limited, so whether this technique can be finally promoted is unknown. (3) Most patients with primary MI have a certain degree of annulus dilatation. This catheter-based artificial chord technique does not solve the problem of annulus expansion, so the durability of the device remains to be seen.

Among the different types of TMVr technologies, each method puts forward higher requirements for patient anatomical analysis, indication screening, and individualization schemes. Meanwhile, 3D printing technology is beneficial to the development of TMVr technology as follows:

1. 3D models printed using materials with a variety of hardnesses and colors can help preoperative screening, doctor–patient communication, more intuitive observation of lesions, and more detailed operative planning.
2. The 3D-printed mitral valve complex structure can help the surgeon to select the most suitable instrument for the specific patient from the plethora of interventional and valvuloplastic instruments, to ensure the success and clinical efficacy of the operation.
3. Currently, a single device is unlikely to perfectly solve MI with different causes. The cardiac team evaluates the preoperative 3D printing simulation model, which helps the surgeon decide whether to choose one or more interventional instruments to perform the operation and to strive for perfection in the treatment of mitral regurgitation, thereby reducing the chances of rehospitalization and reoperation.

4. The TMVr technique for capturing the mitral valve leaflets or annulus is very complicated. The preoperative practice using the 3D model can help the surgeon to assess the operational difficulties in advance and develop targeted intraoperative measures to reduce the operating time and radiation intake.
5. At present, some instruments require a transapical path, and the path from the apex to the mitral valve is not a straight line. The 3D-printed left heart model helps the surgeon to select the precise puncture point, thereby avoiding the coronary artery and the left ventricular papillary muscle and tendon to reduce surgical complications; it can also guide the medical device company representative to shape and adjust the new interventional device.
6. The 3D model combined with in vitro surgical simulation equipment not only helps the surgeon to increase the speed of his or her learning curve for this technique but also assists him or her in the preoperative estimation of intraoperative conditions and treatment effects, thus leading to corresponding adjustments and risk plans.

At present, the application of 3D printing technology to TMVr is still in its infancy. In the preclinical experimental design of many instruments, collisions among various interdisciplinary technologies are expected to produce sparks. On the one hand, 3D printing technology can provide theoretical and practical guidance for TMVr through model printing and practical simulation, helping the surgeon to screen patients, master and improve the operative technology, and evaluate the efficacy through postoperative 3D printing and help the research and development team to continue to improve the device. On the other hand, the development and widespread promotion of TMVr technology will help accelerate the innovation of 3D technology, such as the introduction of new multihardness materials, the development of new bionic materials, the perfection of complete 3D in vitro simulation devices, and so on.

6.2.7 Three-Dimensional Printing and Transcatheter Mitral Valve Replacement

TMVR has always been considered a difficult problem, but with the increasing amount of research on minimally invasive valve replacement procedures, continuous improvements in the instruments and the surgeon's operative technology have occurred. In 2012, researchers successfully performed a transcatheter mitral valve implant for the first time, marking the advent of the TMVR era. On March 7, 2014, Bapat and his colleagues successfully performed a TMVR using a Fortis valve in a patient with severe mitral regurgitation for whom open surgery was contraindicated. In October of the same year, Banai et al. implanted Tiara valves in two patients with end-stage ischemic cardiomyopathy and severe MI.

Depending on the lesions of the autologous mitral valve, TMVR technology is divided into four categories: (1) valve-in-valve technology for patients with previous surgical mitral bioprosthetic valve decay; (2) valve-in-ring technology for patients with an artificial mitral annulus implant for previous valvuloplasty; (3) valve-in-native ring technology for patients with severe mitral annulus calcification or MI; and (4) valve-in-native valve technology for patients with MI without significant calcification of the annulus, who comprise the majority of patients with mitral valve disease. With the first three techniques, because the artificial bioprosthetic valve, the forming ring, or the calcified mitral annulus can provide good fixed support and the annulus shape is relatively fixed, the current transcatheter aortic valve replacement (TAVR) valve [especially the Sapien valve (Edwards Lifesciences, Irvine, CA USA)] or the approved TMVR valve is safer for TMVR surgery. However, the overall proportion of patients with mitral valve disease is small, and strictly speaking, mitral valve disease is not the true indication for TMVR. The true indication for TMVR is the fourth category, which is also the category with the largest proportion of patients.

Compared with TAVR, TMVR presents more problems and challenges because the anatomy of the mitral valve complex is more complicated: (1) The mitral annulus is saddle-shaped and not in the same plane. The incidence of postoperative paravalvular leakage is high. (2) The mitral annulus is soft. Because the cardiac cycle and conditions are constantly changing, it is hard to provide radial support to the stent valve, which makes the fixation method of the stent valve different from that for TAVR, by relying only on radial support force. (3) Ventricular contraction produces large intracavity pressure, and the mitral valve bears much higher pressure than the aortic valve while closing, so the artificial valve is prone to displacement. (4) The ventricular chord and the structure under the valve may influence the implantation and fixation of the valve. (5) The mitral valve is adjacent to the left ventricular outflow tract (LVOT), so the large size of the valve stent can easily lead to LVOT obstruction. (6) Atrial blood flow is slow, so an implanted mitral valve faces a greater risk of thrombosis. (7) The mitral annulus is larger than the aortic annulus, so the aortic valve stent is generally larger than the aortic valve itself.

Corresponding to the specific anatomical characteristics of the mitral valve complex, the operative difficulties of TMVR include the following: (1) The mitral annulus requires high standards for compliance with the size of the extravalvular stent. (2) The surgeon must reduce the influence of the placement of the neo-valve in relation to the LVOT, the left circumflex branch of the coronary artery, the aortic sinus, and the function of the aortic valve. (3) The lack of accurate imaging references for accurate positioning during the operation makes it difficult to anchor the valve. (4) The accessory structural components of the mitral valve such as the chordae and the papillary muscles cause some interference when the surgeon is expanding, positioning, and anchoring the stent. It is easy to damage the accessory structures, thereby causing a paravalvular leak, aggravating the severe pulmonary edema caused by heart failure, and even resulting in death. If the annulus lacks fibrotic or calcified annular support structures, the surgeon needs greater technical skills to ensure the stability of the inserted valve. Patients who have TMVR are younger than patients who have TAVR, so the durability of the valve and the stent needs to be considered.

To deal with the preceding difficulties, several research teams introduced computer modeling and 3D printing technology to help in the comprehensive preoperative evaluation and screening of patients to determine the optimal surgical strategy. The issues involved selection of the appropriate valve and determination of the appropriate depth of the implant. The improved design of the stent valve D-ring and the reduced ventricular area of the stent helped ameliorate the effect of the procedure on the LVOT. The prosthetic valve was fixed by clamping the leaflet or the chordae, the wide margin on the atrial side was designed to reduce the perivalvular leakage, and so on, all of which led to satisfactory results.

6.2.7.1 Screening of Patients for Transcatheter Mitral Valve Replacement

Because TMVR is currently in the clinical trial stage, there are no hospital clinical admissions, so relatively few clinical operations are performed. TMVR is confined to patients with advanced mitral valve disease who cannot tolerate open surgery. Such patients include (a) those with severe stenosis and valvular calcification who have moderate to severe valvular insufficiency and are not suitable for balloon angioplasty; (b) those with high-risk scores for cardiac surgery who cannot undergo surgery other than TMVR; and (c) those who are anatomically suitable for TMVR (mainly refers to the inner diameter of the mitral annulus and a peripheral artery within a suitable range). In this regard, a research team used 3D printing to produce a left heart model during systole and diastole based on patient-specific cardiac CTA data, which may include complex structures such as the left atrium, the left ventricle, the mitral valve and the chordae under it, the papillary muscle, the LVOT, the aortic valve and sinus, the ascending aorta, and the left coronary circumflex branch of the coronary artery. Through further analysis of this model, the researchers can more accurately screen patients and develop surgical strategies (Fig. 6.23).

6.2.7.2 Selection of the Path for Transcatheter Mitral Valve Replacement

According to a review of the literature, the surgical path for TMVR has two routes: transapical and transfemoral. Due to the large size of the current mitral valve and considering the possible damage to the atrial septum, the most common route is the transapical. The transfemoral route is more complicated: After the femoral vein is punctured, the guidewire is placed through the femoral vein. Then the atrial septum is punctured, and the guidewire reaches the descending aorta through the mitral annulus and the left ventricle. Meanwhile, the arrester is placed into the femoral artery and merges with the femoral vein guidewire to establish an arteriovenous loop. The balloon is delivered and dilated in the left atrium and LVOT. After ensuring that the balloon can be freely moved, the hard guidewire is replaced to reconstruct the arteriovenous circuit. The sheath is placed through the femoral vein; the valve is placed in the left ventricle through the atrial septum and the mitral annulus; then the valve is released and fixed in the plane of the mitral valve. After using angiography and transesophageal echocardiography to determine the position and function of the valve, the delivery sheath is withdrawn and the atrial septal defect is blocked with an atrial septal occluder. The transapical approach is simpler than the transfemoral route, and it facilitates the approach to the optimal position for the delivery system.

Computer 3D modeling analysis and printing of parts for model operations can help the surgeon select the appropriate apical puncture position; avoid damage to important structures such as the coronary artery, the intraventricular chordae, and the papillary muscles; and avoid possible damage to the important anatomical structures from guidewire catheters and the replacement valves during the operation. At the same time, for the angle between the apical puncture or the atrial septal puncture site and the mitral annulus in different patients, 3D printing technology can assist the operator in preshaping the operating instruments and in increasing the passage and coaxiality of the device (Fig. 6.24).

6.2.7.3 Left Ventricular Outflow Tract Obstruction Problems

The temporary interruption of blood flow in the LVOT after TMVR valve implantation is ubiquitous and can lead to arrhythmia, congestive heart failure, and even death, especially in elderly patients with severe mitral valve calcification. At present, there is a lack of large-scale clinical data, and there are no uniform surgical operating guidelines, so this problem has not been definitively solved. Because transesophageal ultrasound and preoperative CTA assessments of this complication are limited, 3D printing technology has shown significant advantages in this area.

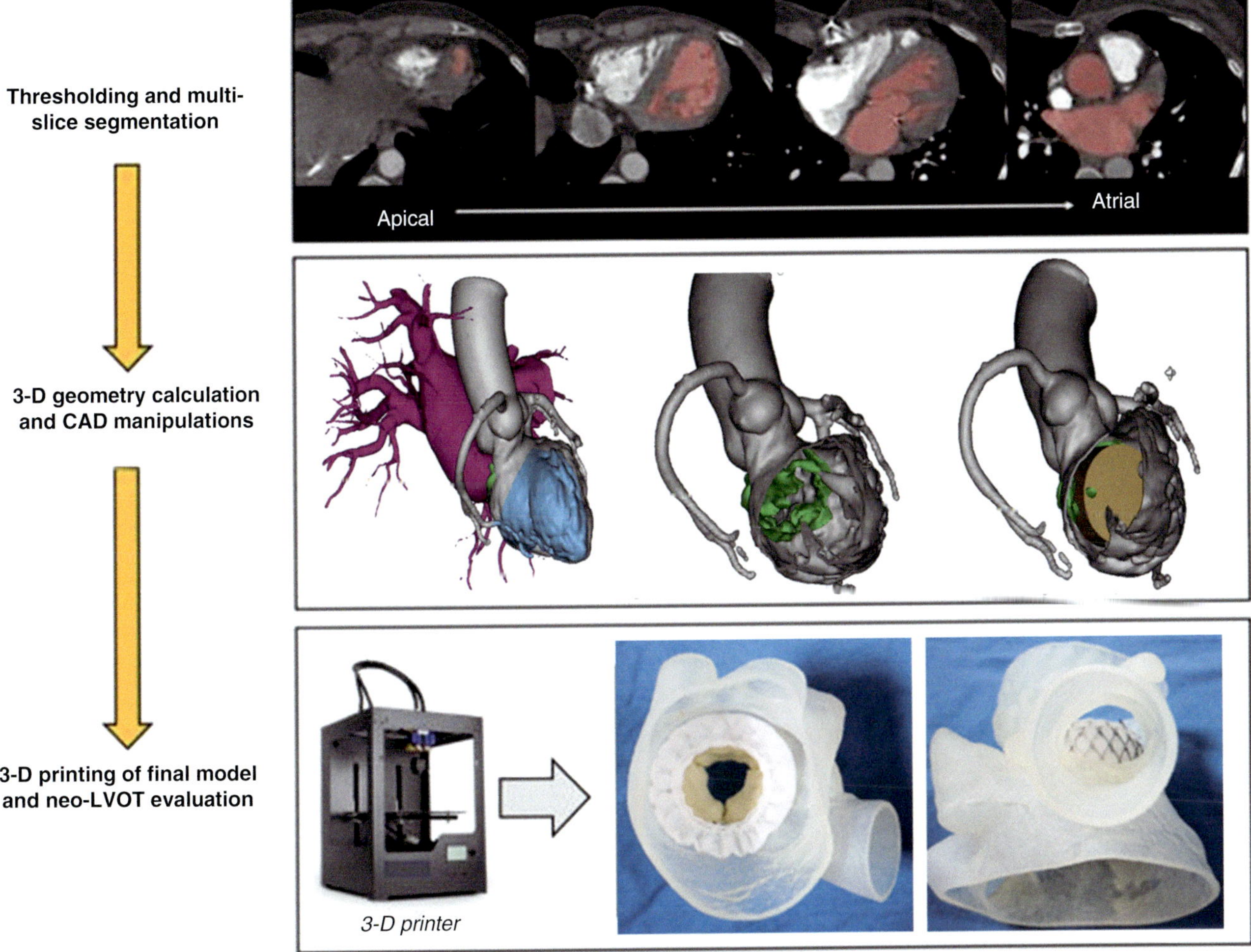

Fig. 6.23 Patient-specific three-dimensional (3D)-printed physical model after 3D modeling based on acquired computed tomography angiography data and in vitro transcatheter mitral valve replacement simulation. Image data and computer 3D reconstruction model from the Department of Cardiovascular Surgery, Xijing Hospital

William O'Neill et al. of the University of Michigan produced a patient-specific 3D-printed model that included important anatomical structures such as the mitral valve complex, the LVOT, and the atrial surface. By simulating the implant of the stented valve prosthesis using a computer-aided design program, they could dynamically analyze the effect of the stent valve on the LVOT after TMVR and further observe the dynamic effect of LVOT by adjusting the inner diameter and the length of the implanted prosthesis, which also contributed feedback about the replacement valve to the research and development team to continuously improve the valve.

Due to changes in the left atrial, left ventricular, and ventricular septal thicknesses caused by mitral valve diseases, the angles of the LVOT and annulus plane of each patient are different. For the interventional mitral valves available on the market, the research team can accurately reflect the risk of LVOT obstruction by establishing and implanting a patient-specific left ventricular 3D model.

6.2.7.4 Replacement Valve Anchoring and Paravalvular Leak

At present, the anchoring principles of the various replacement mitral valves differ and can be divided into a ring-anchoring structure, a double anchoring structure, a reverse leaflet design, and a seal ring design, which use a self-expanding valve design, including a bidirectional, unidirectional, circular, or D-shaped design. The goal is to better position the replacement valve in relation to the mitral annulus and to reduce paravalvular leakage. With the aid of echocardiography and digital subtraction angiography, the mitral valve annulus is maximally fitted in the mitral valve plane without affecting any other functions, such that it is stably fixed on the mitral annulus and forms an effective anchoring structure after endothelialization. However, the active mitral annulus and the mitral annulus with different degrees of calcification do not all allow researchers to do their best. Therefore, in a preclinical study, the research team of Professor Thomas A. Foley of the Mayo Clinic (Rochester,

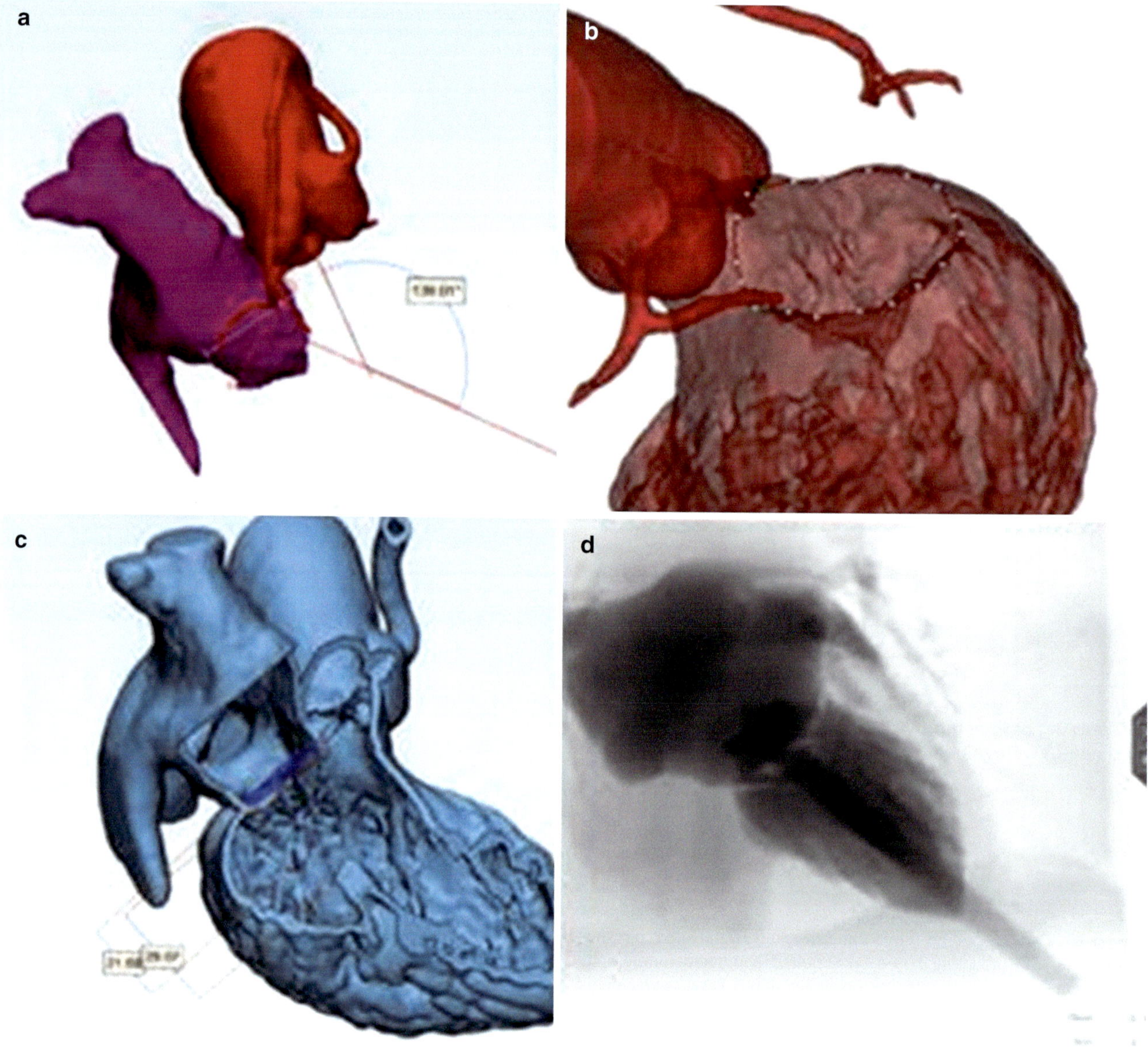

Fig. 6.24 Computer three-dimensional (3D) reconstruction shows the mitral valve and important adjacent structures, guiding the selection of the best transapical path. (**a**) 3D modeling separates the left atrium and aortic root structure. (**b**) 3D modeling shows the relative relationship of the aortic root and the virtual mitral annulus. (**c**) 3D modeling analysis of the left ventricular mitral valve chordae, papillary muscles, and so on. (**d**) 3D modeling simulation of the transapical approach path. Image data and computer 3D reconstruction model from the Department of Cardiovascular Surgery, Xijing Hospital

MN USA) printed heart models of different patients and simulated implanting valvular prostheses. The preoperative and postoperative ultrasound images and the 3D-printed models were used to predict the paravalvular leak. They found that accurate preoperative simulation can effectively reflect the postoperative valve displacement and the location and extent of the paravalvular leak. Using 3D simulation technology, the surgeon can assess the risk of possible valve displacement and paravalvular leakage before surgery and take responsive measures during the operation.

At present, mitral valve intervention still faces challenges, especially when the valves are used in younger patients with a lower risk of surgery, including:

1. Valve thrombosis. To prevent paravalvular leakage, the valve is designed with an atrial rim. There are many artificial structures in the atrium. Because the blood flow velocity in the atrium is very slow, it is easy to form a thrombus there. In addition, the peripheral region of the valve stent on the ventricular side is the blind end, so it is easy to form a thrombus.
2. The resistance of the valve stent to wear and tear. The interventional aortic valve is located at the root of the aorta, where local tissue activity is minimal, so there is rarely a valve tear during TAVR. However, the mitral annulus and chordae tendon tissue contract during the cardiac cycle, and the heart contracts about 100,000 times a

day. The mechanical damage suffered is alarming. Because the current valve follow-up period is short, this problem is not immediately serious, but in the future it will become a prominent problem in patients who have had TMVR.
3. Damage to the heart function. At present, the academic community basically believes that if the mitral valve can be repaired, it should not be replaced. The reason is that the currently used mitral valve replacement procedures damage the mitral valve chordae, which play an important role in ensuring ventricular systolic function. In ventricular systole, on the one hand, the mitral valve is pulled so that it does not prolapse and cause reflux. On the other hand, the tissue of the apex is pulled toward the mitral valve to help the ventricular contraction. Long-term lack of mitral valve chordae will inevitably lead to impaired ventricular function, and severe cases will lead to refractory heart failure and even death.

From the initial rough development of TAVR to now, more than 400,000 patients worldwide have enjoyed the gospel brought by TAVR. The 3-year survival rate after TAVR is presently greater than 90%, which took more than 10 years to achieve. With the introduction of 3D printing technology, advances in materials science, and accumulated experience in interventional cardiology, it is believed that TMVR surgery will make a splash like that of TAVR. Meanwhile, clinicians must be acutely aware of the many problems facing this new technology. The emergence, development, maturity, and promotion of all new technologies and methods need to be constantly explored and monitored. We hope that using 3D printing technology to comprehensively improve upon the difficulties inherent in current TMVR technology and pre- and postoperative simulation and to promote the continuous development of transcatheter valve implantation technology and valve engineering will benefit patients going forward [38–56].

6.3 Transcatheter Tricuspid Valve Replacement and Three-Dimensional Printing

Fanglin Lu, Fang Fang, XiaoKe Shang

The tricuspid valve is located between the right atrium and the right ventricle, also known as the right atrioventricular valve (Fig. 6.25). Although clinical tricuspid lesions are not

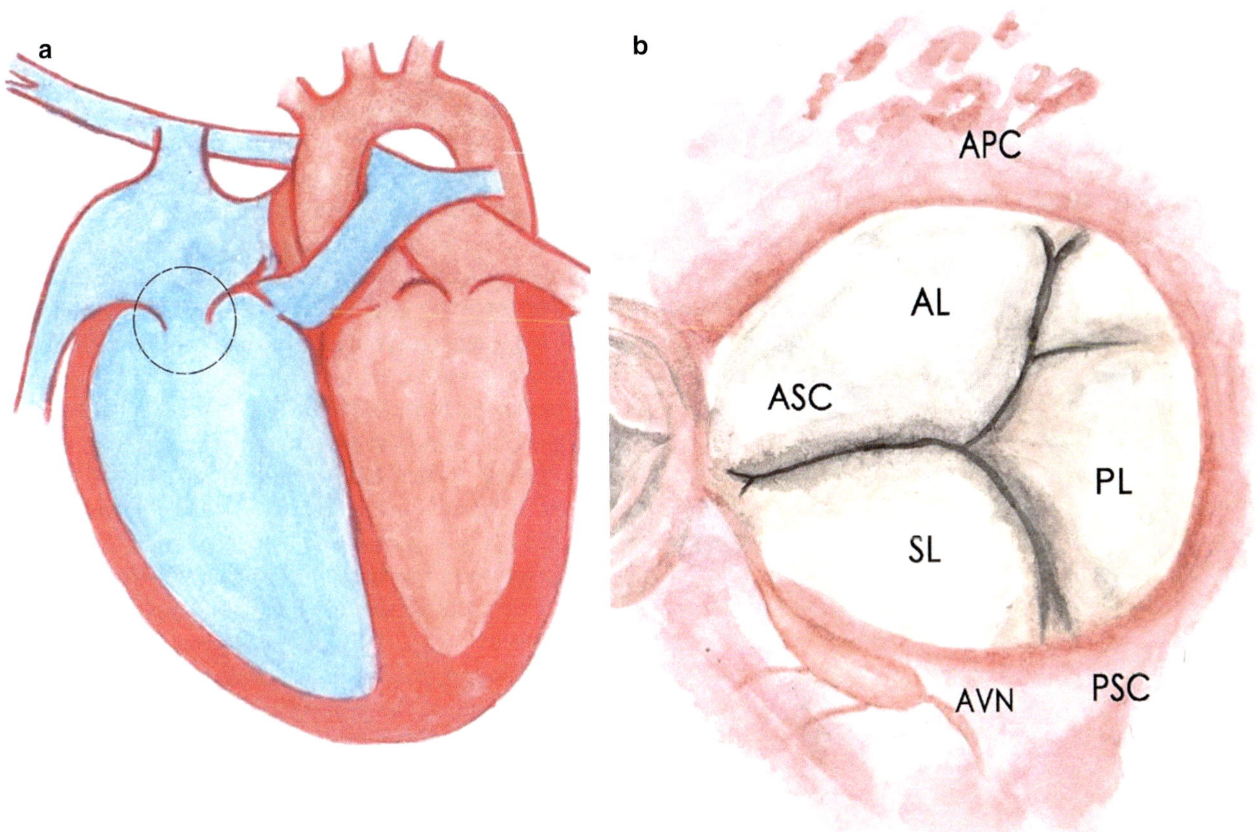

Fig. 6.25 Anatomical schematic of the tricuspid valve. (**a**) Anatomical location of the tricuspid valve; (**b**) Anatomical morphology of the tricuspid valve. *AL* anterior leaflet, *APC* anterior border, *ASC* anterior septum, *AVN* atrioventricular node, *PL* posterior leaflet, *PSC* posterior septal junction, *SL* septum leaflet

as common as mitral or aortic lesions, they can also cause severe clinical symptoms in patients. For example, severe tricuspid regurgitation or stenosis can cause venous blood stasis in the right atrium and in the superior and inferior vena cava. The peripheral venous return is impaired, gradually leading to right heart failure, causing congestion of organs (especially abdominal organs), oxygen insufficiency, symptoms and signs of hepatosplenomegaly, ascites, and lower extremity edema. These symptoms seriously affect patients' quality of life and life expectancy. In patients with severe tricuspid regurgitation, the five-year survival rate is only 50% [57].

Tricuspid regurgitation is the most common form of tricuspid valve disease, and the etiology of tricuspid regurgitation can be divided into two types: organic and functional. The overall incidence of organic tricuspid regurgitation is low, mostly due to rheumatic or carcinoid lesions, perforation or destruction of the leaflets due to tricuspid endocarditis, or associated with device leads [58]. Functional tricuspid regurgitation is a common and difficult problem in clinical practice. It is more common in patients with left heart valvular disease and other pathological changes, such as pulmonary hypertension, atrial fibrillation, myocardial infarction, or myocardial ischemia. In such circumstances, the tricuspid valve leaflets are structurally normal, and tricuspid regurgitation is secondary to enlargement of the right ventricle and tricuspid annulus. In adults with tricuspid regurgitation, the proportion of functional tricuspid regurgitation is high, the condition is complex, the treatment is extremely difficult, and the recommended treatment is controversial, which is an independent risk factor for increasing mortality in cardiac surgery patients [59, 60]. The specific pathogenesis is still unclear, although it is currently believed to be mainly related to the following factors: (1) left ventricular dysfunction leading to high left atrial pressure, causing pulmonary hypertension, and resulting in right heart dysfunction, right ventricular enlargement, and tricuspid annulus enlargement; (2) pulmonary hypertension, left heart valvular disease with a long course often associated with pulmonary hypertension; (3) atrial fibrillation due to irregular ventricular rhythm, leading to tricuspid annulus enlargement; and (4) a left heart valve prosthetic ring causing local deformation of the central fibrous body, which also aggravates deformation of the tricuspid annulus, leading to tricuspid regurgitation. Patients with severe tricuspid regurgitation requiring surgical treatment tend to be older, have more comorbidities, and have a higher risk of surgery. The mortality rate of repeated or multiple tricuspid operations in multicenter registries worldwide is as high as 19%–50%; the mortality rate of tricuspid valve replacement surgery at Xijing Hospital, Fuwai Hospital, and Anzhen Hospital is 13–16%, which is far higher than the mortality rates of other heart surgeries. The results of a previous study showed that nearly half of the patients with left heart valve disease had different degrees of tricuspid valve disease. In the USA, for example, the number of patients with functional tricuspid valve disease is as high as nearly 1.6 million, of which approximately 80% are patients with functional tricuspid regurgitation. Statistics show that the incidence of adult rheumatic valvular heart disease in China is 2.34%–2.72%. Therefore, for a population of 1.3 billion, there are approximately three million adult rheumatic valvular heart disease patients, of which nearly 1.5 million have functional tricuspid valve disease. Approximately 700,000 patients required various valve surgeries, and only one in ten patients underwent surgery each year. Secondary tricuspid regurgitation has become a major issue in the field of cardiovascular surgery [61–63].

Because tricuspid valve disease is often insidious and secondary to left heart valve disease and because the disease progresses slowly, it may be overlooked or masked by pathophysiological changes and clinical manifestations of left heart valve disease. Significant right hemodynamic changes and characteristic clinical manifestations are only apparent when tricuspid valve disease is severe. At this time, the effect of drug treatment is also limited. There are two main types of surgical treatment: tricuspid valvuloplasty and tricuspid valve replacement. Valvuloplasty is much more commonly performed than replacement. However, after the tricuspid valve is repaired, recurrence rate of tricuspid regurgitation is high, and the long-term effect is often not satisfactory. Tricuspid valve replacement, whether with an artificial mechanical heart valve or an artificial biological heart valve, must be permanently implanted into the body by surgical suture. Formation and valve replacement under traditional surgery require extracorporeal circulation and a complicated operation process; the risk of extracorporeal circulation injury is high, surgery requires a long amount of time, bleeding can be extensive, and the rate of complications is high.

Due to the huge market potential and patient needs in this field, new treatment methods with little trauma and reliable effects are urgently needed [64]. Transcatheter interventional techniques can avoid the risks of extracorporeal circulation and reopening, which has become a hot topic of current research. In terms of transcatheter tricuspid valvuloplasty, three new types of techniques have been reported abroad: one is insertion of a transcatheter vena cava artificial valve. This method is not satisfactory for small sample clinical trial results: whether a specially designed vena cava valve or a self-expanding aortic interventional valve is inserted into the vena cava position, the long-term (7–9 months) mortality rate is as high as 80% (4/5) and 90% (9/10) [65, 66]. The second type is transcatheter tricuspid annuloplasty. Among them are Mitralign from mitral valve intervention [67] and TriCinch designed for tricuspid valves. This type of product simulates the Kay or DeVega technique under direct vision. Neither of these products are currently being tested in clinical trials. The third category is a device that increases the leaflet contact area. The use of this technology is the occupational device Forma spacer and the use of MitraClip for "edge-to-edge" shaping [68–70]. However, the reliability of these two types of treatment techniques is still uncertain, and there is still a lack of long-term clinical studies with large sample sizes.

Due to the poor reliability of the interventional treatment, some foreign institutions have turned their attention to the method of tricuspid interventional valve replacement. This will become a hot topic in current interventional therapy for functional tricuspid regurgitation. In recent years, large US medical companies, such as Edwards, Medtronic, etc., have begun research and development of interventional bioprosthetic stent valve systems, and some products have passed European CE and US Food and Drug Administration (FDA) certification [71]. The successful development of the interventional bioprosthetic valve system has led to the transformation of treatment technology for valvular disease. It has become a hot spot in the international market in recent years because of its advantages of simplifying surgery, imposing less trauma, requiring shorter hospital stay, and lowering the surgical risk. European and American scholars begun to try to use existing aortic valve stent devices to treat patients with recurrent tricuspid regurgitation after tricuspid valve replacement or tricuspid annulus repair and have achieved preliminary effects. However, the physiological structure of the tricuspid valve is very complicated, and the annulus is large. After left heart valve replacement, especially mitral valve replacement, the central fibrous body is deformed by the artificial annulus, and the shape of the tricuspid annulus is deformed. Interventional tricuspid valve replacement presents certain difficulties [65, 72, 73].

In recent years, the "LuX" transcatheter tricuspid device jointly developed by Ningbo Jianshi Biotechnology Co., Ltd. and Changhai Hospital has brought new hope for transcatheter artificial tricuspid valve replacement. The "LuX" transcatheter tricuspid valve is composed of a stent, a braided ring, three leaflets, an anchoring needle, and a suture, and the leaflet is fixed on the stent by a suture. The braided ring and the stent are fixed by a suture. The valve is self-expanding, which is released to the tricuspid valve position and secured to the interventricular septum by an anchoring needle. The valve delivery system consists of a tip head, a guidewire tube, an anchoring assembly, a connector, an outer sheath tube, a functional handle, and a fluid injection tube (see Fig. 6.26).

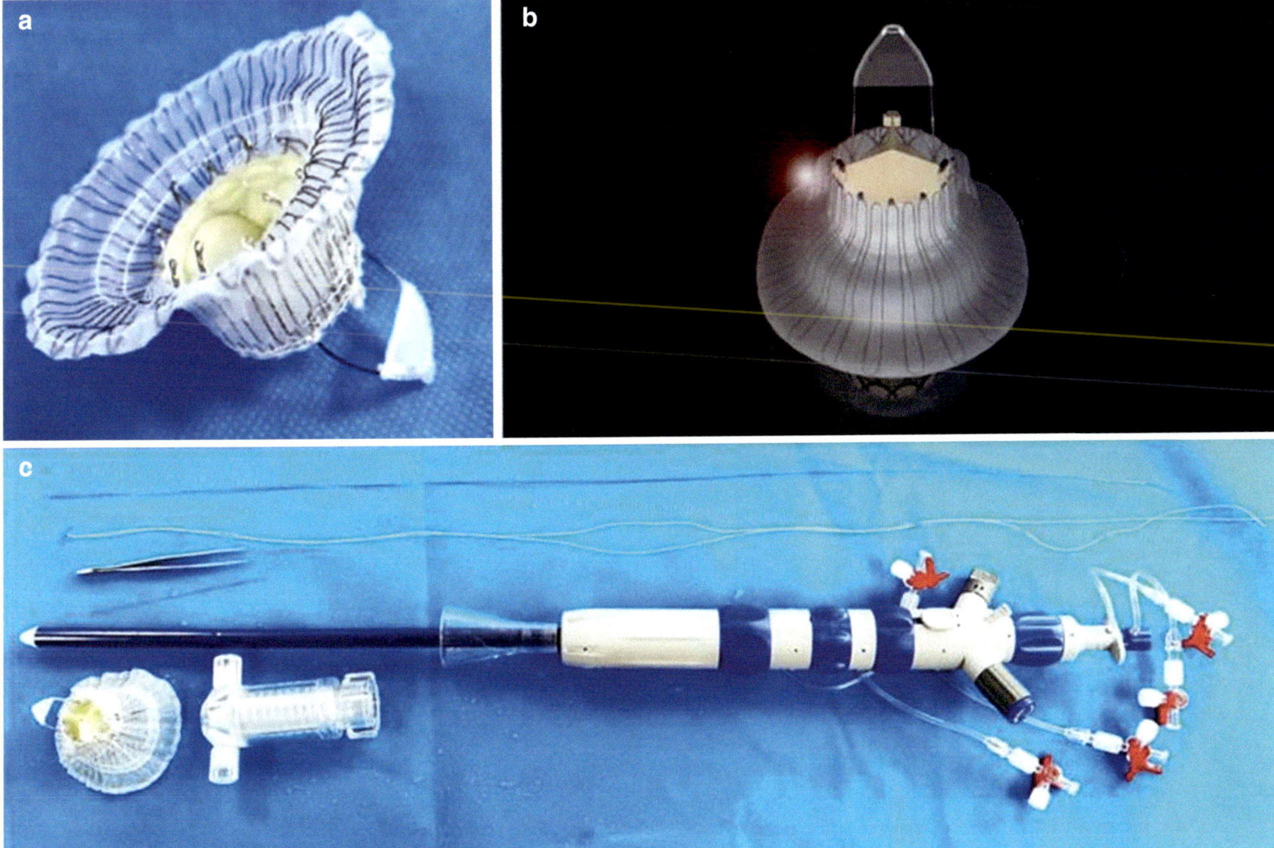

Fig. 6.26 "LuX" transcatheter tricuspid device jointly developed by Ningbo Jianshi Biotechnology Co., Ltd. and Changhai Hospital. (**a**) "LuX" transcatheter tricuspid valve; (**b**) "LuX" transcatheter tricuspid valve Schematic; (**c**) "LuX" transcatheter tricuspid delivery system. Data from the Naval Medical University Changhai Hospital

Surgery is performed through the patient's right atrial approach, and the artificial biological valve is delivered from the catheter to the original native valve position. It replaces the function of the original autologous valve, improves the tricuspid regurgitation of the patient, and maintains the normal function of the valve, thereby ensuring tricuspid hemodynamics, improving cardiac function, and achieving therapeutic goals (Fig. 6.27).

An advanced clinical feasibility study was completed using the device in ten selected patients, with little postoperative paravalvular leakage and satisfactory short-term results. A nationwide multicenter registry study is underway and may become the first approved transcatheter tricuspid device.

Using three-dimensional reconstruction of the anatomy of the tricuspid valve from imaging data such as CTA and echocardiography, the anatomical structure and annulus size around the tricuspid valve can be more accurately evaluated before the interventional replacement of the tricuspid valve. In addition, the 3D printing tricuspid valve model can help the surgeon judge and realize the tricuspid valve and the surrounding anatomical structure. 3D printing can be useful in preoperative surgical simulation to help quickly enter the releasing position during the operation and help with postoperative complication prediction [8].

The author's Department of Cardiovascular Surgery, Xijing Hospital, used computer three-dimensional reconstruction and 3D printing technology to construct a tricuspid regurgitation heart model in vitro for patient education and surgical evaluation. The 3D-printed model can help visualize the important tissue structure around the tricuspid valve,

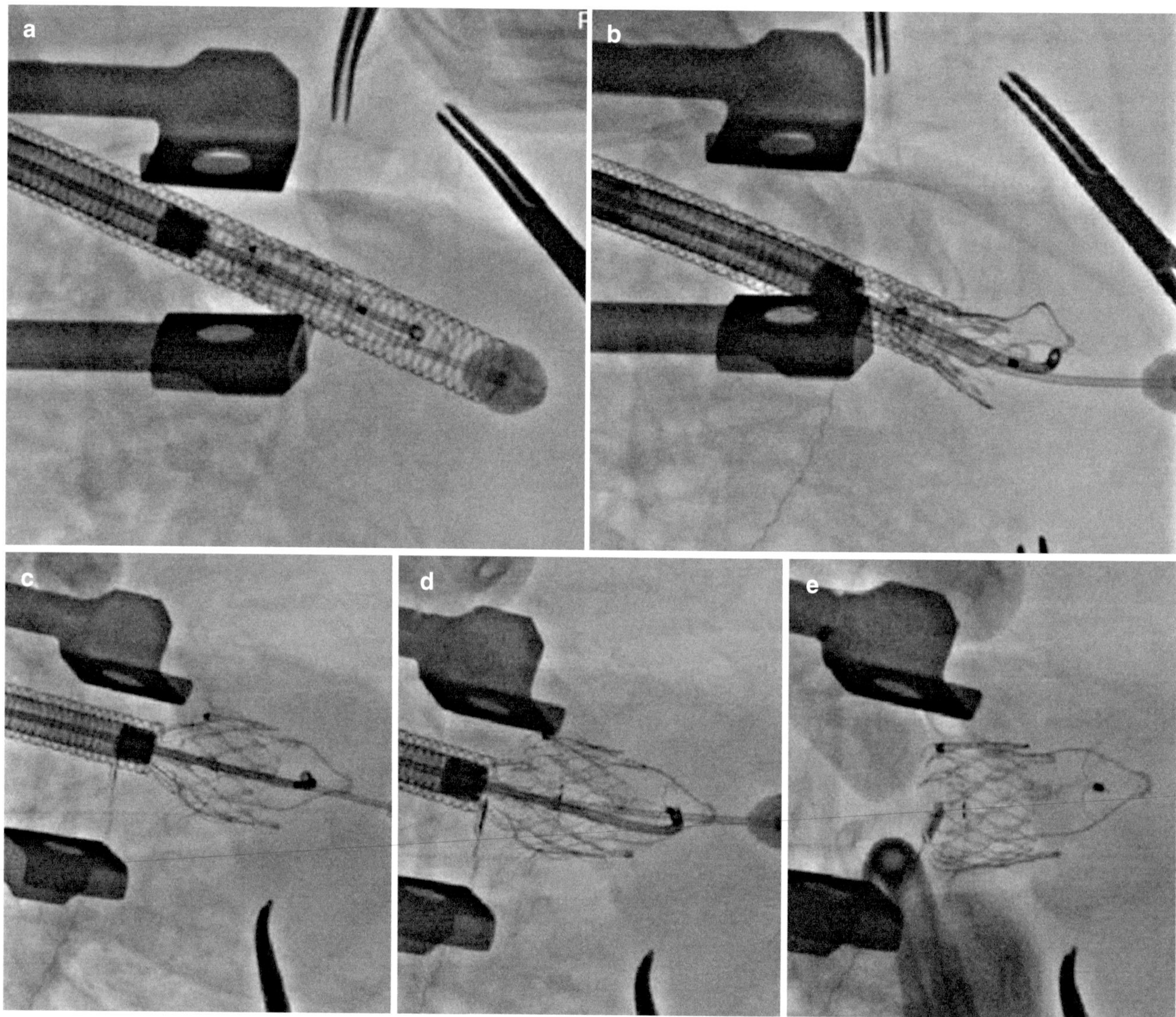

Fig. 6.27 "LuX" transcatheter tricuspid device implantation. (**a**) The "LuX" system to the tricuspid valve; (**b**) the "LuX" front-end release and adjusted position; (**c**) the "LuX" system in the valve positioning release at the ring; (**d**) "LuX" valve anchoring to chamber spacing; (**e**) The delivery system evacuation, "LuX" valve in situ anchoring to the native tricuspid valve. Image data from the Naval Medical University Changhai Hospital

simulate the surgical procedure, and promote the development of young surgeons' understanding of the disease and surgery (Fig. 6.28a, b).

3D printing technology for transcatheter tricuspid valve replacement and other complex interventional procedures can also improve the success rate of surgery, reduce complications, and reduce the cost of surgery. The author's Department of Cardiovascular Surgery, Xijing Hospital, and Changhai Hospital conducted a 3D printing imaging evaluation of the "LuX" transcatheter tricuspid device implantation (Fig. 6.28c, d) and found that the individualized 3D model of the patient is important for selecting the optimal surgical path and for spatial position visualization before catheter tricuspid valve replacement. It can predict the size of the placed

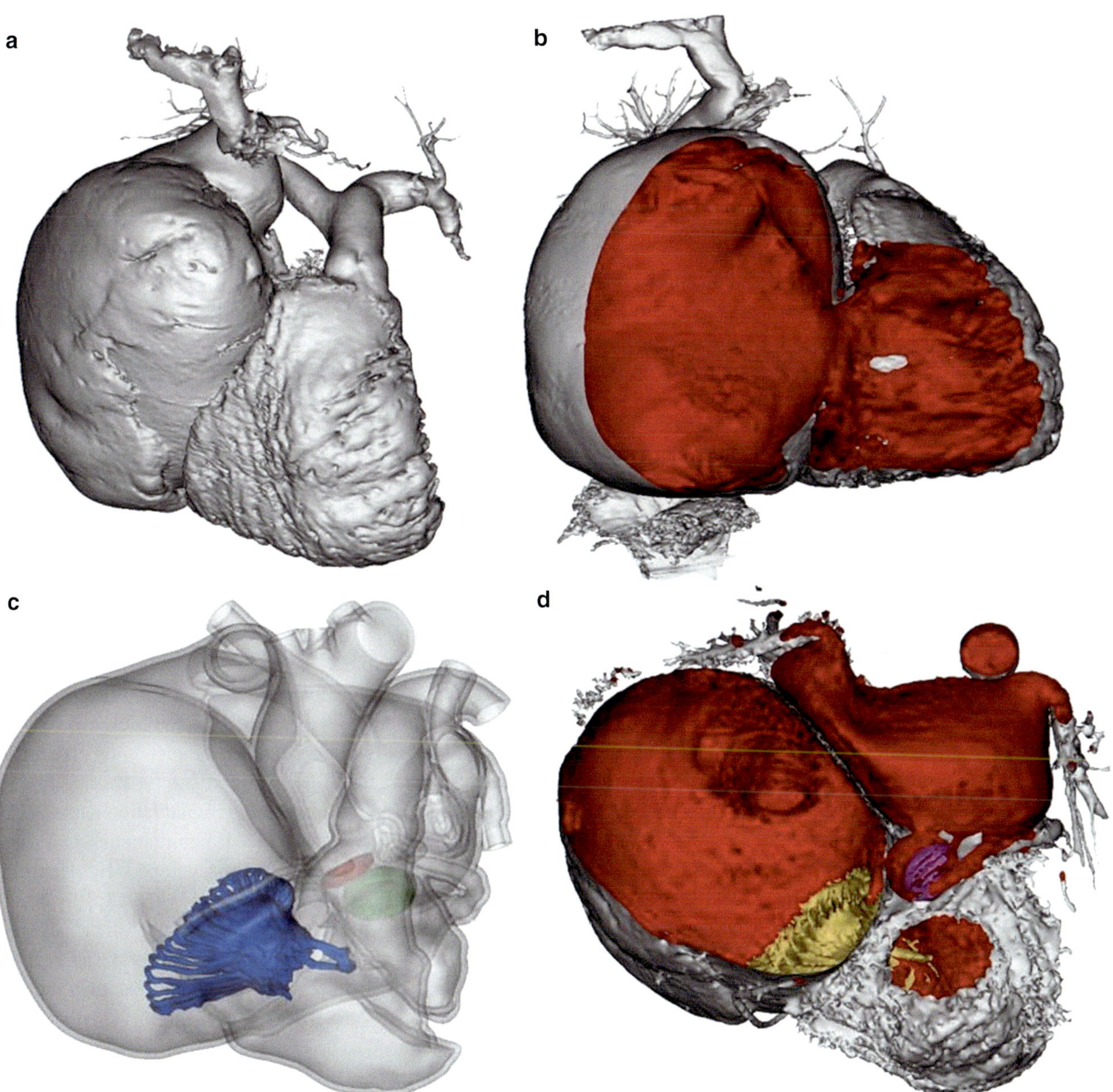

Fig. 6.28 3D image of the transcatheter tricuspid device implanted in patients with tricuspid regurgitation. (**a**) Computer 3D modeling shows tricuspid regurgitation, a huge right atrium; (**b**) a section showing the right atrium, the right ventricle, and three anatomical structures of the cusp; (**c**) The anatomical relationship between the tricuspid valve, the mitral valve, and aortic valve after transcatheter tricuspid device implantation; (**d**) The section shows the tricuspid valve after transcatheter tricuspid device implantation and the anatomical relationship with the mitral and aortic valves. Imaging data and computerized three-dimensional reconstruction from the Naval Medical University Changhai Hospital and Xijing Hospital Cardiovascular Surgery

valve in advance and prevent the occurrence of paravalvular leakage. In addition, 3D printing technology can also be used to evaluate the shape and position of the valve after implantation, the relationship between the prosthetic valve and the surrounding adjacent structures, and the severity of complications such as paravalvular leakage.

In view of the large number of clinical patients with functional tricuspid regurgitation, only one-tenth of the patients undergo surgery each year, there are many high-risk patients requiring minimally invasive surgery, such as transcatheter tricuspid replacement/repair. Unlike tricuspid valve surgery under traditional cardiopulmonary bypass, transcatheter tricuspid valve treatment places extremely high demands on imaging evaluation. With the advent of a new generation of interventional valves, development of domestic and foreign tricuspid interventional valve replacement may bring hope to patients with tricuspid regurgitation. While 3D printing technology is used to guide and evaluate various transcatheter tricuspid valves, it can further advance tricuspid valve surgery and promote the advancement of precision medicine, and it will certainly play a major role [74–76].

6.4 Transcatheter Pulmonary Valve Replacement and Three-Dimensional Printing

XiaoKe Shang, Jian Yang, Yongjian Wu

Pulmonary valve disease is a common heart valve disease. Pulmonary valve disease is mainly divided into pulmonary valve stenosis and pulmonary valve insufficiency. Since the first application of percutaneous balloon pulmonary valvuloplasty by Kan, et al. to treat pulmonary valve stenosis in 1982, the method has gradually matured into a preferred technique for the treatment of pulmonary valve stenosis [77]. Furthermore, 16 out of every 10,000 newborns in the world require surgical correction involving stenosis of the right heart due to congenital heart defects. Right ventricular outflow tract and pulmonary artery patch widening are required in the first operation, and pulmonary valve regurgitation may develop to different degrees in the long-term follow-up. From the pathophysiological mechanism, long-term pulmonary valve insufficiency can lead to extra load and expansion of the right heart, chest tightness, shortness of breath, abdominal distension, anorexia, edema of the lower extremity, decreased activity endurance, and tricuspid regurgitation, which might lead to right heart failure, atrial or ventricular arrhythmia, or even sudden death. In addition, expansion of the right ventricular volume load causes diastolic interventricular septum reverse motion, which leads to left ventricular insufficiency and aggravates the clinical symptoms of the patients. According to long-term prognosis, patients with right ventricular dysfunction have a lower lifetime expectancy than the healthy population [61, 78]. Therefore, recovering pulmonary valve function is critical for patients with right ventricular dysfunction. Surgery has long been the standard treatment for patients with pulmonary valve insufficiency. However, at present, surgical operation has great limitations, including the induction of trauma, slow recovery, high risk, high cost, higher risk of reoperation in the future, and poor acceptance of re-thoracotomy. The preoperative evaluation of pulmonary valve diseases currently depends primarily on transthoracic and transesophageal echocardiography, which can be used to accurately evaluate the types and severity of pulmonary valve insufficiency. It also plays a positive role in the evaluation of hemodynamic indexes in percutaneous pulmonary valve implantation. (Fig. 6.29).

In October 2000, a team of British scholars under Professor Bonhoeffer completed the first case of percutaneous pulmonary valve implantation (PPVI) in the world [79]. This procedure has been used to effectively treat a large number of pulmonary valve regurgitation cases; it improves right ventricular function and perfusion of lung tissues, and there is no need for thoracotomy and cardiopulmonary bypass [80–82]. In addition, trauma from the operation is small, recovery is fast, and the risk of operation is greatly reduced, which provides a new idea for the treatment of patients with severe valvular disease with high surgical risk. In Europe and the USA, a series of Edwards SAPIEN valves and the Medtronic Inc. Melody (TM) commercial interventional pulmonary valve system (Fig. 6.30) have been used for pulmonary valve implantation [83–87]. Based on data from the multicenter clinical trial COMPASSION and the European study, the US FDA approved the Edwards Inc. transcatheter cardiac valve SAPIEN XT for pulmonary valve replacement in 2016 [88, 89]. In 2017, the Melody (TM) artificial pulmonary artery valve produced by Medtronic Company was also certified by the FDA [90].

Percutaneous pulmonary valve implantation has also been attempted in China. The Venus P percutaneous pulmonary valve replacement system was developed by Hangzhou Qiming Medical device Co., Ltd. in May 2013. It is the first self-expandable interventional pulmonary valve to enter a clinical trial worldwide. The valve is shaped like a double horn, a fixed stent does not need to be placed in the right ventricular outflow tract (RVOT) before implantation, a balloon does not need to be expanded, and it is more convenient and economical to use. The valve can be used in the autologous right ventricular outflow tract of transvalvular patches and is suitable for most patients in China (Fig. 6.31a, b, e).

In April 2015, the first percutaneous pulmonary valve replacement in Northwest China was completed in the Department of Cardiovascular Surgery of Xijing Hospital. The patient underwent open-heart correction of tetralogy of Fallot 10 years prior. The patient had long-term right heart

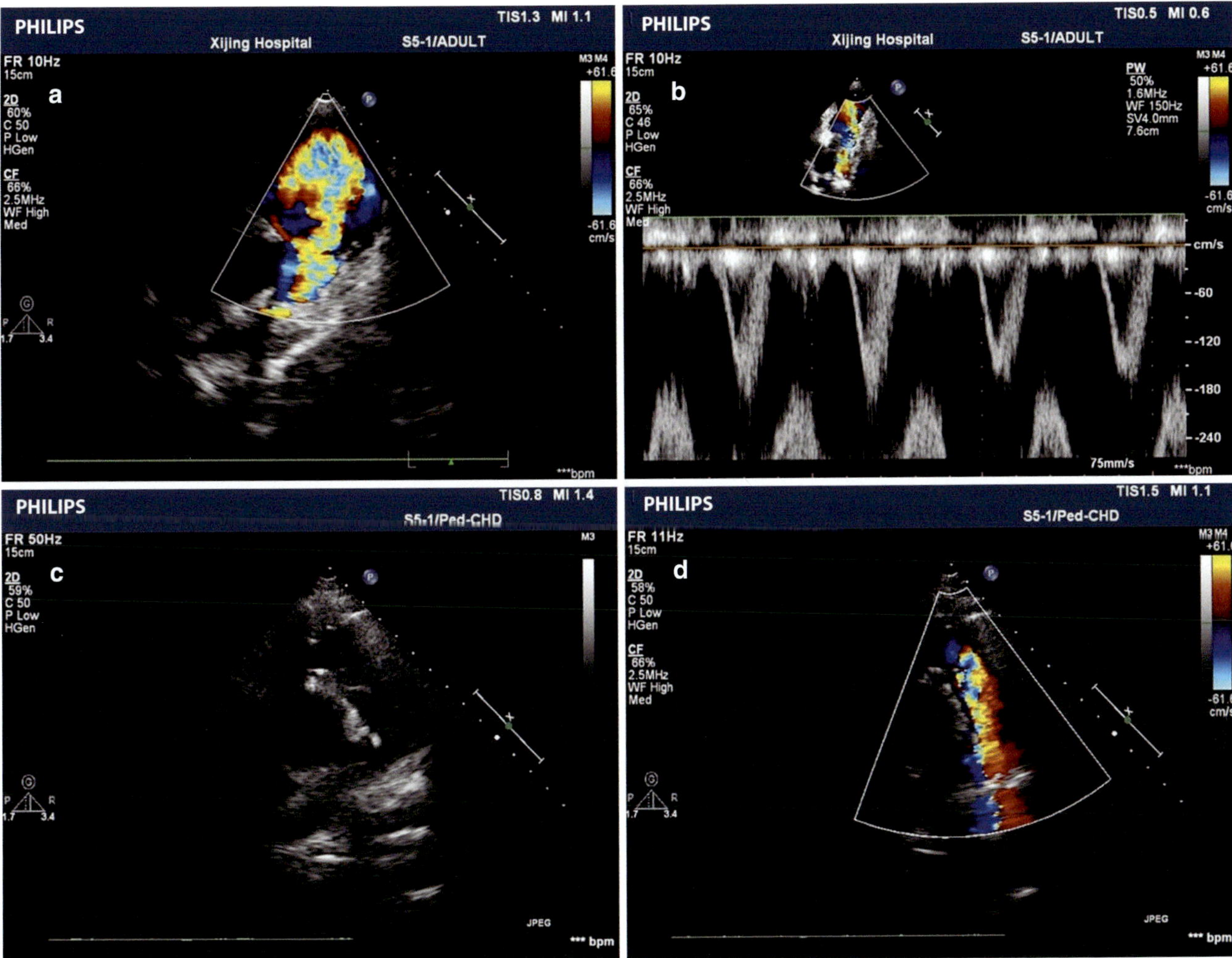

Fig. 6.29 Diagnosis of pulmonary valve insufficiency by echocardiography and evaluation of the efficacy of percutaneous pulmonary valve implantation. (**a**) Observation of pulmonary valve regurgitation on the pulmonary artery plane; (**b**) Evaluation of pressure difference and velocity of pulmonary valve regurgitation by blood flow Doppler; (**c**) Strong echo of pulmonary artery stents can be seen by ultrasound after percutaneous pulmonary valve implantation; (**d**) After percutaneous pulmonary valve implantation, the forward blood flow and reflux disappear. Imaging data from the Department of Cardiovascular Surgery, Xijing Hospital

insufficiency, obvious symptoms of heart failure and chest tightness, shortness of breath, abdominal distension, anorexia, decreased exercise endurance, severe regurgitation of pulmonary valve insufficiency, and tricuspid insufficiency. Under the guidance of radiation and transesophageal echocardiography, a 32 mm Venus P pulmonary valve stent was successfully implanted through the right femoral vein puncture. Postoperative angiography and ultrasound examination showed that the position of the stent valve was good and reflux disappeared, and the operation was completed successfully. The patient recovered well after the operation and was discharged from the hospital 3 days after the operation in good condition. By June 2018, more than 220 cases of Venus P-valve had been implanted in 27 centers in 16 countries and regions around the world [91]. The average follow-up time was more than 2 years, and the curative effect was remarkable. The product will soon carry out FDA-licensed IDE research in 2019. Currently, a clinical trial of the pulmonary valve PT-Valve ®, developed and produced by Beijing Med-Zenith Company in March 2018, is being carried out. The product is designed to realize anatomical and hemodynamic correction of the right heart system. The product is designed with a dumbbell shape: the ends are enlarged, and the middle waist is sutured in the valve, which is beneficial for maintaining the normal working form of the flap (Fig. 6.31c, d, f). More than ten cases have been carried out in a preliminary clinical research study in Wuhan Union Hospital and Xijing Hospital thus far, and the short-term follow-up for half a year has been completed (Fig. 6.31c, d, f).

It has been reported that most patients with tetralogy of Fallot who underwent pulmonary valve implantation were not completely cured because of the wide and irregular outflow tract of the right ventricle, which led to shedding of the valve. To a certain extent, expansion of the applica-

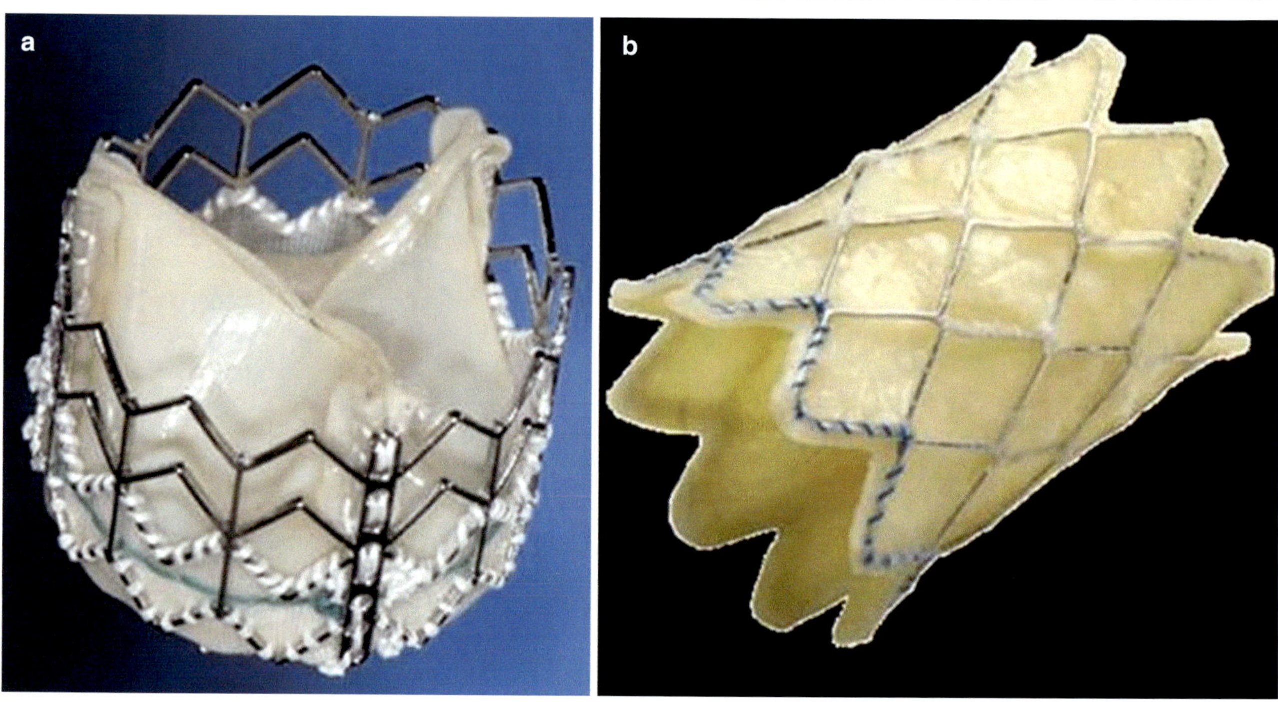

Fig. 6.30 Interventional pulmonary valve system used in Europe and the USA. (**a**) Transcatheter Heart Valve SAPIEN XT, Edwards Life Sciences Company, USA; (**b**) Melody (TM) artificial biological pulmonary valve system, Medtronic Company

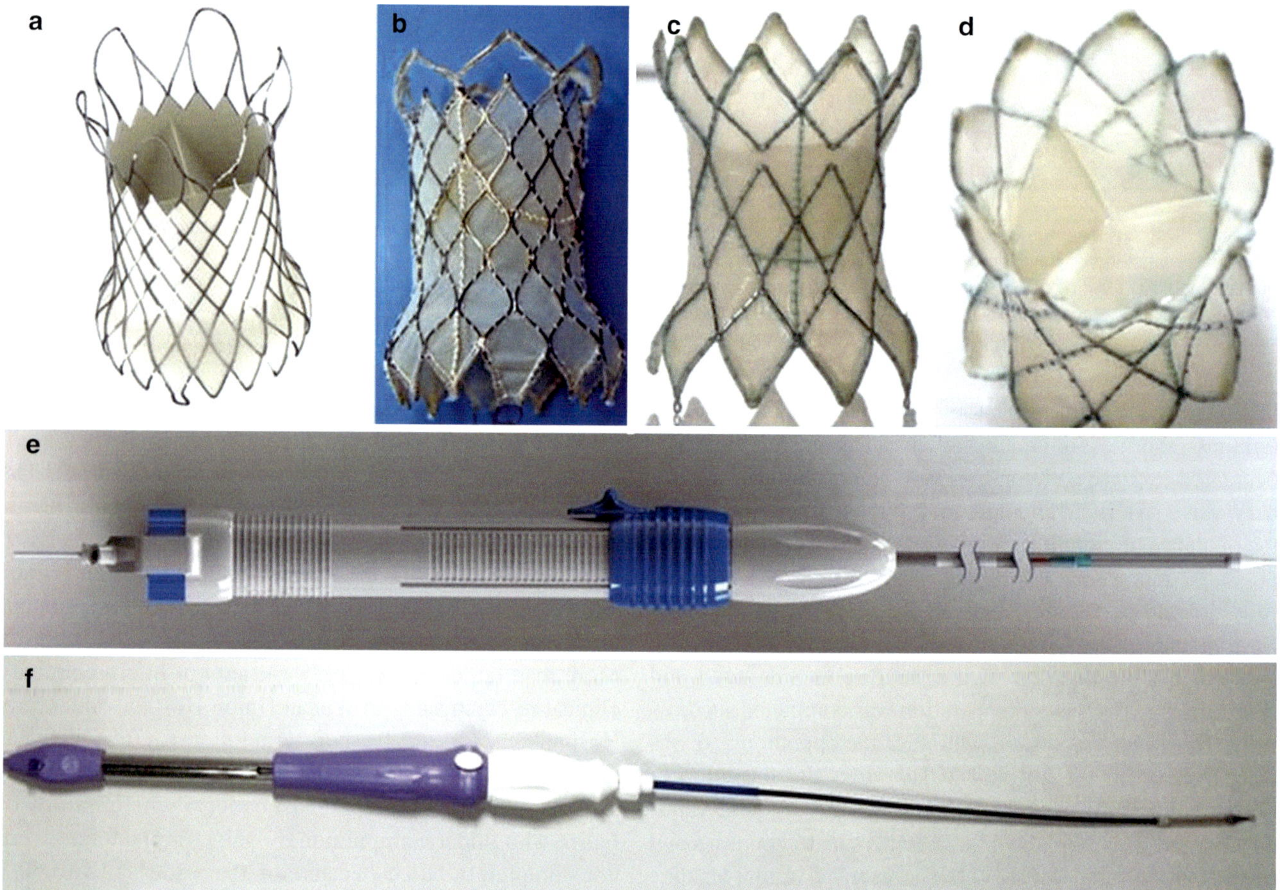

Fig. 6.31 Chinese interventional pulmonary artery valve and its transducing system. (**a**) Schematic diagram of Qiming medical Venus P-Valve; (**b**) A figure of the Venus P-valve (lateral view); (**c**) Interventional pulmonary valve from Med-Zenith Medical Scientific Co., Beijing (lateral view); (**d**) Interventional pulmonary valve from Med-Zenith Medical Scientific Co. (superior view); (**e**) Qiming Medical Venus P-Valve transducing system; (**f**) Med-Zenith interventional pulmonary valve transducing system

tion of this surgical method is limited. To gain a deeper understanding of the anatomical structure of the right heart and pulmonary valve, a 1:1 3D-printed model can play an intuitive and accurate guiding role. Phillips et al. used CTA images for three-dimensional reconstruction. The 3D model of the right ventricular outflow tract was printed for eight patients with tetralogy of Fallot. The related surgical simulation was carried out before pulmonary valve implantation, and the best anchoring area of the right ventricular outflow tract was found to increase the stability of the pulmonary valve, which greatly helped lead to the success of the operation [92]. It was found that when the diameter of the narrowest part of the right ventricular outflow tract was longer than 26 mm, one or more covered stents should be used to implant the anchoring area at the same time, and then, the interventional pulmonary valve could be released. Finally, an Amplatzer Plug II (St. Jude Medical) was implanted into the lumen of the adjacent covered stent. A 3D model can help the whole multidisciplinary R&D team visualize interventional surgery simulation and practice. It can also ensure the success of the operation by allowing different surgical strategies to be considered and providing a more intuitive and individualized view of the anatomical structures of the heart.

Combined with CTA data before the operation, the anatomical structure of the right heart and the pulmonary valve were reconstructed by a computer at Xijing Hospital to accurately evaluate the size of the pulmonary valve, the distance from the pulmonary valve ring to the pulmonary artery branch, the size of the right ventricular outflow tract, and the general location of pulmonary valve release. The reconstruction was also helpful in evaluating the size of the right ventricle and the appropriate pulmonary artery stents for use (Fig. 6.32) [93].

Printing the model reconstructed by computer at a 1:1 size ratio allows the operator to directly view the anatomical structure of the right heart and the pulmonary artery of the patient, and the model can be simulated in vitro according to the transparent 3D model so that the surgical plan can be more accurately and effectively determined (Fig. 6.33) [93–95].

At present, percutaneous pulmonary valve implantation is usually performed through the pigtail catheter of the femoral vein to the main pulmonary artery to show pulmonary valve insufficiency. Then, the balloon is placed to evaluate the type

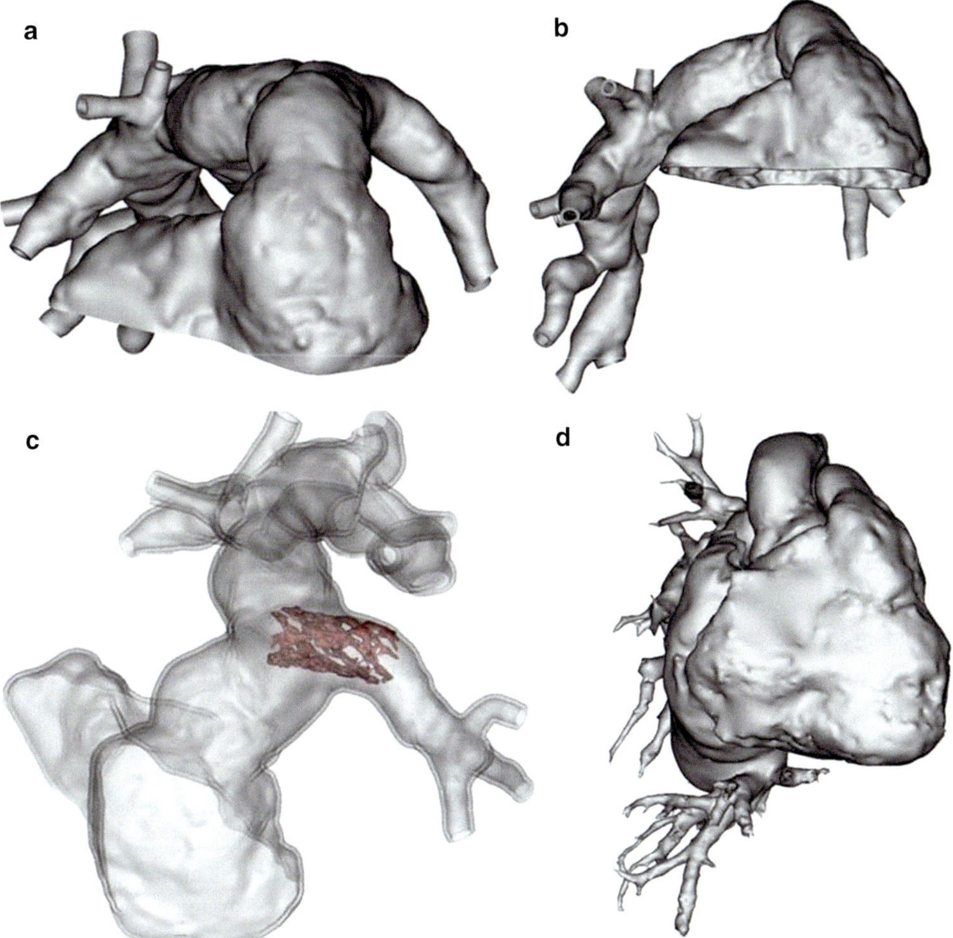

Fig. 6.32 3D modeling of a 3D reconstruction of CTA in patients with pulmonary valve insufficiency in the Department Cardiovascular Surgery, Xijing Hospital. (**a**) Anterior view shows severe widening of the main pulmonary artery and the left and right pulmonary arteries; (**b**) Norma lateralis shows a severely widened right pulmonary artery; (**c**) A profile view of stents previously implanted in the left main pulmonary artery; (**d**) The anterior view shows a severely enlarged right ventricle. Imaging data and three-dimensional reconstruction were from the Department of Cardiovascular Surgery, Shanghai Chest Hospital, and the Department of Cardiovascular Surgery of Xijing Hospital

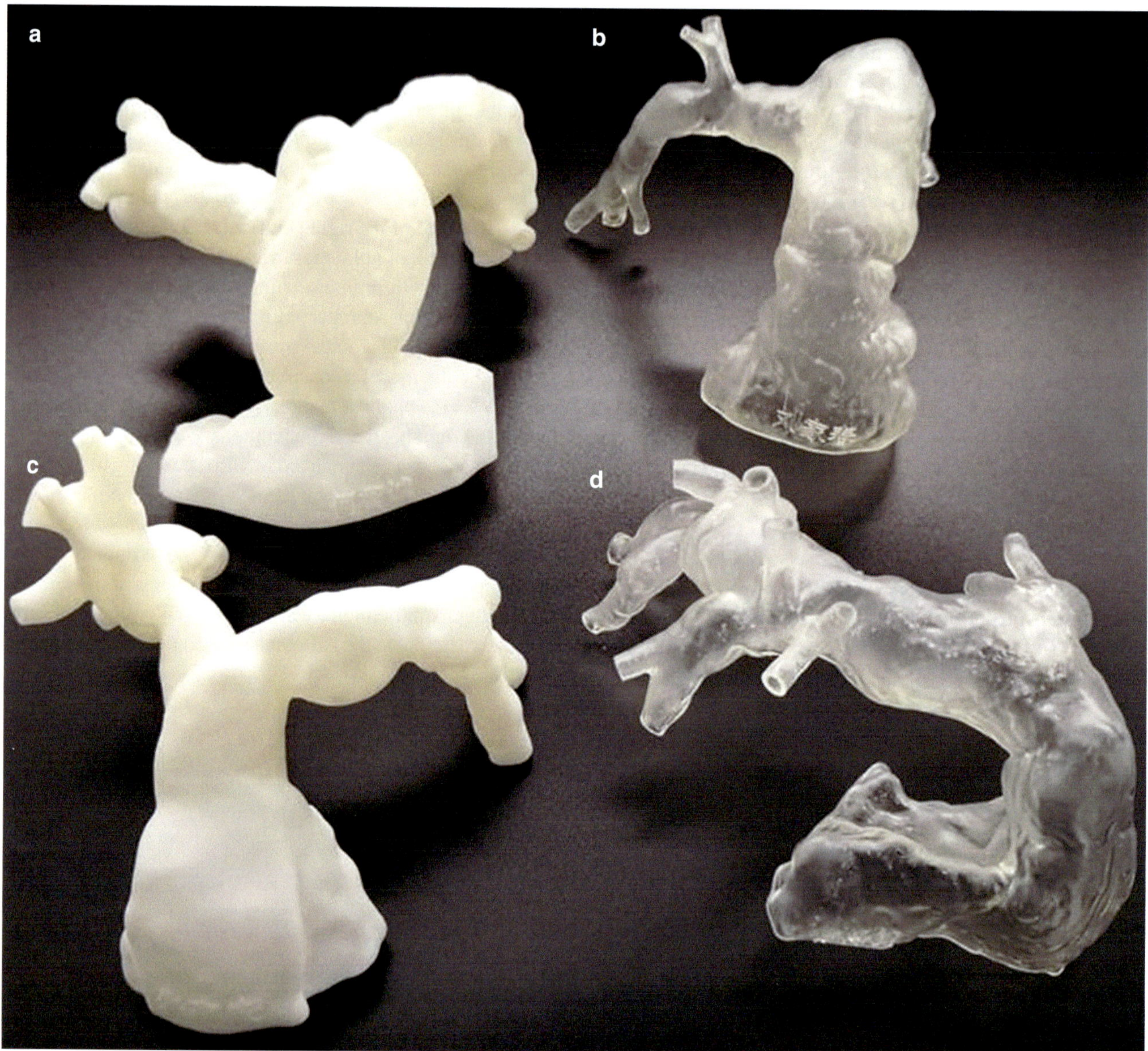

Fig. 6.33 3D-printed models before operation in patients with pulmonary valve insufficiency. (**a, b, c**), and (**d**) correspond to four different patients. The 3D-printed models are from Shanghai Chest Hospital and the Department of Cardiovascular Surgery of Xijing Hospital

of selected valve and the risk of coronary artery compression, and the compressed stent valve crosses the autologous pulmonary valve through the delivery system. Part of the stent valve is spread out in the pulmonary artery to observe the shape and position of the valve. Finally, after complete release of the stent valve, the morphology, position, and paravalvular leakage of the valve can be observed, and the operation is completed (Fig. 6.34).

After percutaneous pulmonary valve implantation, the heart team can also print a 3D model with a computer 3D reconstruction of CTA data after operation to understand the shape and position of the interventional pulmonary valve, whether there is paravalvular leakage, the influence of the stent valve on the surrounding structure, the relationship with the pulmonary artery and the right ventricular outflow tract, and so on, to more intuitively evaluate the shape and position of the valve after operation. Understanding its long-term effect is important and has guiding significance (Fig. 6.35).

3D printing technology will become an auxiliary means in addition to traditional radiography. It will guide preoperative evaluation, surgical simulation, the development of surgical strategies, and postoperative evaluation of transcatheter pulmonary valve replacement in many ways. The further

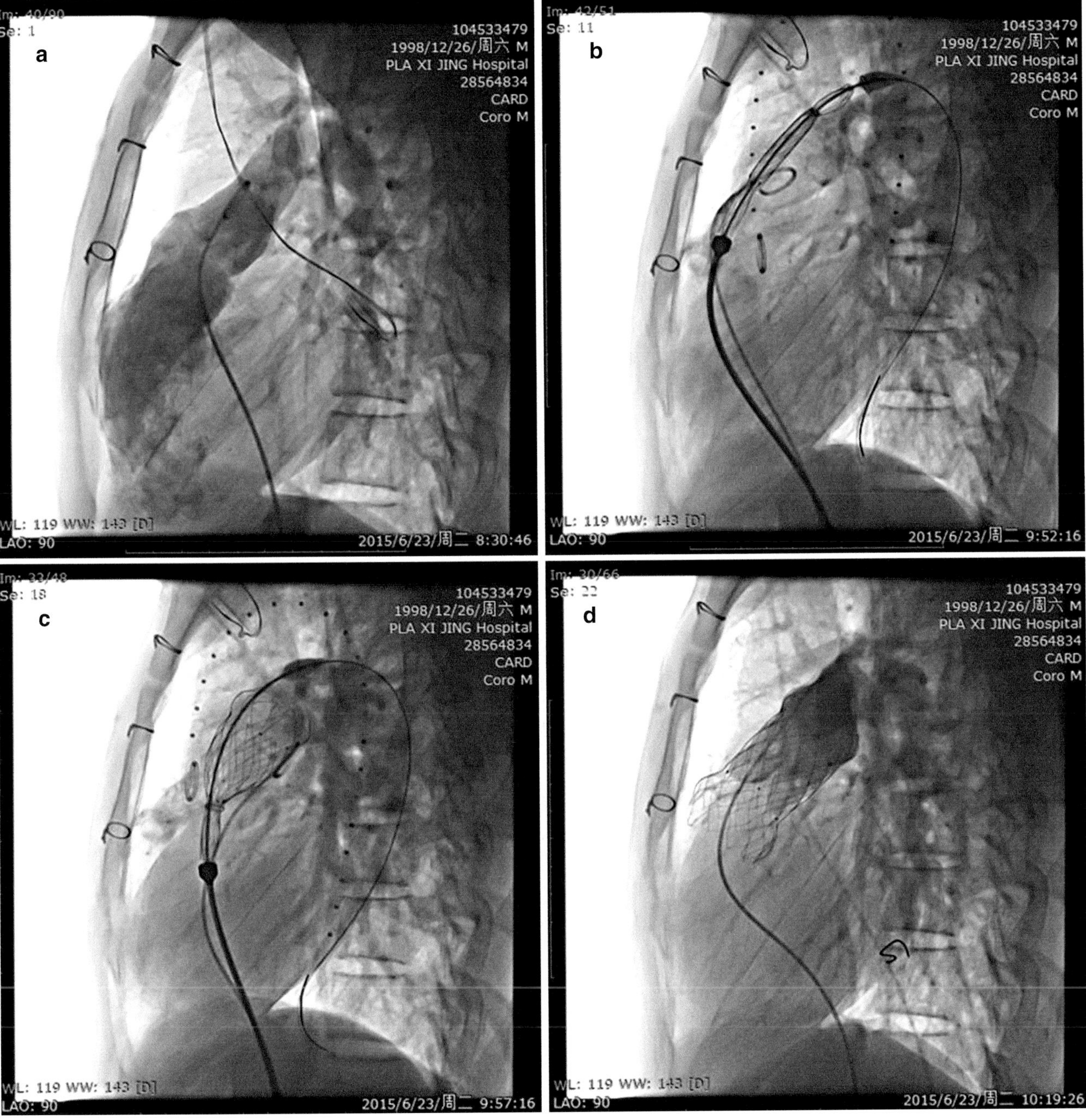

Fig. 6.34 The step diagram of transcatheter valve replacement of insufficiency or regurgitation. (**a**) Pulmonary valve insufficiency shown by angiography from the pigtail catheter to the main pulmonary artery via the femoral vein; (**b**) The compressed stent valve straddles the autologous pulmonary valve through the delivery system; (**c**) Part of the stent valve spreads in the pulmonary artery; (**d**) After complete release of the stent valve, the morphology, position, and paravalvular leakage of the valve can be observed. The imaging data are from the Department of Cardiovascular Surgery at Xijing Hospital

development of 3D printing technology requires extensive cooperation across various disciplines, including radiologists, clinical cardiovascular intervention doctors, surgeons, and medical engineers. With the accumulation of experience, the profound impact of 3D printing technology in the treatment of transcatheter pulmonary valve replacement will continue to expand [92, 94].

6.5 Perivalvular Leakage and Three-Dimensional Printing

Yang Liu, Xin Pan, Haibo Zhang

Paravalvular leakage (PVL) is a unique complication after artificial heart valve replacement. Its incidence is low, but its

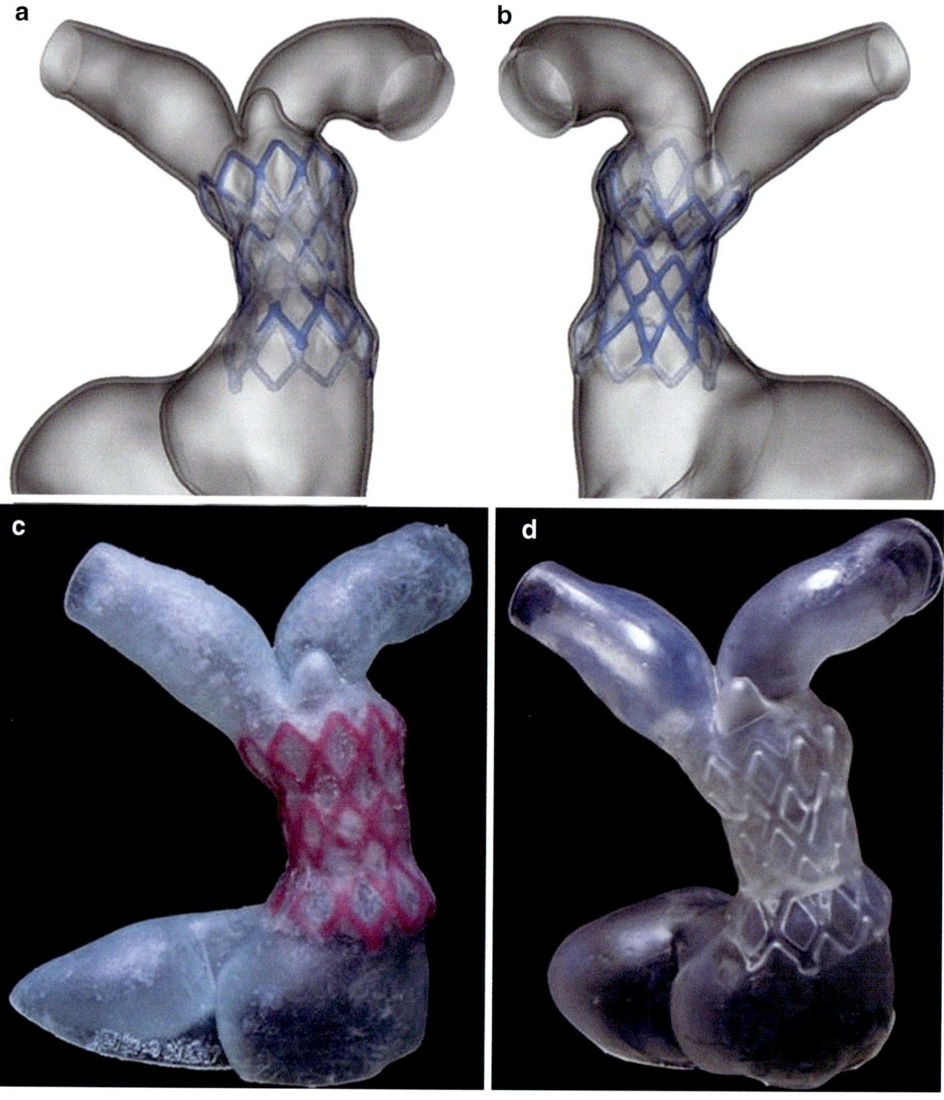

Fig. 6.35 Postoperative model of interventional pulmonary valve replacement in patients who underwent cardiovascular surgery at Xijing Hospital. (**a**) A view of the anterior and posterior position of interventional pulmonary valve model after three-dimensional reconstruction by a computer; (**b**) Three-dimensional computer reconstruction of the posterior–anterior view of the pulmonary valve model after interventional pulmonary valve surgery; (**c**) Colored soft and hard material combined with 3D printing in the interventional pulmonary valve model; (**d**) Rigid monochromatic 3D-printed model after interventional pulmonary valve surgery. The image data, 3D reconstruction, and 3D-printed model are from Wuhan Union Hospital and the Department of Cardiovascular Surgery of Xijing Hospital

outcome is serious. In recent years, the occurrence of paravalvular leakage has increased with the widespread development of transcatheter valves. Although most patients with paravalvular leakage have no clinical symptoms and develop slowly, approximately 1%–5% of patients with paravalvular leakage have severe clinical symptoms and poor prognosis. To date, surgical treatment is still the main treatment for these patients with symptoms of paravalvular leakage. Interventional therapy, which has been widely used in congenital heart disease, is also used to address paravalvular leakage and has shown some advantages [96, 97]. Three-dimensional reconstruction of computer and 3D printing models will have great guiding significance for preoperative evaluation and surgical treatment, which can help clinicians identify a definite target.

Many factors are known to be associated with paravalvular leakage, including degenerative changes in proprioceptive annular tissue, annular calcification, inappropriate surgical suturing, infective endocarditis, connective tissue disease, and other causes such as aging, giant left atrium, renal insufficiency, immunological abnormalities, systemic malnutrition, etc. Clinically, paravalvular leakage is not usually caused by a single factor but may be caused by a combination of multiple factors. Multimodal imaging technology plays an important role in the diagnosis and treatment of paravalvular leak. The diagnosis of paravalvular leak mainly depends on echocardiography, which can clearly show the regurgitation flow, blood flow velocity, and gradient of paravalvular leak. Three-dimensional echocardiography displays well the effects of the location, size, and number of paravalvular leaks [98] (Fig. 6.36).

Echocardiography and computed tomography (CTA) are the main imaging techniques used to evaluate and guide the occlusion of paravalvular leaks [99]. Since interventional catheterization has been used to treat paravalvular leaks, paravalvular leaks have been treated with an additional, less

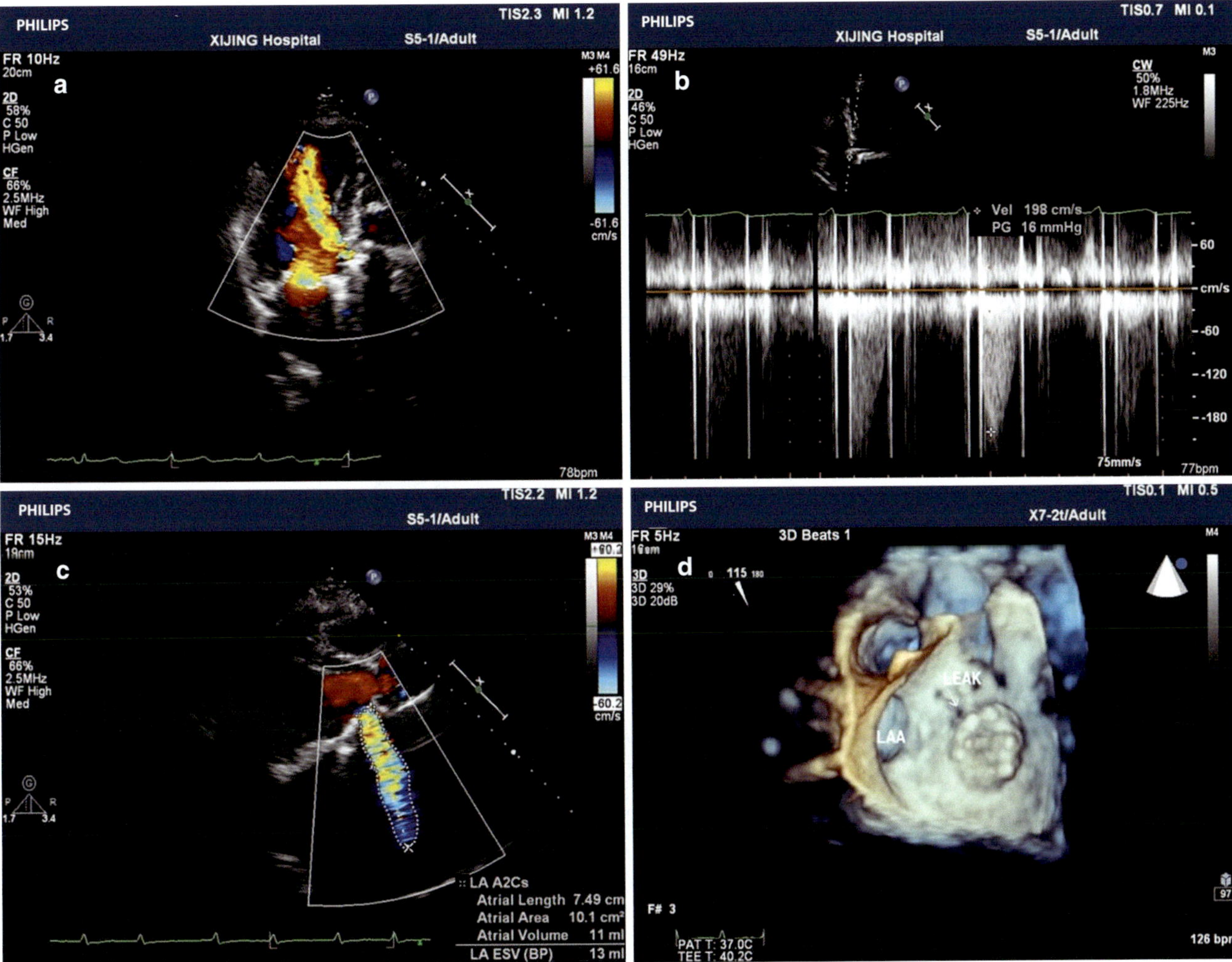

Fig. 6.36 Echocardiography diagnosis of aortic and mitral regurgitation. (**a**) Color Doppler of aortic regurgitation; (**b**) flow Doppler of aortic regurgitation gradient and flow velocity; (**c**) color Doppler of mitral regurgitation; (**d**) three-dimensional echocardiography showing the location, size, and number of mitral regurgitation. Images were obtained from the Department of Cardiovascular Surgery at Xijing Hospital

traumatic option. Interventional treatment of paravalvular leak is the most difficult operation in structural heart disease. It often takes a long time and is associated with a steep learning curve. Interventional techniques, such as catheter and guide wire manipulation, are widely performed, and special types of equipment are needed to successfully complete occlusion. In addition, multidisciplinary collaboration is an important factor in the success of catheter intervention. The heart team may include cardiac interventional doctors, echocardiographers, CTA imaging assessment doctors, cardiac surgeons, and anesthesiologists. The main problem of interventional treatment for paravalvular leakage is the lack of a special percutaneous delivery system and occluding devices. Currently available occluding devices are designed for other heart diseases, such as atrial septal defects, ventricular septal defects, patent ductus arteriosus occlusion, vascular occlusion, etc., but they are not completely suitable for the treatment of paravalvular leakage. Initial interventional devices included umbrella devices, vascular occluders, and coils. The Amplatzer series of congenital heart disease occluders are the mainstream devices for paravalvular leak occlusion treatment, especially the second-generation patent ductus arteriosus occluder and the second-generation vascular plug, which are the most widely used in the world. The square and rectangular paravalvular leak occluders produced by Occlutech have also been certified by CE mark. They are used in Europe but have not yet entered the Chinese market (Fig. 6.37). Domestic Amplatzer-like congenital heart disease occluders are often used in the interventional treatment of paravalvular leakage [100, 101].

Choosing the appropriate occlusion equipment is key to a successful operation. Most plugs are circular except for the AVP III plug, which is elliptical. Paravalvular leaks vary in size and shape; some are crescent-shaped, and some are cylindrical. In addition, paravalvular leaks may be irregular channels, which make it difficult for the guide

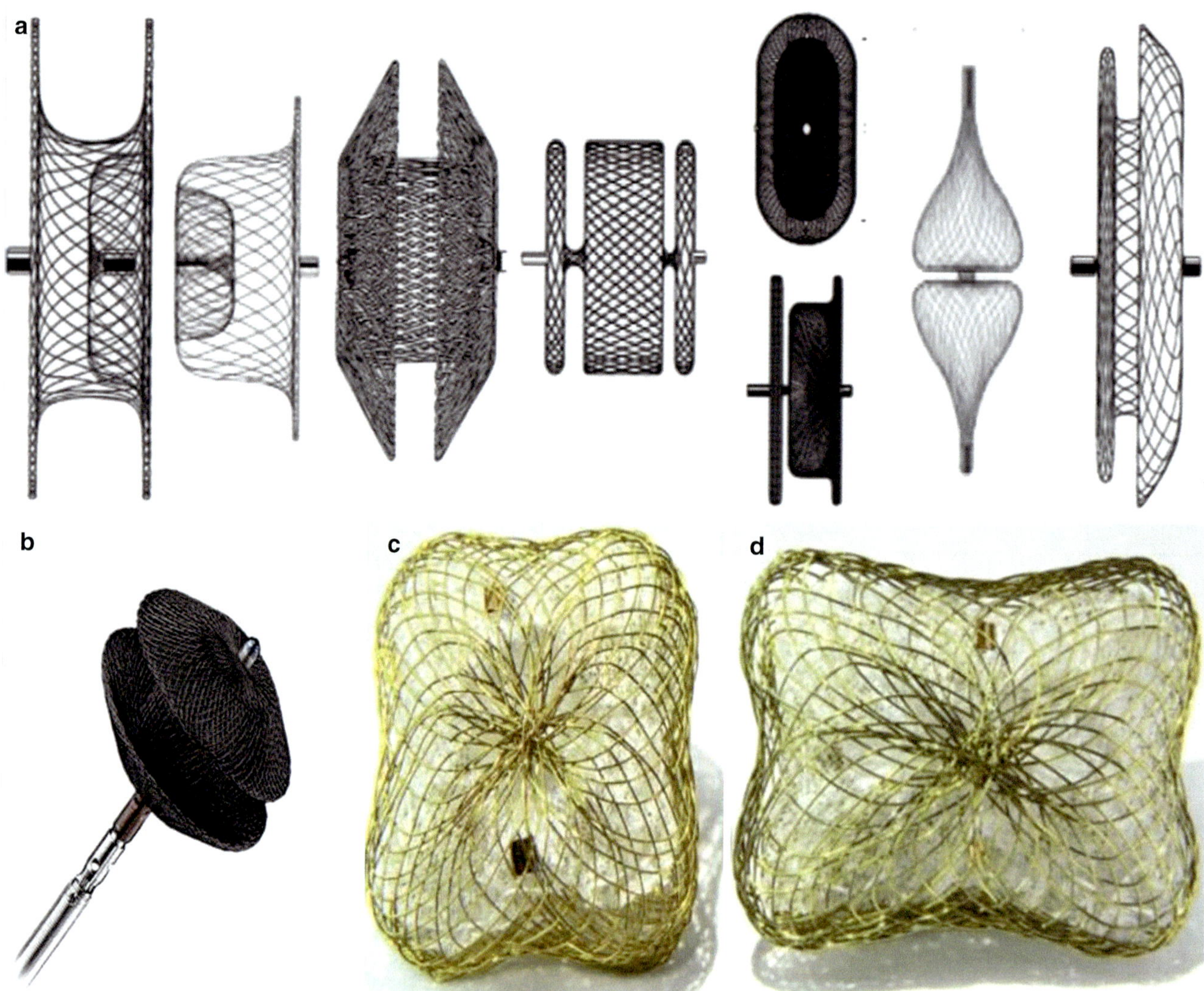

Fig. 6.37 (**a**) Amplatzer series congenital heart disease occluders for paravalvular leaks (from left to right: ventricular septal defect occluder, patent ductus arteriosus occluder, second-generation patent ductus arteriosus occluder, second-generation occlusion, third-generation occlusion, fourth-generation vascular plug, and atrial septal defect occluder; (**b**) Second-generation patent ductus arteriosus occluder; rectangle produced by (**c**) Occlutech rectangular paravalvular leak occluder; (**d**) Occlutech square paravalvular leak occluder

wire to pass through. When a circular plug is used to address the irregular shape of the leakage, a relatively larger plug is needed to achieve a satisfactory plugging effect. However, this may increase the risk of artificial valve interference, especially in mechanical valves. This situation may require the use of multiple small occluders to adequately occlude paravalvular leaks while effectively avoiding secondary prosthetic valve dysfunction. It was reported that the Oval AVP III occluder can also be used for crescent paravalvular leak occlusion [102].

Interventional treatment of aortic paravalvular leak is relatively easy, which can be accomplished by a retrograde femoral artery approach. The usual procedures are as follows: (1) puncture of the bilateral femoral artery: one side is used for implantation of the occluder, and the other side is used for angiography to judge the effect of occlusion; (2) systemic heparinization to maintain ACT >300 seconds; (3) coronary angiography to evaluate the coronary artery and the relationship between aortic leakage and the prosthetic valve; (4) multi-angle retrograde aortic root angiography to show the shape, size, and location of the paravalvular leakage; (5) establish the guide wire and catheter orbit through the paravalvular leakage; (6) select the appropriate occluder (size, shape) and sheath for delivery to the paravalvular leakage; (7) fluoroscopy and ultrasonography imaging to judge the effect of the occlusion and the effect on valve function; and (8) repeated aortic root angiography to show the immediate effect of aortic paravalvular leak occlusion and the relationship between the occluder and coronary ostium before the operation is completed (Fig. 6.38).

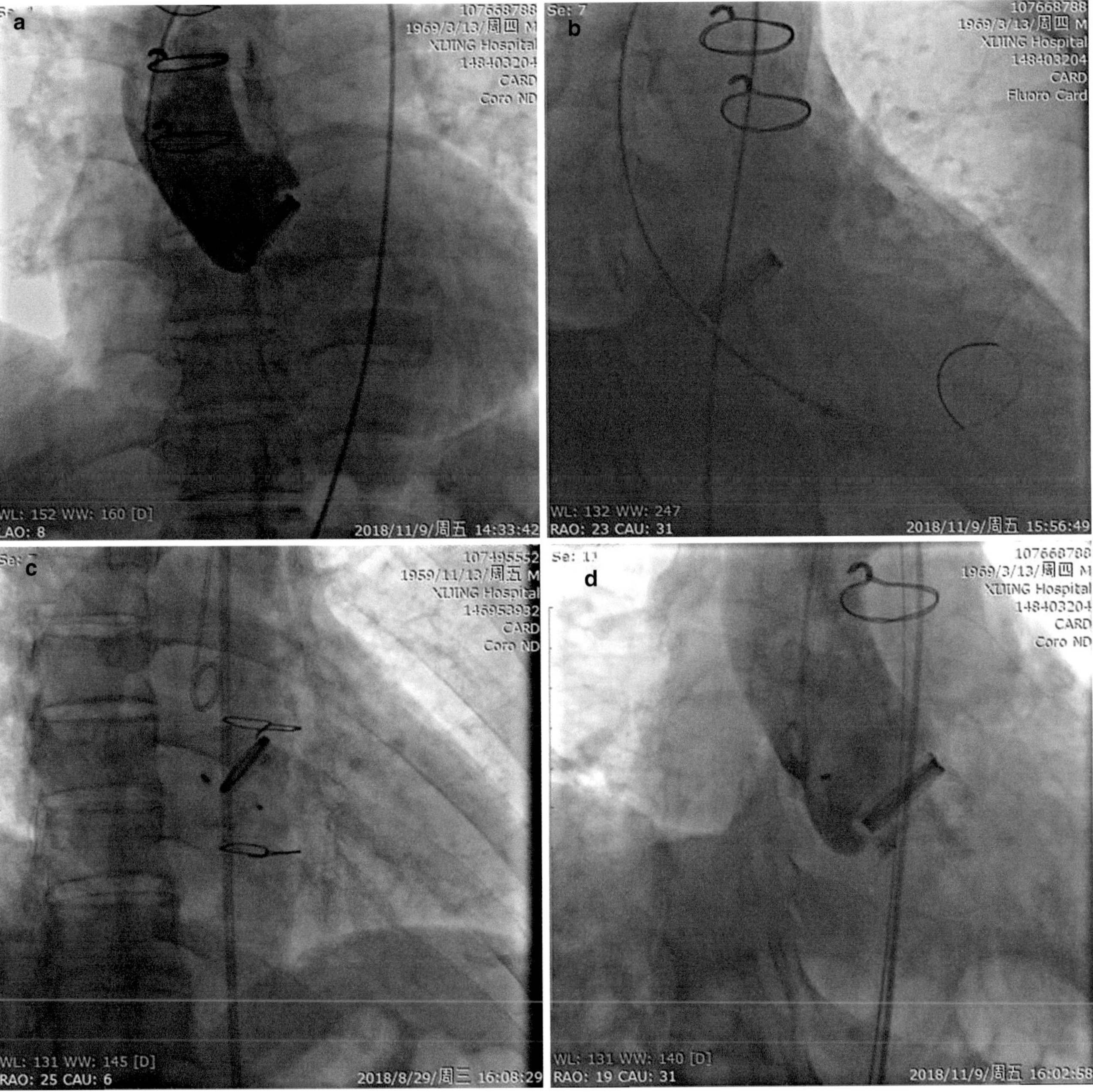

Fig. 6.38 Procedure of interventional treatment for aortic valve circumferential leakage. (**a**) The location, shape, and size of the aortic valve circumferential leakage are shown through the tail catheter from the femoral artery to ascending aorta angiography; (**b**) The guide wire and delivery system pass through the circumferential leakage of the aortic valve; (**c**) The occluder is released in the circumferential leakage location; (**d**) The ascending aorta angiography shows the results of aortic circumferential leakage closure. Image data were obtained from Beijing Anzhen Hospital affiliated with Capital Medical University

In addition to preoperative diagnosis and planning, the application of 3D printing technology to establish the model of aortic paravalvular leak is of great value in evaluating the shape and location of the occluder and the relationship between the occluder and the prosthetic valve (Fig. 6.39).

Interventional treatment of mitral leakage is similar to that of aortic leakage, but the approaches are relatively complex [103]. These approaches include the anterograde femoral vein left atrium approach, the retrograde femoral artery left ventricle approach, and/or the direct apical puncture approach, which are more difficult than aortic leak (Fig. 6.40). The chosen approach depends on the location, size, and adjacent relationship of the paravalvular leakage, valve calcification, and the personal preference of the surgeon.

Paravalvular leakage intervention via the apical approach usually requires exposure of the apex and left ventriculogra-

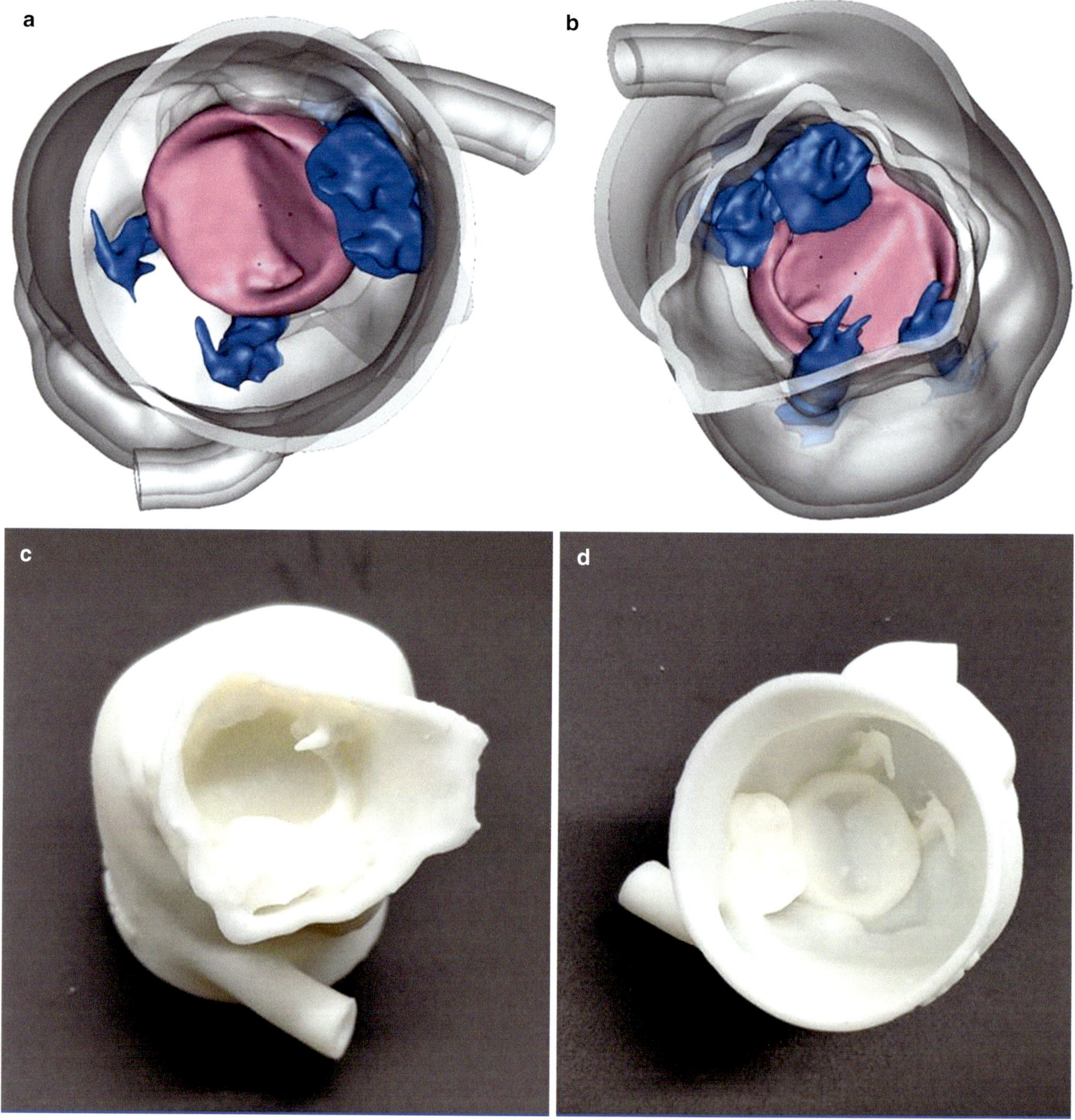

Fig. 6.39 3D-printed image of paravalvular leakage of the aorta after interventional treatment with four occluders. (**a**) Computer modeling diagram from the left ventricular view; (**b**) Computer modeling diagram from the aortic view; (**c**) 3D-printed model from the left ventricular view; (**d**) 3D-printed model from the aortic view. The image data, three-dimensional computer reconstruction, and three-dimensional printing model are from the Department of Cardiovascular Surgery of Xijing Hospital

phy to show the location, shape, and size of the mitral valve leakage. Then, a catheter is used to transport the occluder through mitral valve circumferential leakage. The occluder is released at the leakage site, and the entrance site of the left ventricle is closed before the completion of the operation (Fig. 6.41).

In recent years, it has been gradually recognized that interventional occlusion is safe and feasible for surgical high-risk patients with PVL [103, 104]. With the development of interventional devices and the accumulation of surgical experience, interventional occlusion of PVL has received increasing attention. In the 2014 and 2017 editions of the AHA/ACC

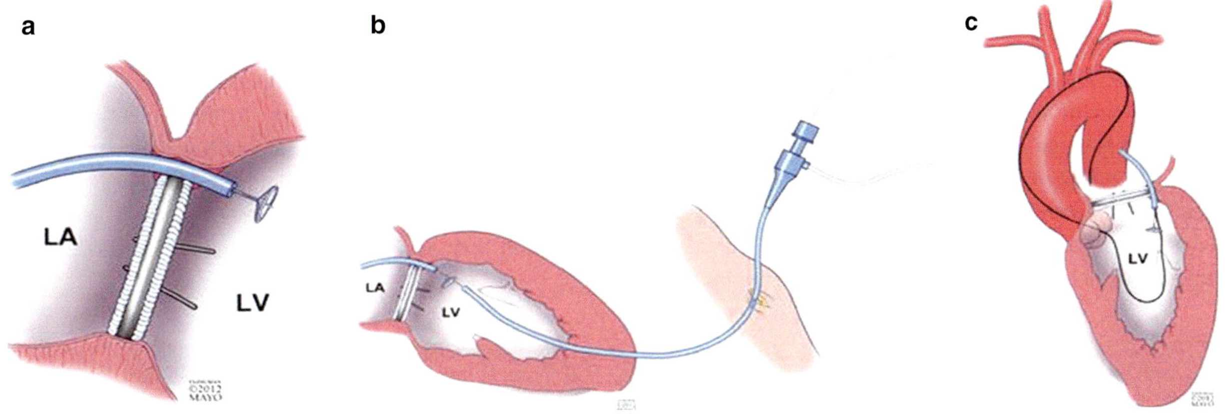

Fig. 6.40 Schematic diagram of interventional therapy for mitral leakage. (**a**) trans-atrial septal approach; (**b**) direct apical approach; (**c**) trans-femoral left ventricular retrograde approach

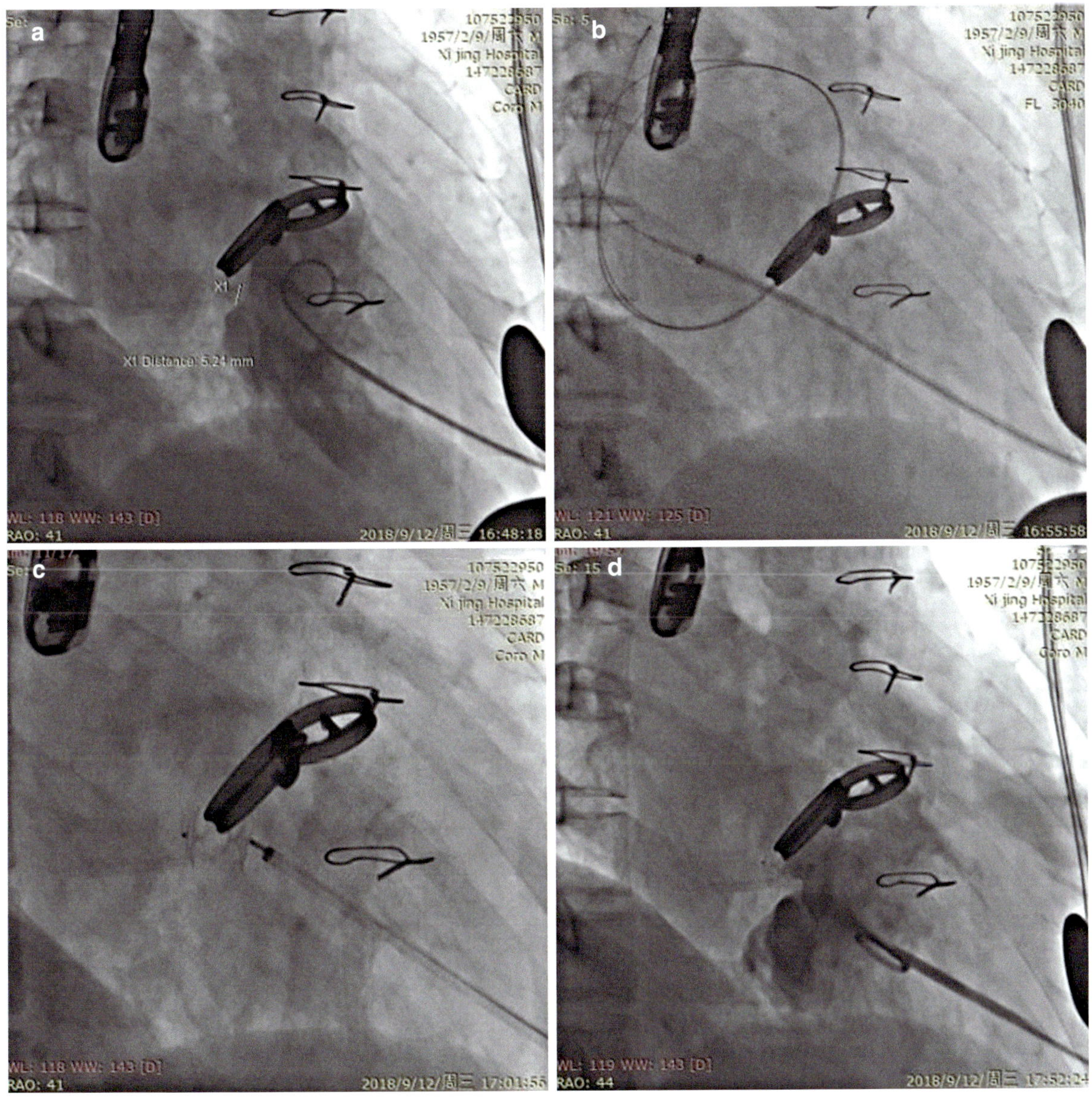

Fig. 6.41 Procedure diagram of interventional treatment for mitral leakage. (**a**) The position, shape, and size of mitral valve circumferential leakage revealed by the left ventriculography of a pig tail catheter via the transapical approach; (**b**) The guide wire and conveying system passing through mitral valve leakage; (**c**) The occluder is released at the periventricular leakage site; (**d**) Left ventricular reangiography showing the results of mitral valve leakage occlusion. Images were obtained from the Department of Cardiovascular Surgery at Xijing Hospital

Guidelines for Valvular Disease Treatment, it was noted that there was a high risk of reoperation due to cardiac insufficiency and/or repeated mechanical hemolysis of PVL after valve replacement and that if the anatomical morphology of paravalvular leakage met the requirements of interventional therapy, transcatheter closure was recommended as the first choice for the treatment of PVL [105–107]. PVL interventional therapy requires high-level surgical skills and proficiency. It is difficult for the guide wire to reach multiple, small leaks, and the radiation time and radiation dose increase significantly. With the maturity of 3D printing technology, the author's department is able to construct and print 1:1 anatomical structural models according to the patient's CTA data. These models are very helpful in guiding the operator regarding the location of the paravalvular leakage, providing shape information, formulating the operation strategy, reducing the operation time and the amount of radiation exposure during

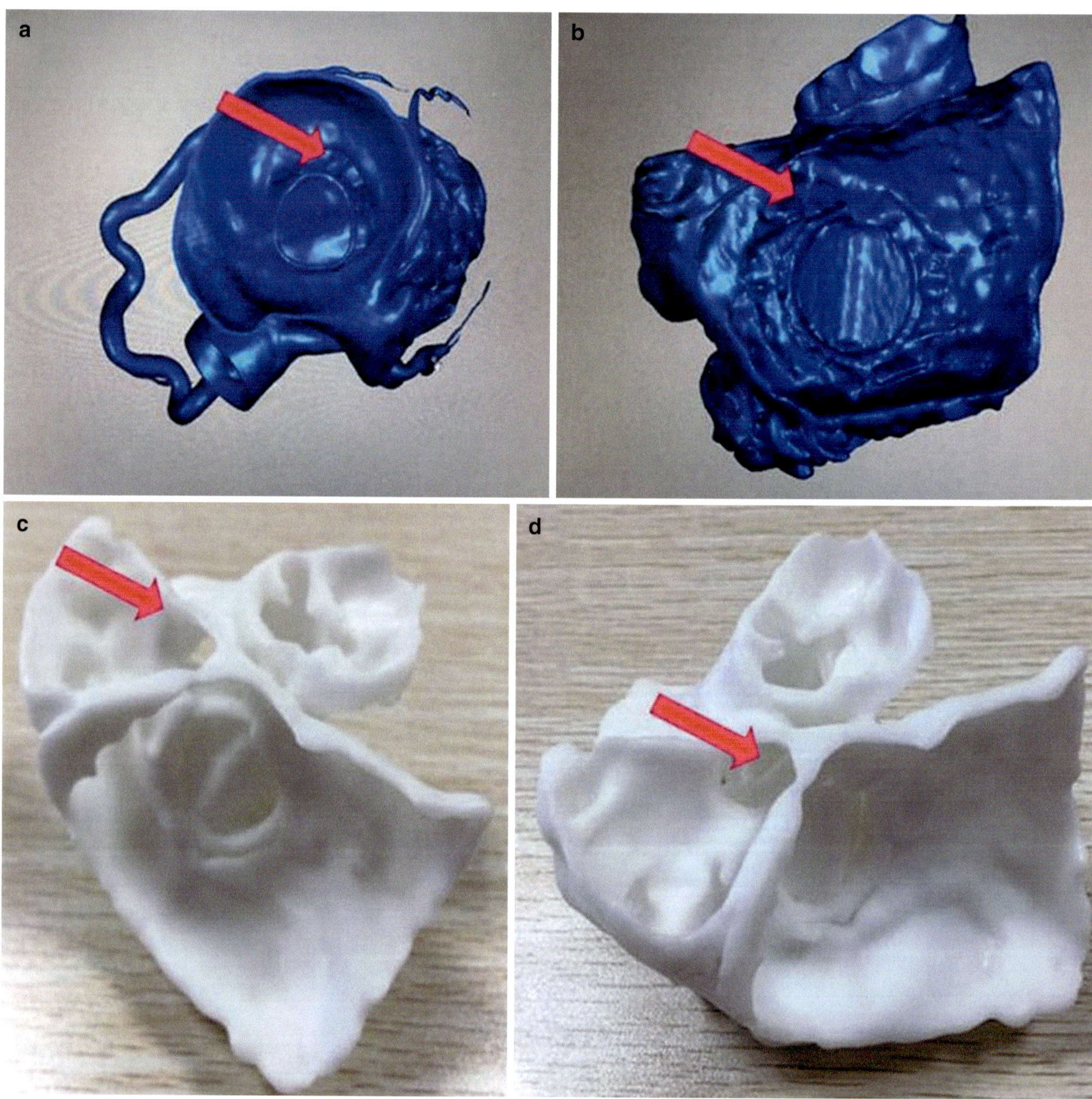

Fig. 6.42 Models and photographs of real products fabricated by 3D printing technology at the Department of Cardiovascular Surgery of Xijing Hospital showing the position and morphology of the paravalvular leak. (**a**) Mitral leak computer modeling of the left atrial view; (**b**) Mitral leak computer modeling of the left ventricular view; (**c**) left atrial view of the 3D-printed paravalvular leak; (**d**) left ventricular view of the 3D-printed paravalvular leak. The image data, three-dimensional computer reconstruction, and three-dimensional printing model are from the Department of Cardiovascular Surgery of Xijing Hospital

the operation, and ensuring the success of the operation (Fig. 6.42).

Current clinical data show that interventional occlusion is safe and effective for patients with high-risk paravalvular leaks [108]. In a group of reports from Shanghai Thoracic Hospital, the closure efficiency of aortic PVL was close to 100% in patients with small or medium leaks, both in mechanical or bioprosthetic valves. One-year follow-up showed that cardiac function, motor ability, and a quality of life index were significantly improved, and there were no obvious complications. Multimodal imaging diagnosis, especially transesophageal dynamic three-dimensional echocardiography (3D TEE) and/or three-dimensional CTA reconstruction (3D CTA), is important for the establishment of complete morphology of PVL if the leak is large or located in the mitral valve position. In clinical practice, multimodal imaging diagnosis can help to accurately select an occluder and approach, increase the success rate of the operation, and reduce complications. In 2011, JACC reported that 57 patients with paravalvular leak received interventional occlusion. The technical success rate was 86%. After the operation, 80% of patients had improved cardiac function above grade I, and the survival rate was 91.9% at 42 months [108–110].

Transcatheter aortic valve replacement (TAVR) is an effective method for the treatment of moderate to severe aortic stenosis. With the rapid development of TAVR, paravalvular leakage is one of the main complications of balloon dilatation. In the Partner IA clinical trial, the incidence of paravalvular leakage in the two-year Edwards SAPIEN valve implantation group (348 cases) was much higher than that in the surgical group (6.9% vs. 0.9%, $p < 0.001$). The survival rate study showed that paravalvular leakage above moderate was an independent predictor of death (risk factor 2.11). Another group reported a retrospective review of 667 patients with immediate paravalvular leakage, regardless of whether they were implanted with Edwards SAPIEN or Core Valve valves via catheter, with an immediate incidence of 21% [111–113]. Upon further analysis, reasons for the high incidence of paravalvular leakage after TAVR are as follows: (1) preoperative examination underestimates the diameter of the original annulus; (2) placement of artificial aortic valve stent is inaccurate, mostly biased to the aortic side or the left ventricular side; and (3) severe calcification of the original aortic valve affects the adherence of the stent valve. The main treatment methods for paravalvular leakage after TAVR are currently (1) accurate positioning of stent valves during operation; (2) posterior dilatation of large balloon stent valves; (3) reimplantation of stent valves in stent valves; and (4) local occlusion with transcatheter occluder.

Multi-slice CT (MDCT) imaging and careful preoperative image evaluation, especially preoperative 3D printing, are helpful for preoperative surgical strategy formulation, optimization of valve type selection, and reducing postoperative PVL. Balloon dilation during TAVR is used for smaller margins and annular calcification to reduce possible complications. Therefore, local anatomy is essential to determine the appropriate size of the valve. In addition, Asian patients have aortic root dysplasia, resulting in a smaller annulus, a smaller valve orifice area, and possibly Watt sinus malformation. Among them, female patients have a higher incidence of complications. Asian patients with TAVR have five times more complications than European patients. The patient's CTA data can be used for three-dimensional reconstruction of the anatomical structure. Maragiannis et al. demonstrated that 3D-printed models can accurately reproduce the anatomical structure and the approach of severe degenerative aortic stenosis and assist in the prediction of paravalvular leak after TAVR and the functional characteristics of pacemaker implantation. Relevant 3D printing studies have used micro-CT to measure the frame area and mismatch area and have clarified the efficacy of stent valves and the mechanism of PVL postexpansion.

Thus far, few heart centers in China have performed interventional closure of paravalvular leaks. Since 2011, the author's Department of Cardiovascular Surgery of Xijing Hospital has reported transcatheter closure of aortic and mitral leaks through different interventional approaches. The success rate of the operation reached more than 90% [114]. To date, more than 150 operations have been successfully completed. In addition, the Department of Cardiovascular Surgery of Xijing Hospital has also explored CTA computer three-dimensional reconstruction and digital image three-dimensional printing technology to assist in the interventional treatment of paravalvular leakage and to evaluate the clinical efficacy of paravalvular leakage after interventional closure. Therefore, preliminary experience using three-dimensional printing technology for assisting in the treatment of paravalvular leakage was obtained (Fig. 6.43).

3D-printed PVL models can also be applied for in vitro simulations to select the right type and size of the occluder. As paravalvular leakage intervention is the most complex type of structural heart disease, with high technical difficulty and long operation time, in vitro simulation by 3D printing technology will undoubtedly greatly reduce the irradiation time, improve the surgical efficiency, and improve the prognosis of patients (Fig. 6.44).

The author collaborated with Professor Wu Yongjian's team from Fuwai Hospital to study a case of an elderly patient with paravalvular leak complicated with aortic stenosis and insufficiency after mitral valve replacement using 3D printing. Preoperative computer modeling and 3D printing revealed that simultaneous paravalvular leak intervention and TAVR could be considered in this patient. Because of the complex anatomy of this patient, the following factors should be considered: (1) the location, size, and interventional treat-

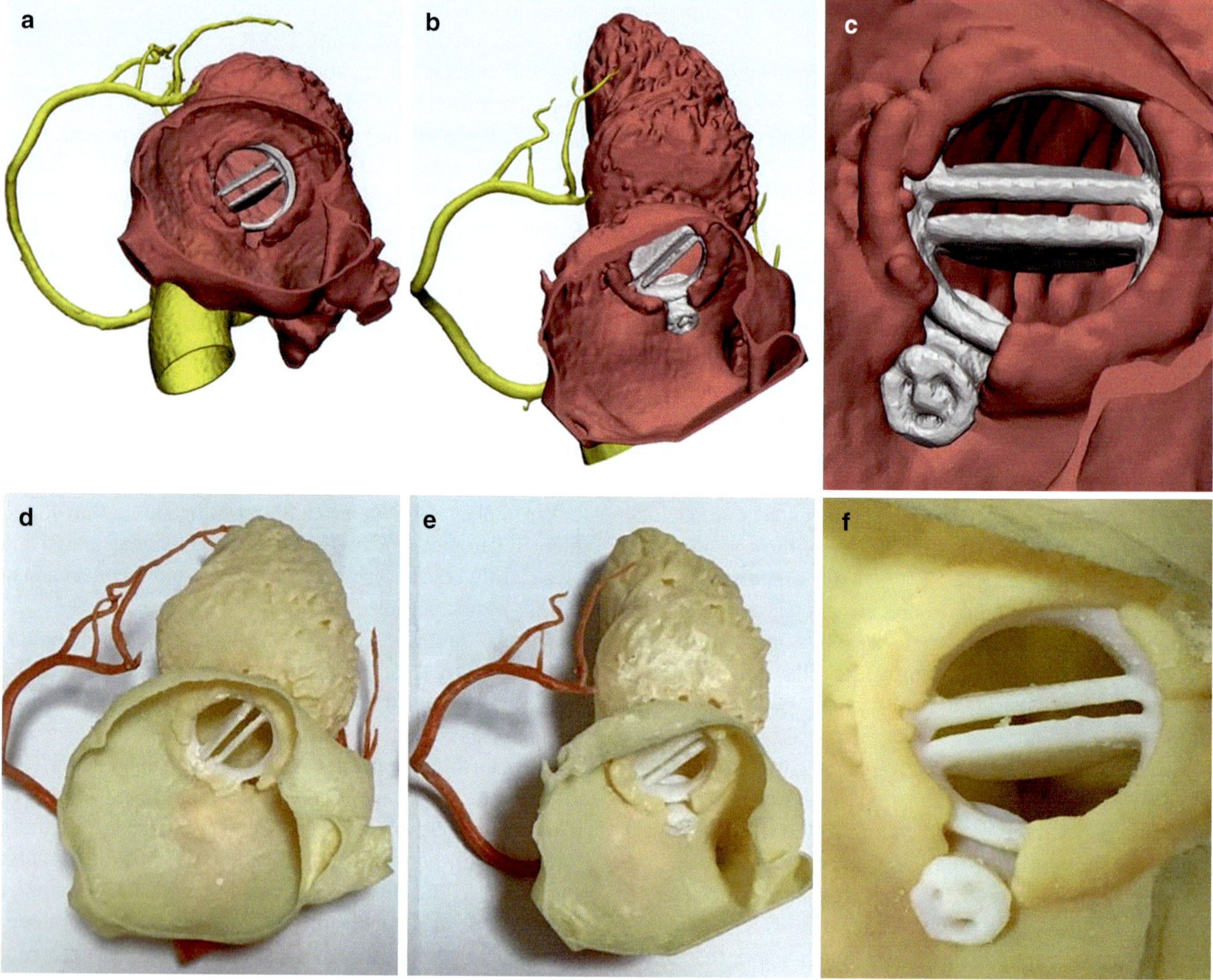

Fig. 6.43 Three-dimensional printing technology of the Department of Cardiovascular Surgery of Xijing Hospital was used to evaluate the clinical efficacy of interventional closure of paravalvular leak. (**a**) Computer-generated mitral PVL model from the left atrial view before leak occlusion; (**b**) Computer-generated mitral PVL model from the left atrial view after mitral PVL occlusion; (**c**) Computer-generated locally magnified view after mitral PVL occlusion; (**d**) 3D-printed mitral PVL model from the left atrial view before mitral leak occlusion.; (**e**) 3D-printed mitral PVL model from the left atrial view after mitral leak occlusion; (**f**) 3D-printed mitral PVL model with local magnification after mitral PVL occlusion. The image data, three-dimensional computer reconstruction, and three-dimensional printing model are from the Department of Cardiovascular Surgery of Xijing Hospital

ment approach of mitral PVL; (2) the distance between the aortic valve and the mitral valve to avoid placing the transcatheter valve too deep such that it interferes with the mechanical mitral valve; (3) selection of the kind of occluder to reach a full occlusion effect without affecting the opening and closing of mechanical valves; (4) choosing an appropriate size of transcatheter valves; and (5) the depth of the transcatheter valve implantation, which is directly related to risks to the coronary artery, conduction block, and so on. Faced with such a complicated and difficult clinical case, the two teams discussed the plan in detail by using 3D printing technology. The occluder and stent valves were also used to simulate the release in vitro. The first step was to occlude the mitral PVL retrograde via the femoral artery under local anesthesia. Then, the patient was switched to general anesthesia, and TAVR was performed through the carotid artery. The stent valve was precisely placed 4 mm below the aortic annulus plane, which ensured the coaxial of the stent valve and the aortic annulus and avoided interaction between the stent aortic valve and the mitral mechanical valve. Postoperative angiography showed that the stent aortic valve and the mitral mechanical valve were all in appropriate positions. The occluder was well positioned and did not affect the opening and closing of the mechanical valves. This challeng-

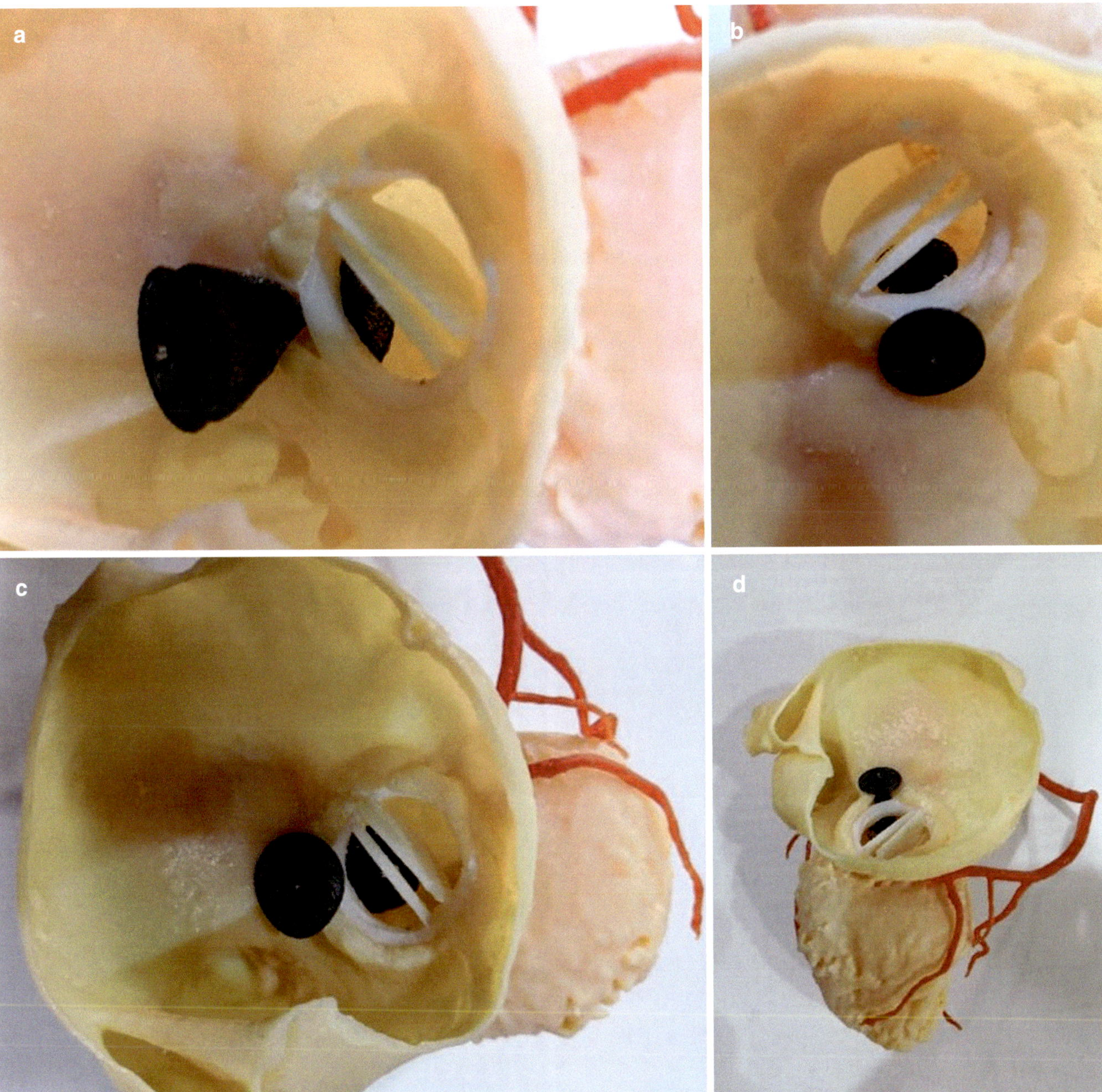

Fig. 6.44 In vitro simulation of PVL occlusion using a 3D-printed model of mitral paravalvular leakage at the Department of Cardiovascular Surgery of Xijing Hospital. (**a**) Selection of a large-sized occluder for mitral paravalvular leakage occlusion affects mitral mechanical valves; (**b**) Selection of the appropriate size of occluder does not affect mitral mechanical valves; (**c**) Placement of the occluder at the waist of the paravalvular leakage; (**d**) General view of the simulated PVL occlusion using a 3D-printed model. The 3D-printed model of the occlusion and the image data are from the Department of Cardiovascular Surgery of Xijing Hospital

ing complex structural heart disease was successfully treated (Fig. 6.45).

After surgery, the team reapplied 3D printing technology to reconstruct the patient's local anatomy, showing good adjacency of the mitral valve mechanical valve, the occluder, and the aortic valve stent (Fig. 6.46). This challenging case also confirms the important role of 3D printing technology in precise guidance, in vitro simulation, and postoperative evaluation for the treatment of complex valvular diseases.

Nevertheless, the interventional treatment of paravalvular leak still has some limitations: the efficacy of interventional closure of paravalvular leaks larger than a quarter of the annulus is uncertain, and because of the different shapes of paravalvular leaks, there is currently no special occluder for paravalvular leaks in China; the long-term efficacy of PVL occlusion remains to be followed up. However, as a new technology, interventional therapy of PVL has been gradually developed and popularized. Interventional therapy has

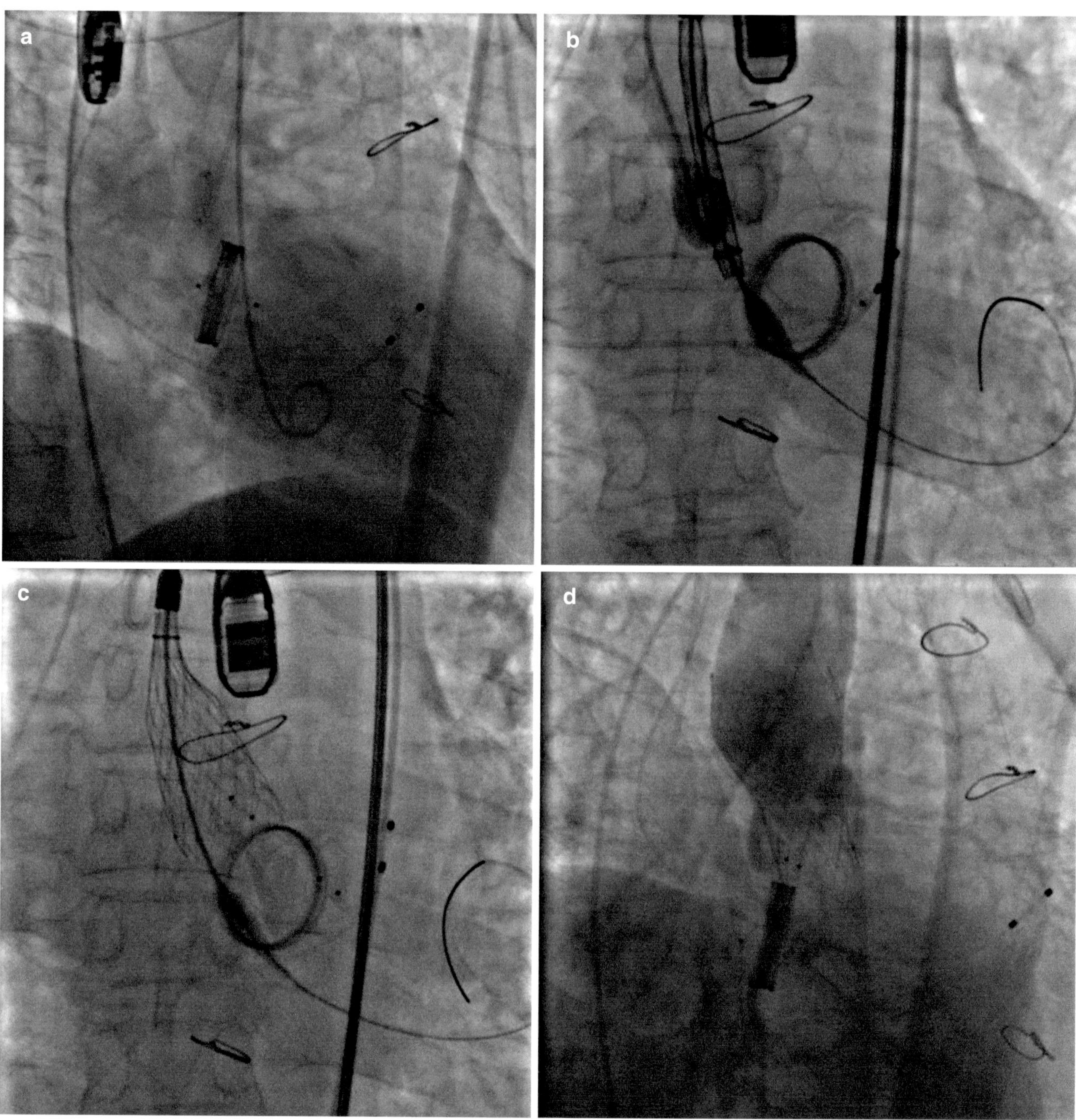

Fig. 6.45 Paravalvular leak occlusion + TAVR angiographic images. (**a**) Mitral leak occlusion via retrograde femoral artery under local anesthesia; (**b**) TAVR via the carotid artery approach; (**c**) Deployment of the stent valve; (**d**) Postoperative angiography showed that there was no interference between the stent aortic valve and the mitral valve mechanical valve, and the occluder position was good, which did not affect the opening and closing of the mechanical valve. The imaging data were obtained from the Cardiovascular Surgery Department of Fuwai Hospital, Chinese Academy of Medical Sciences, and Xijing Hospital

obvious advantages in safety and effectiveness, especially for high-risk patients with paravalvular leaks undergoing reoperation. Current clinical data show that interventional occlusion for paravalvular leak achieves satisfactory results, relieves patients' pain, simplifies treatment methods, and reduces medical costs [105, 115, 116]. In the future, more centers in China will collaborate to further improve the technology and improve the success rate and effectiveness of treatment. We should also note that paravalvular leaks have a certain randomness, high variation, and strong demand for individualized treatment. According to the 3D-printed paravalvular leak model, the location of the paravalvular leak can

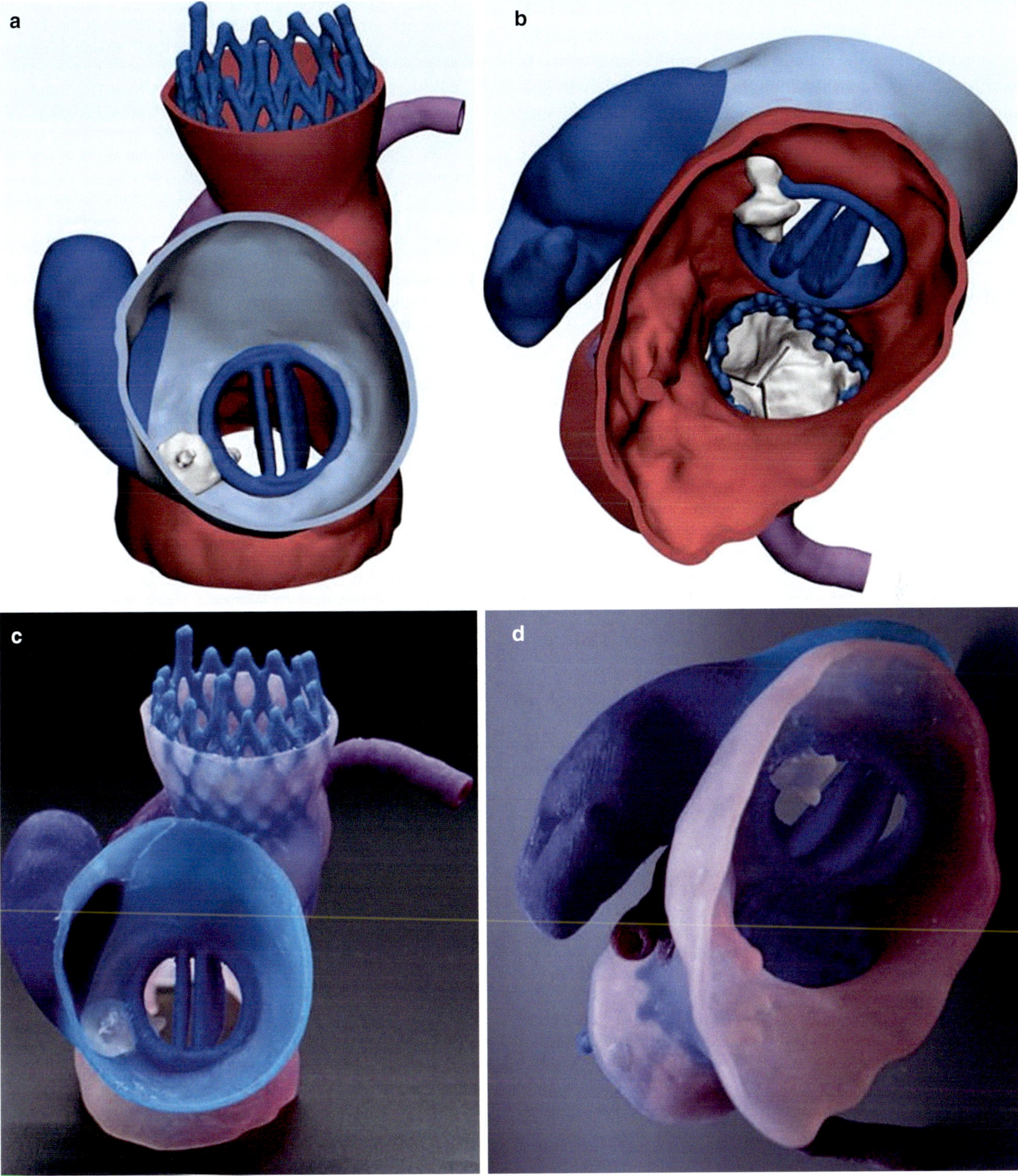

Fig. 6.46 Three-dimensional printing technology for cardiovascular surgery was used to evaluate the clinical efficacy of paravalvular leak occlusion plus TAVR. (**a**) Computer model from the left atrial view after operation; (**b**) Computer model from the left ventricular view after operation; (**c**) 3D model from the left atrial view after operation; (**d**) 3D model from the left ventricular view after operation. The image data, computer three-dimensional reconstruction, and three-dimensional printing model were obtained from the Cardiovascular Surgery Department of Fuwai Hospital, Chinese Academy of Medical Sciences, and Xijing Hospital

be determined, the time of passing through paravalvular leak can be shortened, and the appropriate type of occluder can be selected to reduce the occurrence of complications, which is worthy of further consideration. In the near future, individualized occluders based on different shapes of paravalvular leaks could be manufactured by 3D printing technology, which may provide new avenues for the treatment of paravalvular leaks, the most complex and intractable structural heart disease [11].

References

Section 6.1

1. Bonow RO, Carabello BA, Chatterjee K, JAC DL, Faxon DP, Freed MD, Gaasch WH, Lytle BW, Nishimura RA, O'Gara PT, O'Rourke RA, Otto CM, Shah PM, Shanewise JS, JSC S, Jacobs AK, Adams CD, Anderson JL, Antman EM, Faxon DP, Fuster V, Halperin JL, Hiratzka LF, Hunt SA, Lytle BW, Nishimura R, Page RL, Riegel B. ACC/AHA 2006 practice guidelines for the management of patients with valvular heart disease: executive summary: a report of the American College of Cardiology/American Heart Association Task Force on Practice Guidelines (writing committee to revise the 1998 guidelines for the management of patients with valvular heart disease) developed in collaboration with the society of cardiovascular anesthesiologists endorsed by the society for cardiovascular angiography and interventions and the society of thoracic surgeons. J Am Coll Cardiol. 2006;48:598–675.
2. Vahanian A, Alfieri O, Andreotti F, Antunes MJ, Baron-Esquivias G, Baumgartner H, Borger MA, Carrel TP, De Bonis M, Evangelista A, Falk V, Iung B, Lancellotti P, Pierard L, Price S, Schafers HJ, Schuler G, Stepinska J, Swedberg K, Takkenberg J, Von Oppell UO, Windecker S, Zamorano JL, Zembala M. Guidelines on the management of valvular heart disease (version 2012). Eur Heart J. 2012;33:2451–96.
3. Nishimura RA, Otto CM, Bonow RO, Carabello BA, Erwin JP 3rd, Guyton RA, O'Gara PT, Ruiz CE, Skubas NJ, Sorajja P, Sundt TM 3rd, Thomas JD. American College of Cardiology/American Heart Association Task Force on Practice G. 2014 AHA/ACC guideline for the management of patients with valvular heart disease: a report of the American College of Cardiology/American Heart Association Task Force on Practice Guidelines. J Am Coll Cardiol. 2014;63:e57–185.
4. Baumgartner H, Falk V, Bax JJ, De Bonis M, Hamm C, Holm PJ, Iung B, Lancellotti P, Lansac E, Munoz DR, Rosenhek R, Sjogren J, Tornos Mas P, Vahanian A, Walther T, Wendler O, Windecker S, Zamorano JL, Group ESCSD. 2017 ESC/EACTS guidelines for the management of valvular heart disease. Eur Heart J. 2017;38:2739–91.
5. Cribier A, Eltchaninoff H, Bash A, Borenstein N, Tron C, Bauer F, Derumeaux G, Anselme F, Laborde F, Leon MB. Percutaneous transcatheter implantation of an aortic valve prosthesis for calcific aortic stenosis: first human case description. Circulation. 2002;106:3006–8.
6. Popma JJ, Deeb GM, Yakubov SJ, Mumtaz M, Gada H, O'Hair D, Bajwa T, Heiser JC, Merhi W, Kleiman NS, Askew J, Sorajja P, Rovin J, Chetcuti SJ, Adams DH, Teirstein PS, Zorn GL 3rd, Forrest JK, Tchetche D, Resar J, Walton A, Piazza N, Ramlawi B, Robinson N, Petrossian G, Gleason TG, Oh JK, Boulware MJ, Qiao H, Mugglin AS, Reardon MJ. Evolut low risk trial I. Transcatheter aortic-valve replacement with a self-expanding valve in low-risk patients. N Engl J Med. 2019;380:1706–15.
7. Mack MJ, Leon MB, Thourani VH, Makkar R, Kodali SK, Russo M, Kapadia SR, Malaisrie SC, Cohen DJ, Pibarot P, Leipsic J, Hahn RT, Blanke P, Williams MR, McCabe JM, Brown DL, Babaliaros V, Goldman S, Szeto WY, Genereux P, Pershad A, Pocock SJ, Alu MC, Webb JG, Smith CR, Investigators P. Transcatheter aortic-valve replacement with a balloon-expandable valve in low-risk patients. N Engl J Med. 2019;380:1695–705.
8. O'Neill B, Wang DD, Pantelic M, Song T, Guerrero M, Greenbaum A, O'Neill WW. Transcatheter caval valve implantation using multimodality imaging: roles of TEE, CT, and 3D printing. J Am Coll Cardiol Img. 2015;8:221–5.
9. Jilaihawi H, Kashif M, Fontana G, Furugen A, Shiota T, Friede G, Makhija R, Doctor N, Leon MB, Makkar RR. Cross-sectional computed tomographic assessment improves accuracy of aortic annular sizing for transcatheter aortic valve replacement and reduces the incidence of paravalvular aortic regurgitation. J Am Coll Cardiol. 2012;59:1275–86.
10. Farooqi KM, Sengupta PP. Echocardiography and three-dimensional printing: sound ideas to touch a heart. J Am Soc Echocardiogr. 2015;28:398–403.
11. Qian Z, Wang K, Liu S, Zhou X, Rajagopal V, Meduri C, Kauten JR, Chang YH, Wu C, Zhang C, Wang B, Vannan MA. Quantitative prediction of paravalvular leak in transcatheter aortic valve replacement based on tissue-mimicking 3D printing. J Am Coll Cardiol Img. 2017;10:719–31.
12. Wei L, Liu H, Zhu L, Yang Y, Zheng J, Guo K, Luo H, Zhao W, Yang X, Maimaiti A, Wang C. A new transcatheter aortic valve replacement system for predominant aortic regurgitation implantation of the j-valve and early outcome. JACC Cardiovasc Interv. 2015;8:1831–41.
13. Zhu D, Hu J, Meng W, Guo Y. Successful transcatheter aortic valve implantation for pure aortic regurgitation using a new second generation self-expanding j-valve(tm) system – the first in-man implantation. Heart Lung Circ. 2015;24:411–4.
14. Liao YB, Zhao ZG, Wei X, Xu YN, Zuo ZL, Li YJ, Zheng MX, Feng Y, Chen M. Transcatheter aortic valve implantation with the self-expandable venus A-valve and CoreValve devices: preliminary experiences in China. Catheter Cardiovasc Interv. 2017;89:528–33.
15. Zhu Y, Liu J, Wang L, Guan X, Luo Y, Geng J, Geng Q, Lin Y, Zhang L, Li X, Lu Y. Preliminary study of the application of transthoracic echocardiography-guided three-dimensional printing for the assessment of structural heart disease. Echocardiography. 2017;34:1903–8.
16. Ripley B, Kelil T, Cheezum MK, Goncalves A, Di Carli MF, Rybicki FJ, Steigner M, Mitsouras D, Blankstein R. 3D printing based on cardiac CT assists anatomic visualization prior to transcatheter aortic valve replacement. J Cardiovasc Comput Tomogr. 2016;10:28–36.
17. Gallo M, D'Onofrio A, Tarantini G, Nocerino E, Remondino F, Gerosa G. 3d-printing model for complex aortic transcatheter valve treatment. Int J Cardiol. 2016;210:139–40.
18. Hernandez-Enriquez M, Brugaletta S, Andreu D, Macia-Munoz G, Castrejon-Subira M, Fernandez-Suelves S, Hernandez-Obiols M, Dantas AP, Freixa X, Martin-Yuste V, Camara O, Sabate M. Three-dimensional printing of an aortic model for transcatheter aortic valve implantation: possible clinical applications. Int J Cardiovasc Imaging. 2017;33:283–5.
19. Maragiannis D, Jackson MS, Igo SR, Schutt RC, Connell P, Grande-Allen J, Barker CM, Chang SM, Reardon MJ, Zoghbi WA, Little SH. Replicating patient-specific severe aortic valve stenosis with functional 3D modeling. Circ Cardiovasc Imaging. 2015;8:e003626.

20. Leon MB, Smith CR, Mack M, Miller DC, Moses JW, Svensson LG, Tuzcu EM, Webb JG, Fontana GP, Makkar RR, Brown DL, Block PC, Guyton RA, Pichard AD, Bavaria JE, Herrmann HC, Douglas PS, Petersen JL, Akin JJ, Anderson WN, Wang D, Pocock S. Transcatheter aortic-valve implantation for aortic stenosis in patients who cannot undergo surgery. N Engl J Med. 2010;363:1597–607.
21. Kodali SK, Williams MR, Smith CR, Svensson LG, Webb JG, Makkar RR, Fontana GP, Dewey TM, Thourani VH, Pichard AD, Fischbein M, Szeto WY, Lim S, Greason KL, Teirstein PS, Malaisrie SC, Douglas PS, Hahn RT, Whisenant B, Zajarias A, Wang D, Akin JJ, Anderson WN, Leon MB. Two-year outcomes after transcatheter or surgical aortic-valve replacement. N Engl J Med. 2012;366:1686–95.
22. Reardon MJ, Van Mieghem NM, Popma JJ, Kleiman NS, Sondergaard L, Mumtaz M, Adams DH, Deeb GM, Maini B, Gada H, Chetcuti S, Gleason T, Heiser J, Lange R, Merhi W, Oh JK, Olsen PS, Piazza N, Williams M, Windecker S, Yakubov SJ, Grube E, Makkar R, Lee JS, Conte J, Vang E, Nguyen H, Chang Y, Mugglin AS, Serruys PW, Kappetein AP, Investigators S. Surgical or transcatheter aortic valve replacement in intermediate-risk patients. N Engl J Med. 2017;376:1321–31.
23. Toggweiler S, Stortecky S, Holy E, Zuk K, Cuculi F, Nietlispach F, Sabti Z, Suciu R, Maier W, Jamshidi P, Maisano F, Windecker S, Kobza R, Wenaweser P, Luscher TF, Binder RK. The electrocardiogram after transcatheter aortic valve replacement determines the risk for post-procedural high-degree AV block and the need for telemetry monitoring. JACC Cardiovasc Interv. 2016;9:1269–76.
24. Urena M, Rodes-Cabau J. Permanent pacemaker implantation following transcatheter aortic valve replacement: still a concern? JACC Cardiovasc Interv. 2015;8:70–3.
25. Pilgrim T, Kalesan B, Wenaweser P, Huber C, Stortecky S, Buellesfeld L, Khattab AA, Eberle B, Gloekler S, Gsponer T, Meier B, Juni P, Carrel T, Windecker S. Predictors of clinical outcomes in patients with severe aortic stenosis undergoing TAVI: a multistate analysis. Circ Cardiovasc Interv. 2012;5:856–61.
26. Virk SA, Tian DH, Liou K, Pathan F, Villanueva C, Akhunji Z, Cao C. Systematic review of percutaneous coronary intervention and transcatheter aortic valve implantation for concomitant aortic stenosis and coronary artery disease. Int J Cardiol. 2015;187:453–5.
27. Sarangi S, Rihal CS, Bruce CJ, Greason KL, Gossl M, Nishimura RA, Suri RM. Left main coronary artery protection during transcatheter aortic valve deployment. J Am Coll Cardiol. 2014;63:1583.
28. So CY, Fan Y, Wu EB, Lee AP. 3d printing in transcatheter aortic valve implantation: anticipating coronary obstruction in high risk aortic root anatomy. EuroIntervention. 2019;15 https://doi.org/10.4244/EIJ-D-19-00609.
29. Kanjanahattakij N, Horn B, Vutthikraivit W, Biso SM, Ziccardi MR, Lu MLR, Rattanawong P. Comparing outcomes after transcatheter aortic valve replacement in patients with stenotic bicuspid and tricuspid aortic valve: a systematic review and meta-analysis. Clin Cardiol. 2018;41:896–902.
30. Kong WKF, Regeer MV, Poh KK, Yip JW, van Rosendael PJ, Yeo TC, Tay E, Kamperidis V, van der Velde ET, Mertens B, Ajmone Marsan N, Delgado V, Bax JJ. Inter-ethnic differences in valve morphology, valvular dysfunction, and aortopathy between Asian and European patients with bicuspid aortic valve. Eur Heart J. 2018;39:1308–13.
31. Kim MS, Hansgen AR, Wink O, Quaife RA, Carroll JD. Rapid prototyping: a new tool in understanding and treating structural heart disease. Circulation. 2008;117:2388–94.

Section 6.2

32. Alfieri O, Maisano F, Colombo A. Future of transcatheter repair of the mitral valve. Am J Cardiol. 2005;96(12A):71L–5L.
33. Al-Lawati A, Cheung A. Transcatheter mitral valve replacement. Interv Cardiol Clin. 2016;5(1):109–15.
34. Babaliaros VC, Greenbaum AB, Khan JM, Rogers T, Wang DD, Eng MH, et al. Intentional percutaneous laceration of the anterior mitral leaflet to prevent outflow obstruction during transcatheter mitral valve replacement: first-in-human experience. JACC Cardiovasc Interv. 2017;10(8):798–809.
35. Bagur R, Cheung A, Chu MWA, Kiaii B. 3-dimensional-printed model for planning transcatheter mitral valve replacement. JACC Cardiovasc Interv. 2018;11(8):812–3.
36. Capretti G, Urena M, Himbert D, Brochet E, Goublaire C, Verdonk C, et al. Valve thrombosis after transcatheter mitral valve replacement. J Am Coll Cardiol. 2016;68(16):1814–5.
37. Chiam PT, Ruiz CE. Percutaneous transcatheter mitral valve repair: a classification of the technology. JACC Cardiovasc Interv. 2011;4(1):1–13.
38. El Sabbagh A, Eleid MF, Matsumoto JM, Anavekar NS, Al-Hijji MA, Said SM, et al. Three-dimensional prototyping for procedural simulation of transcatheter mitral valve replacement in patients with mitral annular calcification. Catheter Cardiovasc Interv. 2018;92(7):E537–E49.
39. Guerrero M, Eleid M, Foley T, Said S, Rihal C. Transseptal transcatheter mitral valve replacement in severe mitral annular calcification (transseptal valve-in-MAC). Ann Cardiothor Surg. 2018;7(6):830–3.
40. Izzo RL, O'Hara RP, Iyer V, Hansen R, Meess KM, Nagesh SVS, et al. 3D printed cardiac phantom for procedural planning of a transcatheter native mitral valve replacement. Proc SPIE Int Soc Opt Eng. 2016;9789
41. Kohli K, Wei ZA, Yoganathan AP, Oshinski JN, Leipsic J, Blanke P. Transcatheter mitral valve planning and the neo-LVOT: utilization of virtual simulation models and 3D printing. Curr Treat Options Cardiovasc Med. 2018;20(12):99.
42. Lim DS, Reynolds MR, Feldman T, Kar S, Herrmann HC, Wang A, et al. Improved functional status and quality of life in prohibitive surgical risk patients with degenerative mitral regurgitation after transcatheter mitral valve repair. J Am Coll Cardiol. 2014;64(2):182–92.
43. Muller DWM, Farivar RS, Jansz P, Bae R, Walters D, Clarke A, et al. Transcatheter mitral valve replacement for patients with symptomatic mitral regurgitation: a global feasibility trial. J Am Coll Cardiol. 2017;69(4):381–91.
44. Rasla S, El Meligy A, Marmoush F. The feasibility of transcatheter mitral valve replacement for patients with symptomatic mitral regurgitation. J Am Coll Cardiol. 2017;69(25):3123–4.
45. Sorajja P, Mack M, Vemulapalli S, Holmes DR Jr, Stebbins A, Kar S, et al. Initial experience with commercial transcatheter mitral valve repair in the United States. J Am Coll Cardiol. 2016;67(10):1129–40.
46. Stone GW, Lindenfeld J, Abraham WT, Kar S, Lim DS, Mishell JM, et al. Transcatheter mitral-valve repair in patients with heart failure. N Engl J Med. 2018;379(24):2307–18.
47. Takagi H, Hari Y, Kawai N, Kuno T, Ando T, Group A. Transcatheter mitral valve replacement for mitral regurgitation-a meta-analysis. J Card Surg. 2018;33(12):827–35.
48. Vaquerizo B, Theriault-Lauzier P, Piazza N. Percutaneous transcatheter mitral valve replacement: patient-specific three-dimensional computer-based heart model and prototyping. Revista Espanola de Cardiologia. 2015;68(12):1165–73.

49. Vukicevic M, Puperi DS, Jane Grande-Allen K, Little SH. 3D printed modeling of the mitral valve for catheter-based structural interventions. Ann Biomed Eng. 2017;45(2):508–19.
50. Wang DD, Eng M, Greenbaum A, Myers E, Forbes M, Pantelic M, et al. Predicting LVOT obstruction after TMVR. J Am Coll Cardiol Img. 2016;9(11):1349–52.
51. Wang DD, Eng MH, Greenbaum AB, Myers E, Forbes M, Karabon P, et al. Validating a prediction modeling tool for left ventricular outflow tract (LVOT) obstruction after transcatheter mitral valve replacement (TMVR). Catheter Cardiovasc Interv. 2018;92(2):379–87.
52. Li P. 3D printing contributes to high-risk transcatheter mitral valve implantation. Chin J Cardiovasc Med. 2017;22(06):381.
53. Liu XB, Pu ZX, Yu L, Feng Y, He W, Lin JJ, et al. A single center experience of transcatheter mitral valve repair. Chin J Intervent Cardiol. 2014;22(07):448–51.
54. Pan WZ, Zhou DX, Ge JB. Transcatheter mitral regurgitation therapeutics: state-of-art 2018. Chin J Front Med Sci. 2018;10(01):1–5.
55. Qin Y, Xu CN, Yang J. Clinical application and prospect of transapical mitral valve replacement. Chin J Intervent Cardiol. 2019;27(02):115–8.
56. Yang DT, He XJ, Yang J. Development of transcatheter mitral valve implantation. Chin Heart J. 2017;29(04):482–6.

Section 6.3

57. Rogers JH, Bolling SF. The tricuspid valve: current perspective and evolving management of tricuspid regurgitation. Circulation. 2009;119:2718–25.
58. Looi JL, Lee AP-W, Wong RHL, Yu C-M. 3D echocardiography for traumatic tricuspid regurgitation. JACC Cardiovasc Imaging. 2012;5:1285–7.
59. Latib A, Grigioni F, Hahn RT. Tricuspid regurgitation: what is the real clinical impact and how often should it be treated? EuroIntervention. 2018;14:AB101–11.
60. Lauten A, Figulla HR. Tricuspid valve interventions in 2015. EuroIntervention. 2015;11:W133-6.
61. Vahanian A, Alfieri O, Andreotti F, Antunes MJ, Barón-Esquivias G, Baumgartner H, Borger MA, Carrel TP, Bonis MD, Evangelista A, Falk V, Lung B, Lancellotti P, Pierard L, Price S, Schäfers H-J, Schuler G, Stepinska J, Swedberg K, Takkenberg J, UOV O, Windecker S, Zamorano JL, Zembala M. Guidelines on the management of valvular heart disease (version 2012): the joint task force on the management of Valvular heart disease of the European Society of Cardiology (ESC) and the European Association for Cardio-Thoracic Surgery (EACTS). Eur J Cardiothorac Surg. 2012;42:S1–S44.
62. Iung B, Baron G, Butchart EG, Delahaye F, Gohlke-Bärwolf C, Levang OW, Tornos P, Vanoverschelde J-L, Vermeer F, Boersma E, Ravaud P, Vahanian A. A prospective survey of patients with valvular heart disease in Europe: the euro heart survey on valvular heart disease. Eur Heart J. 2003;24:1231–43.
63. Nishimura RA, Otto CM, Bonow RO, Carabello BA, Erwin JP 3rd, Guyton RA, O'Gara PT, Ruiz CE, Skubas NJ, Sorajja P, Sundt TM 3rd, Thomas JD, Members AATF. 2014 AHA/ACC Guideline for the Management of Patients with Valvular Heart Disease: executive summary: a report of the American College of Cardiology/American Heart Association Task Force on Practice Guidelines. Circulation. 2014;129:2440–92.
64. Rogers JH. Functional tricuspid regurgitation: percutaneous therapies needed. JACC Cardiovasc Interv. 2015;8:492–4.
65. Lauten A, Doenst T, Hamadanchi A, Franz M, Figulla HR. Percutaneous bicaval valve implantation for transcatheter treatment of tricuspid regurgitation: clinical observations and 12-month follow-up. Circ Cardiovasc Interv. 2014;7:268–72.
66. Lauten A, Figulla HR, Unbehaun A, Fam N, Schofer J, Doenst T, Hausleiter J, Franz M, Jung C, Dreger H, Leistner D, Alushi B, Stundl A, Landmesser U, Falk V, Stangl K, Laule M. Interventional treatment of severe tricuspid regurgitation: early clinical experience in a multicenter, observational, first-in-man study. Circ Cardiovasc Interv. 2018;11:e006061.
67. Besler C, Meduri CU, Lurz P. Transcatheter treatment of functional tricuspid regurgitation using the Trialign device. Interv Cardiol. 2018;13:8–13.
68. Nickenig G, Kowalski M, Hausleiter J, Braun D, Schofer J, Yzeiraj E, Rudolph V, Friedrichs K, Maisano F, Taramasso M, Fam N, Bianchi G, Bedogni F, Denti P, Alfieri O, Latib A, Colombo A, Hammerstingl C, Schueler R. Transcatheter treatment of severe tricuspid regurgitation with the edge-to-edge MitraClip technique. Circulation. 2017;135:1802–14.
69. Andreas M, Russo M, Taramasso M, Zuber M, Mascherbauer J. Novel transcatheter clip device (MitraClip XTR) enables significant tricuspid annular size reduction. Eur Heart J Cardiovasc Imaging. 2019;20:1070.
70. Ledwoch J, Fellner C, Poch F, Schlatterbeck L, Dommasch M, Dirschinger R, Stundl A, Laugwitz KL, Kupatt C, Hoppmann P. Reverse cardiac remodeling after Transcatheter treatment of severe tricuspid regurgitation using the edge-to-edge MitraClip technique. J Invasive Cardiol. 2019;31:89–93.
71. Azeem Latib M, Eustachio Agricola M, Alberto Pozzoli M, Paolo Denti M, Maurizio Taramasso M, Pietro Spagnolo M, Jean-Michel Juliard M, Eric Brochet M, Phalla Ou M, Maurice Enriquez-Sarano M, Francesco Grigioni M, Ottavio Alfieri M, Alec Vahanian M, Antonio Colombo M, Francesco Maisano M. First-in-man implantation of a tricuspid annular remodeling device for functional tricuspid regurgitation. JACC Cardiovasc Interv. 2015;8:E211–4.
72. Lauten A, Ferrari M, Hekmat K, Pfeifer R, Dannberg G, Ragoschke-Schumm A, Figulla HR. Heterotopic transcatheter tricuspid valve implantation: first-in-man application of a novel approach to tricuspid regurgitation. Eur Heart J. 2011;32:1207–13.
73. Laule M, Stangl V, Sanad W, Lembcke A, Baumann G, Stangl K. Percutaneous Transfemoral Management of Severe Secondary Tricuspid Regurgitation with Edwards Sapien XT bioprosthesis first-in-man experience. J Am Coll Cardiol. 2013;61:1929–31.
74. Wang DD, Lee JC, O'Neill BP, O'Neill WW. Multimodality imaging of the tricuspid valve for assessment and guidance of Transcatheter repair. Interv Cardiol Clin. 2018;7:379–86.
75. Asmarats L, Puri R, Latib A, Navia JL, Rodes-Cabau J. Transcatheter tricuspid valve interventions: landscape, challenges, and future directions. J Am Coll Cardiol. 2018;71:2935–56.
76. Borer JS. Application of Transcatheter repair to tricuspid regurgitation: still looking through a dark glass. J Am Coll Cardiol. 2019;73:1916–8.

Section 6.4

77. Chen C, Cheng T, Huang T, Zhou U, Chen J, Huang Y, Li H. Percutaneous balloon valvuloplasty for pulmonic stenosis in adolescents and adults. N Engl J Med. 1996;335:21–5.
78. Nishimura RA, Otto CM, Bonow RO, Carabello BA, Erwin JP, Guyton RA, O'Gara PT, Ruiz CE, Skubas NJ, Sorajja P, Sundt TM, Thomas JD. AHA/ACC guideline for the management of patients with valvular heart disease: executive summary: a report of the American College of Cardiology/American Heart Association Task Force on Practice Guidelines. Circulation. 2014;2014 https://doi.org/10.1161/CIR.0000000000000029.

79. Bonhoeffer P, Boudjemline Y, Saliba Z, Merckx J, Aggoun Y, Bonnet D, Acar P, Le Bidois J, Sidi D, Kachaner J. Percutaneous replacement of pulmonary valve in a right-ventricle to pulmonary-artery prosthetic conduit with valve dysfunction. Lancet. 2000;356:1403–5.
80. Bonhoeffer P, Boudjemline Y, Qureshi SA, Le Bidois J, Iserin L, Acar P, Merckx J, Kachaner J, Sidi D. Percutaneous insertion of the pulmonary valve. J Am Coll Cardiol. 2002;39:1664–9.
81. Khambadkone S, Coats L, Taylor A, Boudjemline Y, Derrick G, Tsang V, Cooper J, Muthurangu V, Hegde SR, Razavi RS, Pellerin D, Deanfield J, Bonhoeffer P. Percutaneous pulmonary valve implantation in humans: results in 59 consecutive patients. Circulation. 2005;112:1189–97.
82. Coats L, Khambadkone S, Derrick G, Hughes M, Jones R, Mist B, Pellerin D, Marek J, Deanfield JE, Bonhoeffer P, Taylor AM. Physiological consequences of percutaneous pulmonary valve implantation: the different behaviour of volume- and pressure-overloaded ventricles. Eur Heart J. 2007;28:1886–93.
83. Kenny D, Hijazi ZM, Kar S, Rhodes J, Mullen M, Makkar R, Shirali G, Fogel M, Fahey J, Heitschmidt MG, Cain C. Percutaneous implantation of the Edwards SAPIEN transcatheter heart valve for conduit failure in the pulmonary position: early phase 1 results from an international multicenter clinical trial. J Am Coll Cardiol. 2011;58:2248–56.
84. Faza N, Kenny D, Kavinsky C, Amin Z, Heitschmidt M, Hijazi ZM. Single-center comparative outcomes of the Edwards SAPIEN and Medtronic melody transcatheter heart valves in the pulmonary position. Catheter Cardiovasc Interv. 2013;82:E535–41.
85. Gillespie MJ, Rome JJ, Levi DS, Williams RJ, Rhodes JF, Cheatham JP, Hellenbrand WE, Jones TK, Vincent JA, Zahn EM, McElhinney DB. Melody valve implant within failed bioprosthetic valves in the pulmonary position: a multicenter experience. Circ Cardiovasc Interv. 2012;5:862–70.
86. Petit CJ, Justino H, Ing FF. Melody valve implantation in the pulmonary and tricuspid position. Catheter Cardiovasc Interv. 2013;82:E944–6.
87. Cheatham JP, Hellenbrand WE, Zahn EM, Jones TK, Berman DP, Vincent JA, McElhinney DB. Clinical and hemodynamic outcomes up to 7 years after transcatheter pulmonary valve replacement in the us melody valve investigational device exemption trial. Circulation. 2015;131:1960–70.
88. Hascoet S, Karsenty C, Tortigue M, Watkins AC, Riou J-Y, Boet A, Tahhan N, Fabre D, Haulon S, Brenot P, Petit J. A modified procedure for percutaneous pulmonary valve implantation of the Edwards SAPIEN 3 valve. EuroIntervention. 2019;14:1386–8.
89. Jones TK, Rome JJ, Armstrong AK, Berger F, Hellenbrand WE, Cabalka AK, Benson LN, Balzer DT, Cheatham JP, Eicken A, McElhinney DB. Transcatheter pulmonary valve replacement reduces tricuspid regurgitation in patients with right ventricular volume/pressure overload. J Am Coll Cardiol. 2016;68:1525–35.
90. Eicken A, Ewert P, Hager A, Peters B, Fratz S, Kuehne T, Busch R, Hess J, Berger F. Percutaneous pulmonary valve implantation: two-Centre experience with more than 100 patients. Eur Heart J. 2011;32:1260–5.
91. Morgan G, Prachasilchai P, Promphan W, Rosenthal E, Sivakumar K, Kappanayil M, Sakidjan I, Walsh KP, Kenny D, Thomson J, Koneti NR, Awasthy N, Thanopoulos B, Roymanee S, Qureshi S. Medium-term results of percutaneous pulmonary valve implantation using the venus p-valve: international experience. EuroIntervention. 2019;14:1363–70.
92. Armillotta A, Bonhoeffer P, Dubini G, Ferragina S, Migliavacca F, Sala G, Schievano S. Use of rapid prototyping models in the planning of percutaneous pulmonary valved stent implantation. Proc Inst Mech Eng H J Eng Med. 2007;221:407–16.
93. Poterucha JT, Foley TA, Taggart NW. Percutaneous pulmonary valve implantation in a native outflow tract: 3-dimensional DynaCT rotational angiographic reconstruction and 3-dimensional printed model. JACC Cardiovasc Interv. 2014;7:E151–2.
94. Valverde I, Sarnago F, Prieto R, Zunzunegui JL. Three-dimensional printing in vitro simulation of percutaneous pulmonary valve implantation in large right ventricular outflow tract. Eur Heart J. 2017;38:1262–3.
95. Schievano S, Migliavacca F, Coats L, Khambadkone S, Carminati M, Wilson N, Deanfield JE, Bonhoeffer P, Taylor AM. Percutaneous pulmonary valve implantation based on rapid prototyping of right ventricular outflow tract and pulmonary trunk from MR data. Radiology. 2007;242:490–7.

Section 6.5

96. Kliger C, Eiros R, Isasti G, Einhorn B, Jelnin V, Cohen H, Kronzon I, Perk G, Fontana GP, Ruiz CE. Review of surgical prosthetic paravalvular leaks: diagnosis and catheter-based closure. Eur Heart J. 2013;34:638–49.
97. Ruiz CE, Hahn RT, Berrebi A, Borer JS, Cutlip DE, Fontana G, Gerosa G, Ibrahim R, Jelnin V, Jilaihawi H, Jolicoeur EM, Kliger C, Kronzon I, Leipsic J, Maisano F, Millan X, Nataf P, O'Gara PT, Pibarot P, Ramee SR, Rihal CS, Rodes-Cabau J, Sorajja P, Suri R, Swain JA, Turi ZG, Tuzcu EM, Weissman NJ, Zamorano JL, Serruys PW, Leon MB, Paravalvular Leak Academic Research C. Clinical trial principles and endpoint definitions for paravalvular leaks in surgical prosthesis: an expert statement. J Am Coll Cardiol. 2017;69:2067–87.
98. Spoon DB, Malouf JF, Spoon JN, Nkomo VT, Sorajja P, Mankad SV, Lennon RJ, Cabalka AK, Rihal CS. Mitral paravalvular leak: description and assessment of a novel anatomical method of localization. JACC Cardiovasc Imaging. 2013;6:1212–4.
99. Lesser JR, Kelly B, Newell M, Schwartz RS, Pedersen W, Sorajja P. Use of cardiac ct angiography to assist in the diagnosis and treatment of aortic prosthetic paravalvular leak: a practical guide. J Cardiovasc Comput Tomogr. 2015;9:159–64.
100. Hourihan M, Perry SB, Mandell VS, Keane JF, Rome JJ, Bittl JA, Lock JE. Transcatheter umbrella closure of valvular and paravalvular leaks. J Am Coll Cardiol. 1992;20:1371–8.
101. Backer OD, Piazza N, Banai S, Lutter G, Maisano F, Herrmann HC, Franzen OW, Søndergaard L. Percutaneous transcatheter mitral valve replacement: an overview of devices in preclinical and early clinical evaluation. Circ Cardiovasc Interv. 2014;7:400–9.
102. Gossl M, Rihal CS. Percutaneous treatment of aortic and mitral valve paravalvular regurgitation. Curr Cardiol Rep. 2013;15:388.
103. Reed GW, Tuzcu EM, Kapadia SR, Krishnaswamy A. Catheter-based closure of paravalvular leak. Expert Rev Cardiovasc Ther. 2014;12:681–92.
104. Jilaihawi I. Complex transcatheter paravalvular leak repair. Catheter Cardiovasc Interv. 2010;76:194–7.
105. Ruiz CE, Jelnin V, Kliger C, Kronzon I, Leipsic J, Maisano F, Millan X, Nataf P, O'Gara PT, Pibarot P, Rodes-Cabau J, Ramee SR, Rihal CS, Sorajja P, Hahn RT, Leon MB, Suri R, Tuzcu EM, Swain JA, Turi ZG, et al. Clinical trial principles and endpoint definitions for paravalvular leaks in surgical prosthesis: an expert statement. J Am Coll Cardiol. 2017;69:2067–87.
106. Nishimura RA, Otto CM, Bonow RO, Carabello BA, Erwin JP 3rd, Guyton RA, O'Gara PT, Ruiz CE, Skubas NJ, Sorajja P, Sundt TM 3rd, Thomas JD, Members AATF. 2014 AHA/ACC guideline for the management of patients with valvular heart disease: a report of the American College of Cardiology/American Heart Association Task Force on Practice Guidelines. Circulation. 2014;129:e521–643.
107. Nishimura RA, Otto CM, Bonow RO, Carabello BA, Erwin JP 3rd, Fleisher LA, Jneid H, Mack MJ, McLeod CJ, O'Gara PT, Rigolin VH, Sundt TM 3rd, Thompson A. 2017 AHA/ACC focused update

of the 2014 AHA/ACC guideline for the management of patients with valvular heart disease: a report of the American College of Cardiology/American Heart Association Task Force on Clinical Practice Guidelines. Circulation. 2017;135:e1159–95.

108. Sorajja P, Cabalka AK, Hagler DJ, Rihal CS. Long-term follow-up of percutaneous repair of paravalvular prosthetic regurgitation. J Am Coll Cardiol. 2011;58:2218–24.
109. Sorajja P, Cabalka AK, Hagler DJ, Rihal CS. Percutaneous repair of paravalvular prosthetic regurgitation: acute and 30-day outcomes in 115 patients/clinical perspective. Circ Cardiovasc Interv. 2011;4:314–21.
110. Ruiz CE, Jelnin V, Kronzon I, Dudiy Y, Del Valle-Fernandez R, Einhorn BN, Chiam PTL, Martinez C, Eiros R, Roubin G, Cohen HA. Clinical outcomes in patients undergoing percutaneous closure of periprosthetic paravalvular leaks. J Am Coll Cardiol. 2011;58:2210–7.
111. Toggweiler S, Humphries KH, Lee M, Binder RK, Moss RR, Freeman M, Ye J, Cheung A, Wood DA, Webb JG. 5-year outcome after transcatheter aortic valve implantation. J Am Coll Cardiol. 2013;61:413–9.
112. Mehran R, Sorrentino S, Claessen BE. Paravalvular leak: an interesting interplay of acquired VWF-disease and late bleeding after TAVR. J Am Coll Cardiol. 2018;72:2149–51.
113. Genereux P, Head SJ, Hahn R, Daneault B, Kodali S, Williams MR, van Mieghem NM, Alu MC, Serruys PW, Kappetein AP, Leon MB. Paravalvular leak after transcatheter aortic valve replacement: the new Achilles' heel? A comprehensive review of the literature. J Am Coll Cardiol. 2013;61:1125–36.
114. Xu CN, Li XF, Chen WS, Yang XL, Wang XW, Zhu YS, Li HL, Ma R, Chen M, Yu SQ, Yang J. Efficacy of interventional therapy on paravalvular leakage after mitral valve replacement. Zhonghua Xin Xue Guan Bing Za Zhi. 2016;44:238–43.
115. Sorajja P, Cabalka AK, Hagler DJ, Rihal CS. The learning curve in percutaneous repair of paravalvular prosthetic regurgitation: an analysis of 200 cases. J Am Coll Cardiol Intv. 2014;7:521–9.
116. Mookadam F, Raslan SF, Jiamsripong P, Jalal U, Murad MH. Percutaneous closure of mitral paravalvular leaks: a systematic review and meta-analysis. J Heart Valve Dis. 2012;21:208–17.

3D Printing for LAA Occlusion

7

Yiting Fan, Yat-Yin Lam, and Alex Pui-Wai Lee

The left atrial appendage (LAA) is a narrow, tubular, blind-ended structure extending anterolaterally from the main body of the left atrium (LA). The LAA is located above the LV, on the left side of the pulmonary artery and ascending aorta, between the left superior pulmonary vein and the mitral annulus. With prominent muscular ridges, the LAA has active contraction. The appendage is also an endocrine organ, containing almost 30% of the heart atrial natriuretic factor [1]. Because of its increased distensibility, the LAA may augment hemodynamic function by alleviating pressure rise in the LA and ensure filling of the left ventricle (LV). In cardiovascular diseases, the LAA is the main site of thrombus formation because of its special anatomical structure and functional characteristics. Thrombi originating from the LAA account for 90% of atrial thrombi in nonvalvular atrial fibrillation [2].

The shape of the LAA varies greatly. The length of the LAA is 16–51 mm, the diameter of its opening is 5–40 mm, its volume is 0.77–19.20 mL, and 70% of the main axis is obviously curved or spiral [3, 4]. The orifice of the LAA can be round, elliptical, triangular, and droplet-like. Veinot et al. found in 500 autopsied normal hearts that 44% of LAAs had at least two lobes, existing in different planes of the heart. Most pectinate muscles were > or = 1 mm in width [5]. On clinical imaging, the appendage morphology has been assessed by computed tomography (CT) and classified into four types: chicken wing, cactus, wind sock, and cauliflower (Fig. 7.1). Patients with chicken wing LAA morphology are less likely to have an embolic event even after controlling for comorbidities and CHADS2 score [6].

Y. Fan · A. P.-W. Lee (✉)
Laboratory of Cardiac Imaging and 3D Printing, Li Ka Shing Institute of Health Science; Department of Medicine and Therapeutics, Faculty of Medicine, The Chinese University of Hong Kong, Hong Kong, China

Division of Cardiology, Department of Medicine and Therapeutics, The Chinese University of Hong Kong, Hong Kong, China
e-mail: alexpwlee@cuhk.edu.hk

Y.-Y. Lam
Hong Kong Asia Heart Centre, Hong Kong, China

The LAA is the source of embolism originating from the heart in 90% of patients who had systemic thromboembolism complicating atrial fibrillation (AF). By mechanically excluding the LAA from systemic circulation, percutaneous techniques of LAA occlusion have emerged to be effective alternatives for prophylaxis of systemic thromboembolism in patients with relative or absolute contraindications to long-term oral anticoagulation [7]. Several types of LAA occluder devices are commercially available (Fig. 7.2).

The irregular morphology of the LAA may cause difficulties in implantation of the LAA occluder devices. Recognizing patients with LAA morphology unsuitable for device implantation can avoid implantation failure; inappropriate device sizing and positioning may result in multiple attempts in device deployment which may be complicated by cardiac injury and perforation [8]; in addition, if the device is not implanted optimally, cardiac injury, incomplete occlusion, device embolization, and thrombus formation may occur [9]. Therefore, it is important to accurately evaluate the anatomical shape of the LAA and guide its occlusion correctly before and during the procedure [10]. TEE and fluoroscopic guidance are commonly used for peri-procedurally planning and guidance of LAA occlusion, while CT is increasingly used preprocedurally [11, 12]. Based on CT (Fig. 7.3) or 3D TEE (Fig. 7.4) data sets, a 3D-printed model of the LAA can be created. Although measurements of the LAA can be made accurately on the CT or TEE data, additional information on tissue-device interactions can be obtained from in vitro testing in 3D-printed physical models. The ability to perform "rehearsal" procedure on the 3D-printed models can identify potential problems during the actual implantation, allowing the operators to anticipate and avoid these problems. Such information can be crucial to implantation success and outcomes. Effective implantation of the LAA device relies on precise sizing of the device landing region and coaxial placement of the catheter at the correct depth and orientation prior to release of the device [13]. Anatomic information obtainable from the 3D-printed models includes the appendageal morphology, size of the orifice, depth of the body, and extent

J. Yang et al. (eds.), *Cardiovascular 3D Printing*, https://doi.org/10.1007/978-981-15-6957-9_7

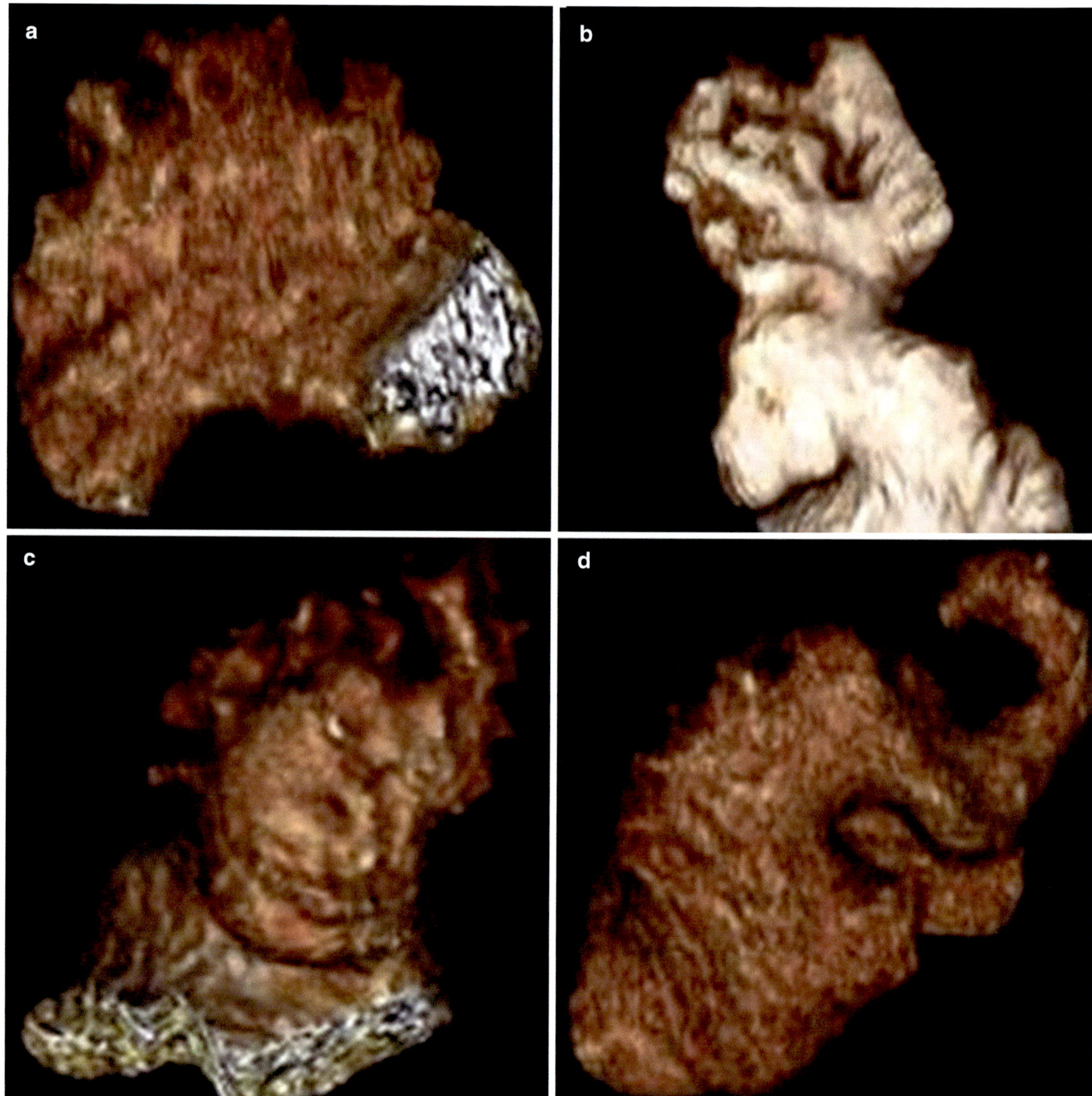

Fig. 7.1 CT images of four different types of LAA morphologies. (**a**) cauliflower; (**b**) wind sock; (**c**) cactus; (**d**) chicken wing

and location of the appendageal trabeculations (Fig. 7.5) [14–16]. More importantly, preprocedural in vitro simulation of LAA occlusion testing different types and sizes of devices may reduce the number of unsuccessful deployment attempts during the actual procedure, hence saving procedural time and potentially reducing complications.

Otton et al. [10] reported a successful case of LAA occlusion guided by 3D printing in a 74-year-old patient. TEE examination showed that the diameter of the LAA opening was 15 mm and 18 mm. CT examination was performed before the operation. The LAA model was printed by 3D printing technology according to the data provided by CT. Three types of occluders, 21 mm, 24 mm, and 27 mm, were selected for test occlusion in vitro. The results showed that occlusion using the 21 mm occluder was incomplete and occlusion using the 27 mm occluder was excessive. The 24 mm occluder was the most suitable occluder and was directly used during the operation to achieve complete occlusion. Jiadan and Zhou et al. [17] applied a 3D-printed model based on 3D TEE to print the LAA of ten patients with non-valvular atrial fibrillation. All ten patients were successfully occluded. It was concluded that 3D-TEE image data can be

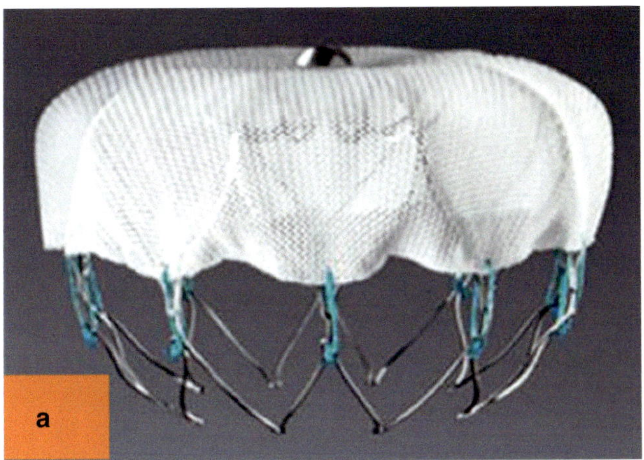

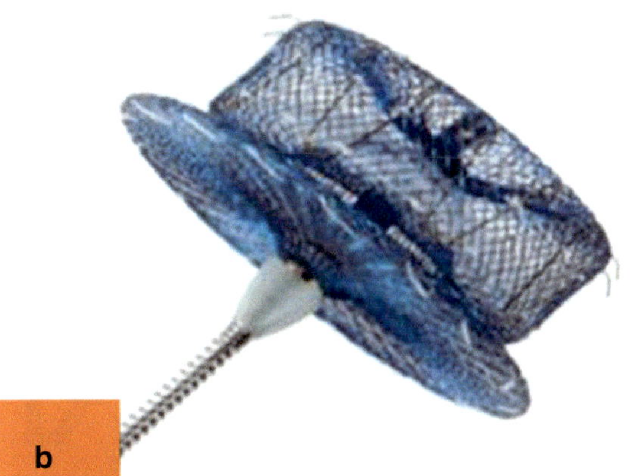

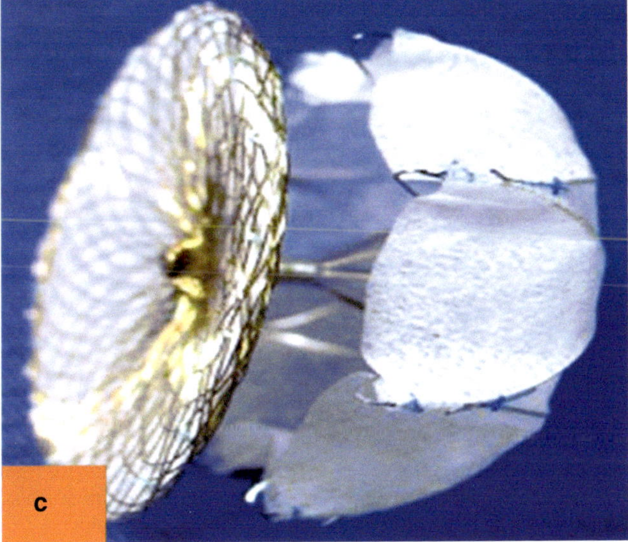

Fig. 7.2 Commercially available LAA occlude devices. (**a**) Watchman™ device; (**b**) Amulet™ device; (**c**) LAmbre™ device

used for 3D modeling and 3D printing of the LAA and can effectively assist in the clinical decision-making related to LAA occlusion. Fan et al. demonstrated in more than a hundred patients undergoing LAA occlusion that device size selection guided by 3D printing is associated with superior acute procedural and long-term clinical outcomes [18, 19]. Computerized 3D deformation analysis of the LAA models during in vitro device implantation may provide quantitative data of device-model interactions [16] and potentially able to identify high-pressure points on the LAA walls that can result in cardiac injury during the procedure. More recently, Robinson et al. reported the feasibility of using 3D printing to fabricate patient-specific LAA devices [20], offering an option for occluding LAA with morphologies deemed unsuitable for occlusion using off-the-shelf devices.

Successful LAA occlusion supported by 3D printing technology requires close cooperation between cardiac imagers, interventional cardiologists, engineers, and other members of the heart team. First, fine scanning images of the LAA must be collected. Then, the model is processed, the preprinting part is selected, and the LAA model is printed using a 3D printer. According to the printed LAA model, a personalized occlusion plan can be developed for the patient. Because of the large variations in the LAA, it is difficult to predict occlusion before the operation for some patients with a complex LAA. If placed too deep, the opening of the umbrella occluder may break the wall of the LAA and cause complications such as pericardial tamponade. If the position of the plug is too shallow, complete plugging will not be achieved, and the stability of the plug will be affected, directly affecting the success rate of LAA occlusion. The 3D-printed LAA model can help the doctor determine the "battle terrain" beforehand, become familiarized with the patient's LAA structure before the operation, and determine the best occlusion strategy for the patient, which may improve the success rate of operations and ease the learning curve of interventional doctors for learning and mastering new clinical skills [21].

When 3D TEE is used to create 3D LAA models, we typically acquire volumetric data sets at mid-esophageal level, with the region of interest including the LAA lobes, orifice, left superior pulmonary vein, and the coumadin ridge, the segment of the left circumflex artery that runs in lateral atrioventricular groove. Acquisition settings are set to maximize the blood-tissue contrast, especially that adjacent to the appendageal trabeculations. Data are then exported in Cartesian DICOM format for segmentation of the LAA at the end systolic phase. Segmentation of the LAA blood volume is performed on a workstation using techniques such as thresholding of pixel intensity, region growing, and manual edition to create a hollow digital geometric mesh model. The model is then converted to a stereolithography file for 3D printing in a 1:1 scale. There are many types of materials that can used to print the LAA models. In order to create models that mimic the physical properties of cardiovascular tissues, flexible, rubber-like translucent photopolymer materials with shore hardness of scale A 30–35, tensile properties of 2.4–3.1 MPa, and tear resistance of 5–7 kg/cm are typically used.

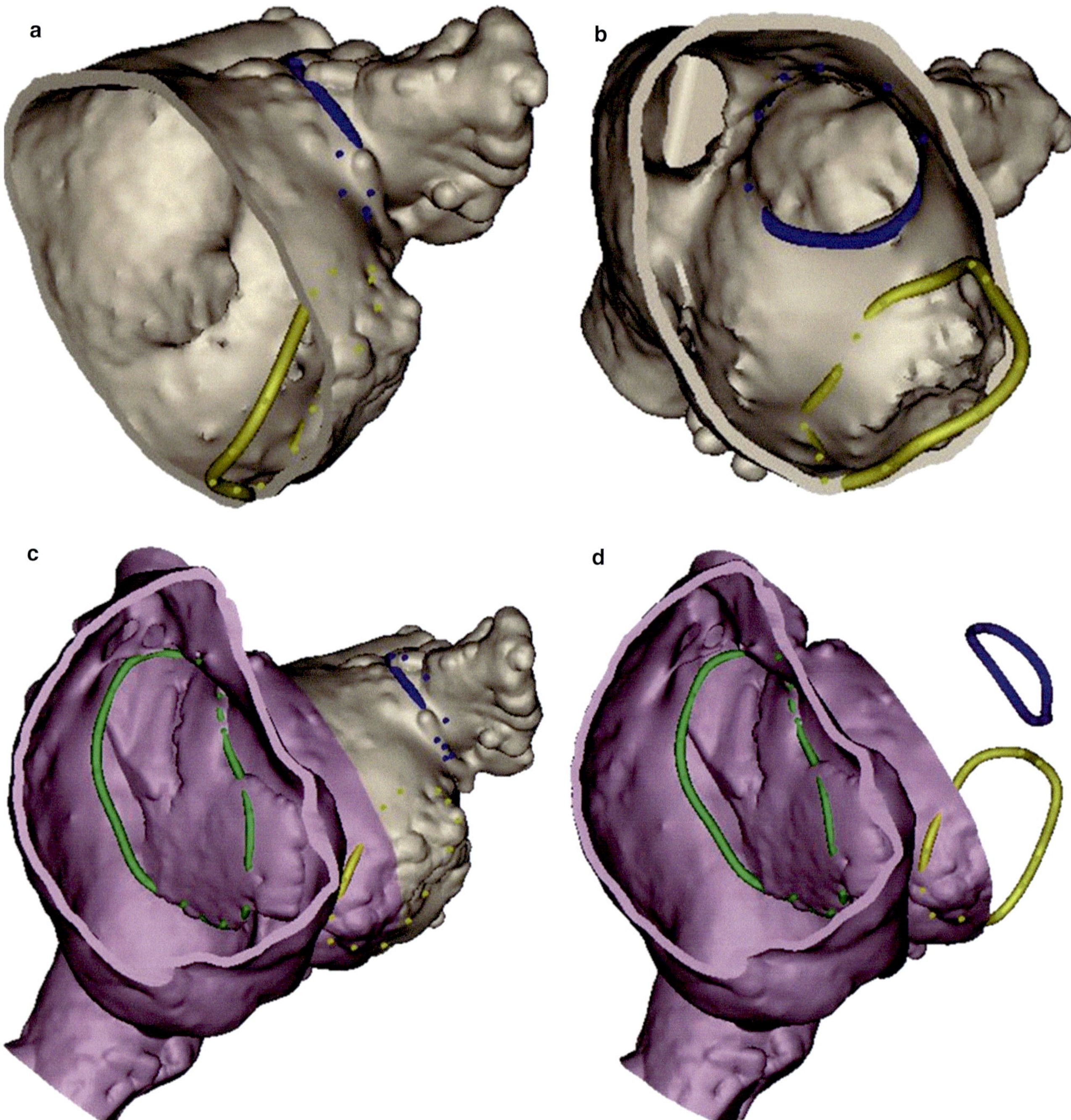

Fig. 7.3 3D digital model based on CT showing the location, size, and shape of the LAA. (**a**, **b**) LA and LAA digital model created by segmentation of CT data. The blue ring denotes the opening of the LAA and yellow ring the mitral valve; (**c**, **d**) Digital model showing the right atrium, interatrial septum (green rings), and the LAA ostium (blue rings). Courtesy of West China Hospital of Sichuan University

With respect to time and monetary cost, segmentation of 3D imaging data sets for each case usually took approximately 30 min. Models are typically printed in batch, with each batching consisting of five to ten models depending on the size of the 3D printing, and typically took 4 h per batch. After printing, removal of supporting materials and model finishing took about 15 min for each model. The material cost for printing each model is approximately $15 to $30. The devices used for in vitro testing are reusable.

In summary, 3D printing technology can be used to reconstruct LAA anatomy based on data provided by cardiac CT or TEE [22]. This technology enables doctors to understand the size and morphological structure of the LAA more intuitively before LAA occlusion, to formulate individualized surgical plans for patients through in vitro simulation operations, and to improve the success rate and clinical efficacy of LAA occlusion, thus having broad application prospects [17, 23].

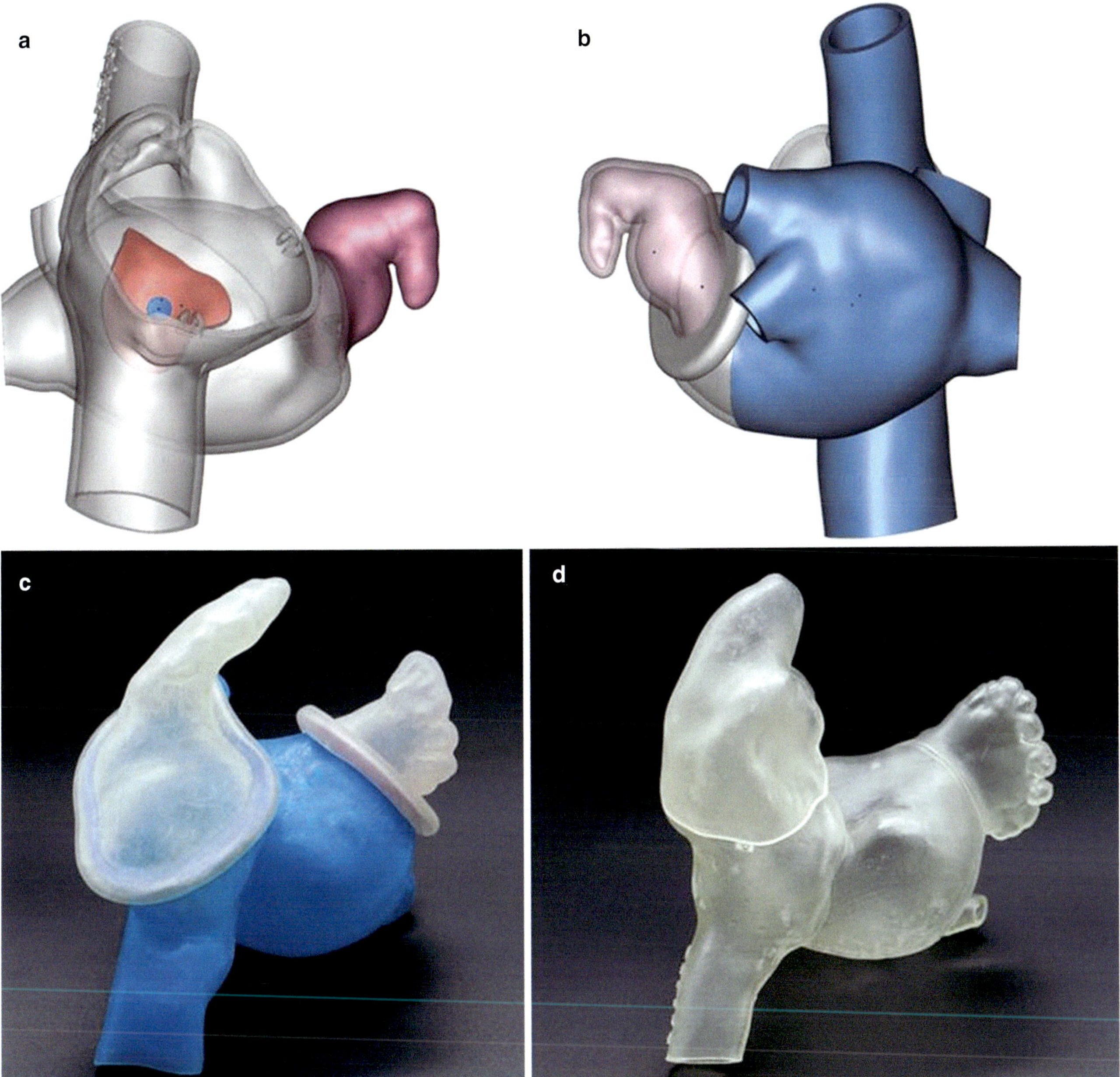

Fig. 7.4 3D printing of the LA and LAA. (**a**) CT-based atrial modeling, RA perspective view; (**b**) LA perspective; (**c**) 3D printing of atrial and LAA model using multicolor materials; (**d**) 3D printing of the atrial and LAA model using transparent materials. Courtesy of Xijing Hospital

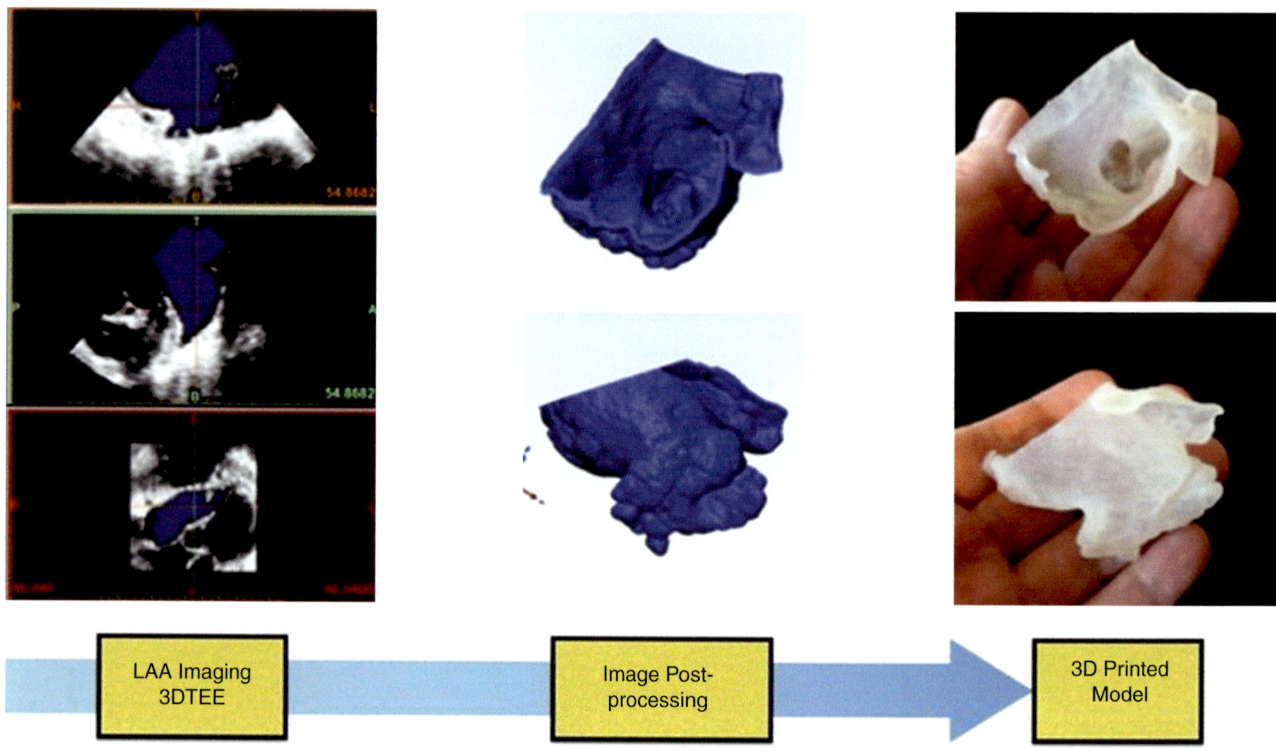

Fig. 7.5 3D printing of LAA based on 3D TEE data. (**a**) Acquisition of 3D TEE image of the LAA. (**b**) Postprocessing of 3D TEE image data, a process known as segmentation, to create the digital model of the LAA. (**c**) 3D printing of the physical model of the LAA using flexible material

References

1. Al-Saady NM, Obel OA, Camm AJ. Left atrial appendage: structure, function, and role in thromboembolism. Heart. 1999;82:547–54.
2. Odell JA, Blackshear JL, Davies E, Byrne WJ, Kollmorgen CF, Edwards WD, Orszulak TA. Thoracoscopic obliteration of the left atrial appendage: potential for stroke reduction? Ann Thorac Surg. 1996;61:565–9.
3. Ernst G, Stollberger C, Abzieher F, Veit-Dirscherl W, Bonner E, Bibus B, Schneider B, Slany J. Morphology of the left atrial appendage. Anat Rec. 1995;242:553–61.
4. Mugge A, Kuhn H, Nikutta P, Grote J, Lopez JA, Daniel WG. Assessment of left atrial appendage function by biplane transesophageal echocardiography in patients with nonrheumatic atrial fibrillation: identification of a subgroup of patients at increased embolic risk. J Am Coll Cardiol. 1994;23:599–607.
5. Veinot JP, Harrity PJ, Gentile F, Khandheria BK, Bailey KR, Eickholt JT, Seward JB, Tajik AJ, Edwards WD. Anatomy of the normal left atrial appendage: a quantitative study of age-related changes in 500 autopsy hearts: implications for echocardiographic examination. Circulation. 1997;96:3112–5.
6. Di Biase L, Santangeli P, Anselmino M, Mohanty P, Salvetti I, Gili S, Horton R, Sanchez JE, Bai R, Mohanty S, Pump A, Cereceda Brantes M, Gallinghouse GJ, Burkhardt JD, Cesarani F, Scaglione M, Natale A, Gaita F. Does the left atrial appendage morphology correlate with the risk of stroke in patients with atrial fibrillation? Results from a multicenter study. J Am Coll Cardiol. 2012;60:531–8.
7. Reddy VY, Sievert H, Halperin J, Doshi SK, Buchbinder M, Neuzil P, Huber K, Whisenant B, Kar S, Swarup V, Gordon N, Holmes D, Committee PAS and Investigators. Percutaneous left atrial appendage closure vs warfarin for atrial fibrillation: a randomized clinical trial. JAMA. 2014;312:1988–98.
8. Reddy VY, Holmes D, Doshi SK, Neuzil P, Kar S. Safety of percutaneous left atrial appendage closure: results from the Watchman left atrial appendage system for embolic protection in patients with AF (PROTECT AF) clinical trial and the continued access registry. Circulation. 2011;123:417–24.
9. Saw J, Lempereur M. Percutaneous left atrial appendage closure: procedural techniques and outcomes. JACC Cardiovasc Interv. 2014;7:1205–20.
10. James M, Otton M, Roberto Spina M, Romina Sulas B, Rajesh N, Subbiah M, Neil Jacobs M, Muller DWM, Gunalingam B. Left atrial appendage closure guided by personalized 3D-printed cardiac reconstruction. JACC Cardiovasc Interv. 2015;8:1004–6.
11. Goitein O, Fink N, Guetta V, Beinart R, Brodov Y, Konen E, Goitein D, Di Segni E, Grupper A, Glikson M. Printed MDCT 3D models for prediction of Left Atrial Appendage (LAA) occluder device size – A feasibility study. EuroIntervention. 2017;13:e1076–9.
12. Boucebci S, Pambrun T, Velasco S, Duboe P-O, Ingrand P, Tasu J-P, Velasco S. Assessment of normal left atrial appendage anatomy and function over gender and ages by dynamic cardiac CT. Eur Radiol. 2016;26:1512–20.
13. Masoudi FA, Calkins H, Kavinsky CJ, Slotwiner DJ, Turi ZG, Drozda JP Jr, Gainsley P, American College of C, Heart Rhythm S, Society for Cardiovascular A and Interventions. 2015 ACC/HRS/SCAI left atrial appendage occlusion device societal overview: a professional societal overview from the American College of Cardiology, Heart Rhythm Society, and Society for Cardiovascular Angiography and Interventions. Catheter Cardiovasc Interv. 2015;86:791–807.

14. Wang DD, Eng M, Kupsky D, Myers E, Forbes M, Rahman M, Zaidan M, Parikh S, Wyman J, Pantelic M, Song T, Nadig J, Karabon P, Greenbaum A, O'Neill W. Application of 3-dimensional computed tomographic image guidance to WATCHMAN implantation and impact on early operator learning curve: single-center experience. JACC Cardiovasc Interv. 2016;9:2329–40.
15. Fan Y, Kwok KW, Zhang Y, Cheung GS, Chan AK, Lee AP. Three-dimensional printing for planning occlusion procedure for a double-lobed left atrial appendage. Circ Cardiovasc Interv. 2016;9:e003561.
16. Otton JM, Spina R, Sulas R, Subbiah RN, Jacobs N, Muller DW, Gunalingam B. Left atrial appendage closure guided by personalized 3D-printed cardiac reconstruction. JACC Cardiovasc Interv. 2015;8:1004–6.
17. Jia D, Zhou Q, Song HN, Zhang L, Chen JL, Liu Y, Kong B, He FZ, Wang YJ, Yang YT. The value of the left atrial appendage orifice perimeter of 3D model based on 3D TEE data in the choice of device size of LAmbre occluder. Int J Card Imaging. 2019;35:1841.
18. Fan Y, Wong RHL, Lee AP-W. Three-dimensional printing in structural heart disease and intervention. Ann Transl Med. 2019;7:579.
19. Fan Y, Yang F, Cheung GS, Chan AK, Wang DD, Lam YY, Chow MC, Leong MC, Kam KK, So KC, Tse G, Qiao Z, He B, Kwok KW, Lee AP. Device sizing guided by echocardiography-based three-dimensional printing is associated with superior outcome after percutaneous left atrial appendage occlusion. J Am Soc Echocardiogr. 2019;32:708–719.e1.
20. Robinson SS, Alaie S, Sidoti H, Auge J, Baskaran L, Aviles-Fernandez K, Hollenberg SD, Shepherd RF, Min JK, Dunham SN, Mosadegh B. Patient-specific design of a soft occluder for the left atrial appendage. Nat Biomed Eng. 2018;2:8–16.
21. Ciobotaru V, Combes N, Martin CA, Marijon E, Maupas E, Bortone A, Bruguiere E, Thambo JB, Teiger E, Pujadas-Berthault P, Ternacle J, Iriart X. Left atrial appendage occlusion simulation based on three-dimensional printing: new insights into outcome and technique. EuroIntervention. 2018;14:176–84.
22. Obasare E, Mainigi SK, Morris DL, Slipczuk L, Goykhman I, Friend E, Ziccardi MR, Pressman GS. CT based 3D printing is superior to transesophageal echocardiography for pre-procedure planning in left atrial appendage device closure. Int J Card Imaging. 2018;34:821–31.
23. Hachulla AL, Noble S, Guglielmi G, Agulleiro D, Muller H, Vallee JP. 3D-printed heart model to guide LAA closure: useful in clinical practice? Eur Radiol. 2019;29:251–8.

3D Printing of Coronary Artery Diseases

8

Alex Pui-Wai Lee, Yiting Fan, Guangyuan Song, and Vladimiro L. Vida

The coronary artery, which divides into the left coronary artery and the right coronary artery, is the first branch of the ascending aorta. The left coronary artery is a short trunk that originates from the left aortic sinus. It passes through the beginning of the pulmonary artery and the left atrial appendage and travels 3–5 mm along the coronary sulcus to the front of the left side of the heart. It is immediately divided into the anterior descending branch and the circumflex branch. The anterior descending branch descends along the anterior interventricular sulcus, bypassing the apical notch to the diaphragm of the heart, and anastomoses with the posterior interventricular branch of the right coronary artery. The right coronary artery originates from the right aortic sinus, travels along the right coronary sulcus between the root of the pulmonary artery and the right auricle, bypasses the right edge of the heart, continues along the coronary sulcus of the diaphragm, and projects into the posterior descending branch near the atrioventricular junction, that is, the posterior interventricular branch.

The blood supply to the heart is received from the coronary artery. Blood enters the heart through two main coronary arteries and then through the vascular network on the surface of the myocardium so that the heart gets nutrients. A problem with the coronary artery will affect the functioning of the heart. Common coronary artery diseases are coronary atherosclerosis [1] and coronary artery fistula. Currently, percutaneous coronary intervention is widely used, and most coronary artery diseases are treated through intervention. Interventional therapies can recanalize narrow or even occluded vessels through angiography, balloon, stent, and other techniques and play a positive role in the diagnosis and treatment of coronary artery diseases (Fig. 8.1).

Surgical coronary artery bypass grafting is also an effective treatment for complex coronary artery diseases. Because of the great variation in coronary artery diseases and obvious individual differences, the specific anatomical structure of coronary artery disease changes rapidly, which has a considerable impact on the success rate of surgery [2]. With the development of medical 3D printing technology, the understanding of coronary artery diseases been improved.

Since its advent, 3D printing technology has been widely used in the medical field, especially for the precise medical treatment of cardiovascular diseases. With the maturity of 3D printing technology in cardiovascular science, medical 3D printing has been increasingly widely applied in the study of cardiovascular diseases [3, 4]. In the study of coronary artery diseases, an individualized model can be printed according to CTA and other imaging data. For example, 1:1 reverse printing of models of the aortic root with the coronary artery will help doctors to determine the location of the coronary artery orifice more easily with higher preciseness, speed up angiography operations, reduce the operational difficulties caused by abnormal coronary artery structure, and enable doctors to treat various coronary artery diseases. By instructing 3D printing technology, doctors can identify the location and degree of the lesion more quickly and accurately so that the operation can be carried out smoothly. In addition, with the combination of 3D printing technology with hydrodynamics, 3D models of the

A. P.-W. Lee · Y. Fan
Laboratory of Cardiac Imaging and 3D Printing, Li Ka Shing Institute of Health Science; Department of Medicine and Therapeutics, Faculty of Medicine, The Chinese University of Hong Kong, Hong Kong, China

Division of Cardiology, Department of Medicine and Therapeutics, The Chinese University of Hong Kong, Hong Kong, China

G. Song
Fuwai Hospital, Chinese Academy of Medical Sciences, Beijing, China

V. L. Vida (✉)
University of Padua, Padua, Italy

J. Yang et al. (eds.), *Cardiovascular 3D Printing*, https://doi.org/10.1007/978-981-15-6957-9_8

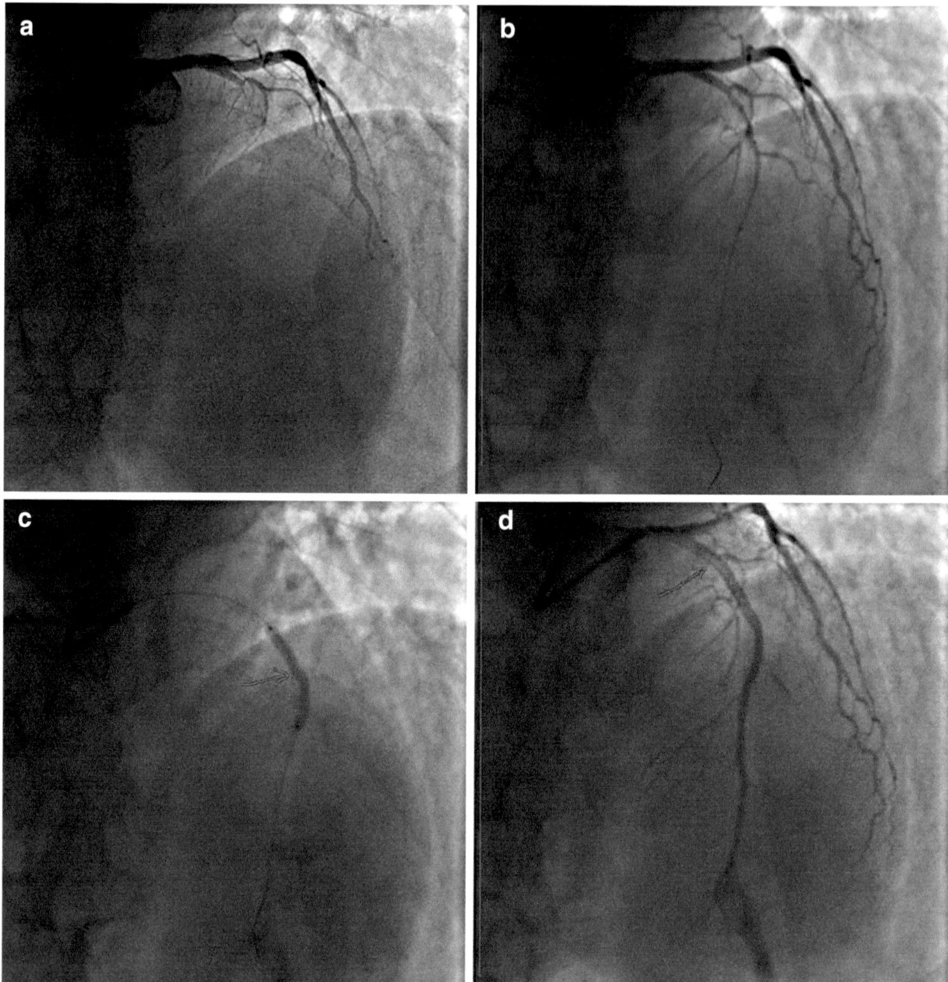

Fig. 8.1 Angiographic images of interventional therapy for coronary heart disease. (**a**) Left coronary angiography showing acute occlusion of the anterior descending branch, with the arrow showing the blind end; (**b**) Guide wire entering the distal end of the vessel through the occluded orifice of the anterior descending branch; (**c**) Expansion of the stenosis with a balloon, pointed by the arrow; (**d**) Angiography after stent implantation showing that the blood flow of the anterior descending branch was restored, the arrow pointing at the stent. Images were obtained from the Department of Cardiovascular Surgery of Xijing Hospital

coronary artery can be reconstructed and printed via a computer based on the patient's image data, and preoperative simulation can be conducted by combining with the hydrodynamic testing platform to accurately evaluate the degree of difficulty of intervention and determine the plan of the operation.

8.1 3D Printing of the Normal Coronary Artery

In contrast to traditional sketches of the coronary arteries anatomy, the coronary artery was reconstructed through the application of CTA and the related Mimics software. After deriving the STL file, 3D models of the coronary artery can be printed with the corresponding 3D printer so that the anatomical structure and the distribution of the coronary artery can be more intuitively observed [5]. The author's Department of Cardiovascular Surgery of Xijing Hospital used the CTA data of patients to reconstruct three-dimensional models of the aortic root with the coronary artery to guide treatment and help teach PCI (Fig. 8.2).

8.2 3D Printing of the Anomalous Anatomical Structure of the Coronary Artery Orifice

In clinic, very few patients have abnormal coronary artery anatomy, which may cause inconvenience when coronary artery intervention is required. The author's Department of Cardiovascular Surgery of Xijing Hospital reconstructed three-dimensional images of the coronary arteries based on patients' CTA images and prepared 3D-printed models of various cases of an abnormal coronary artery opening, including the left and right coronary arteries originating from the same aortic sinus (Fig. 8.3); the coronary artery opening at the sinus-tube junction (Fig. 8.4); and the coronary artery opening at the ascending aorta (Fig. 8.5). Very few coronary arteries have three openings (Fig. 8.6). These abnormal openings are generally not dysfunctional but may cause technical difficulties in coronary artery intervention. 3D printing of abnormal opening of the coronary arteries is helpful for doctors to reasonably select devices, develop the appropriate interventional plan, and shorten the operation time before intervention.

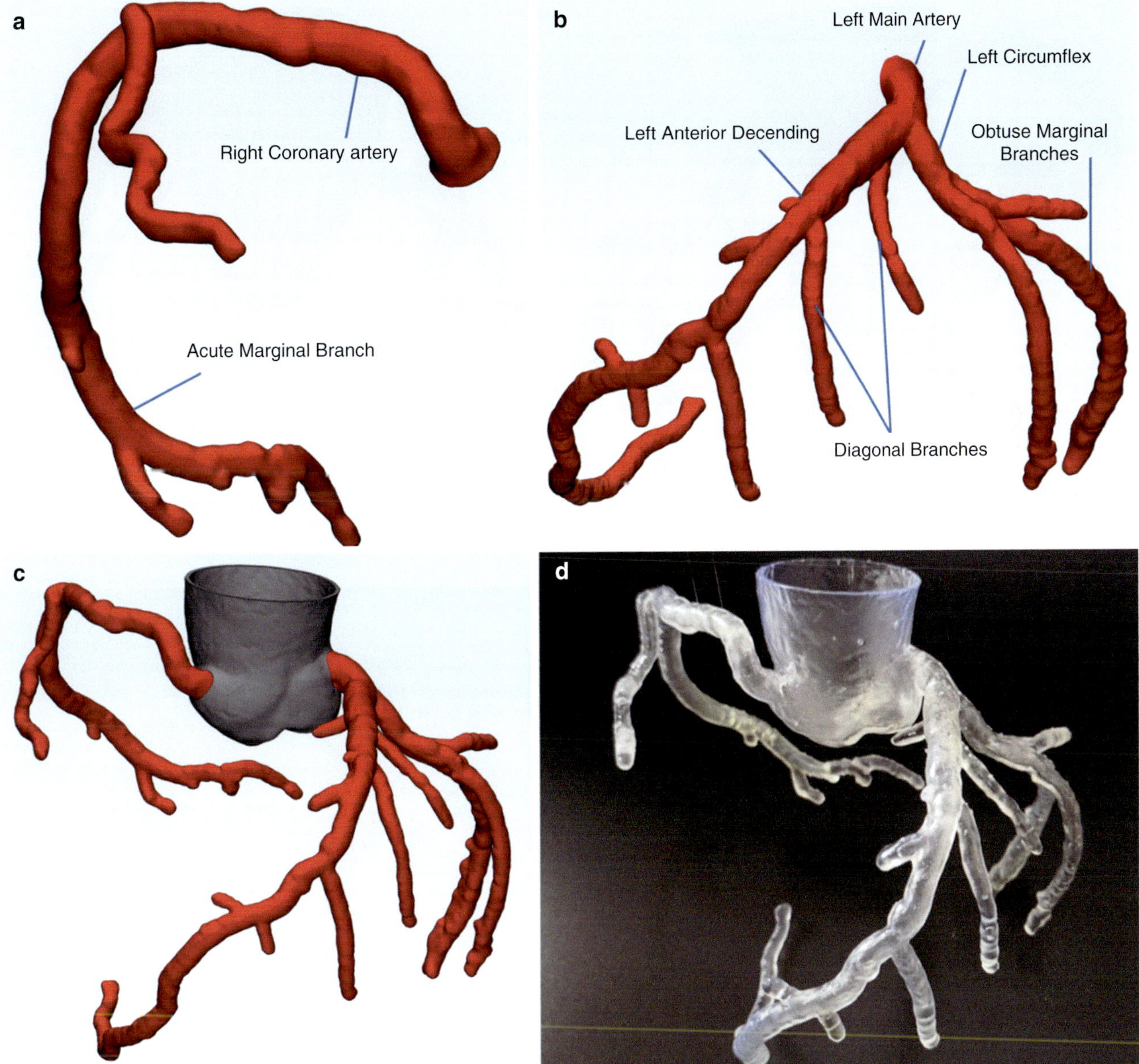

Fig. 8.2 3D printing of the normal coronary artery. (**a**) Computer three-dimensional reconstruction of the right coronary artery and its branches; (**b**) Computer three-dimensional reconstruction of the left coronary artery and its branches; (**c**) Computer three-dimensional reconstruction of the aortic root with the left and right coronary artery; (**d**) 3D printing of the aortic root with the coronary artery model. The image data, computer three-dimensional reconstruction, and 3D-printed model were obtained from the General Hospital of the People's Liberation Army

8.3 Application of 3D Printing in Coronary Heart Diseases

Coronary heart disease (CHD), also known as ischemic heart disease, is a type of heart disease which is caused by the stenosis or the obstruction of coronary arteries (atherosclerosis or dynamic vasospasm), myocardial ischemia, anoxia (angina pectoris), or myocardial necrosis (myocardial infarction). Coronary heart disease is one of the most common heart diseases among middle-aged and elderly people [6] and is mainly caused by abnormal lipid metabolism. The coronary arteries provide nutrition to the myocardium, while cholesterol and fat deposit in the coronary artery, which gradually narrows the coronary artery blood channel, a condition known as coronary atherosclerosis. When stimulated by external environment, the heart beats faster, oxygen consumption increases, and the requirement of nutrients increases, which will then result in the deficiency of coronary artery, with the clinical manifestation

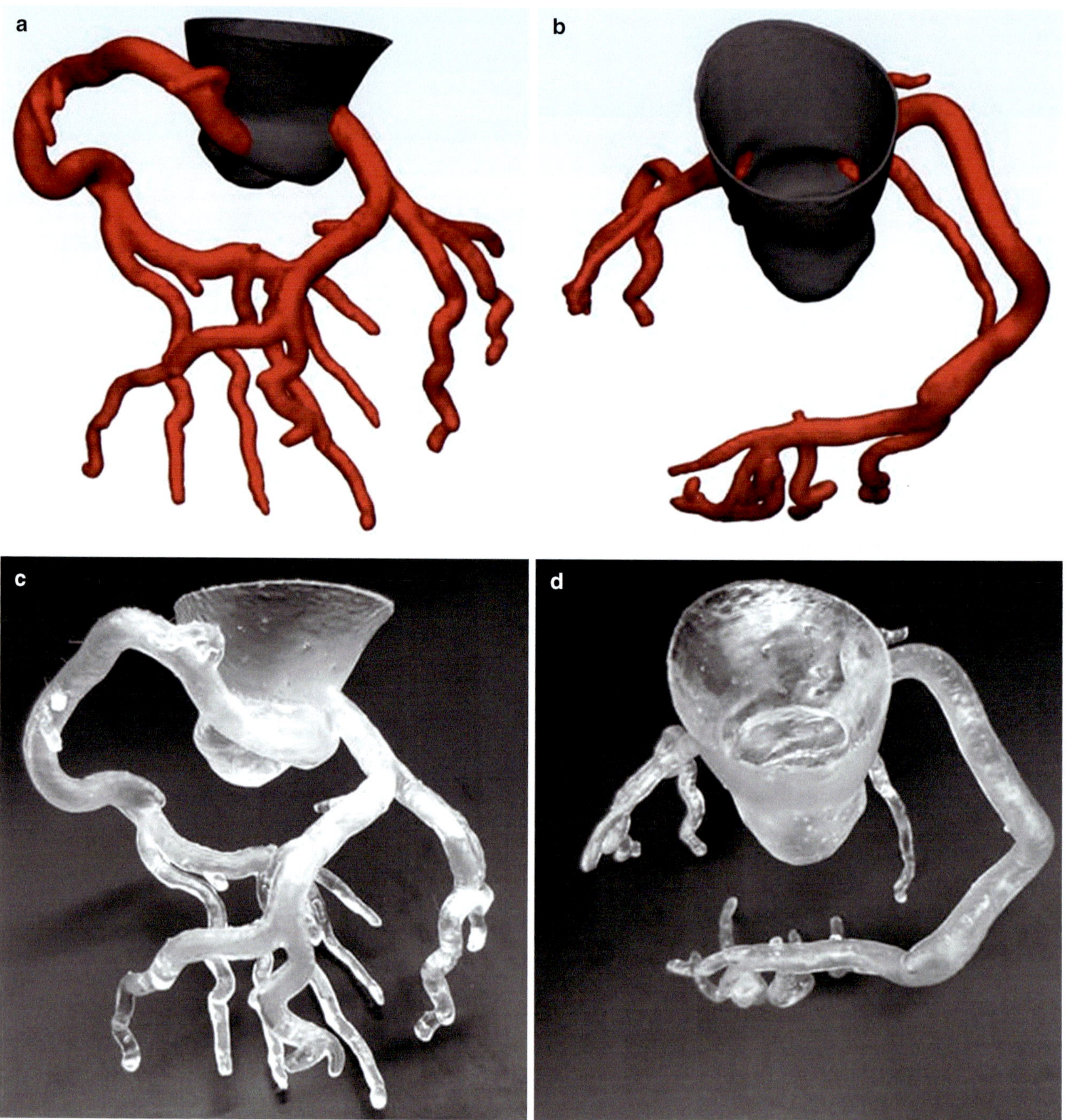

Fig. 8.3 3D printing showing the left and right coronary artery openings to one side of the coronary sinus. (**a**) The left and right coronary artery openings in the same sinus can be seen on the outer wall of the aortic root model reconstructed by the three-dimensional computer model. (**b**) The left and right coronary artery openings in the same sinus can be seen in the inner wall of the aortic root model reconstructed by the three-dimensional computer model. (**c**) The left and right coronary artery openings in the same sinus can be seen on the outer wall of the aortic root model printed in the 3D model. (**d**) 3D printing of the aortic root model showing that the left and right coronary artery openings were in the same sinus. The image data, three-dimensional computer reconstruction, and three-dimensional printing model were obtained from the Department of Cardiovascular Surgery of Xijing Hospital

being myocardial ischemia, angina pectoris, myocardial infarction, heart failure, or sudden cardiac death [7].

Without 3D printing,, doctors can only judge the location and degree of stenosis according to image data of the patients ahead of the intervention surgery [8]. However, with the application of 3D printing technology, a 1:1 3D-printed model of the aortic root with the coronary artery was established in the author's

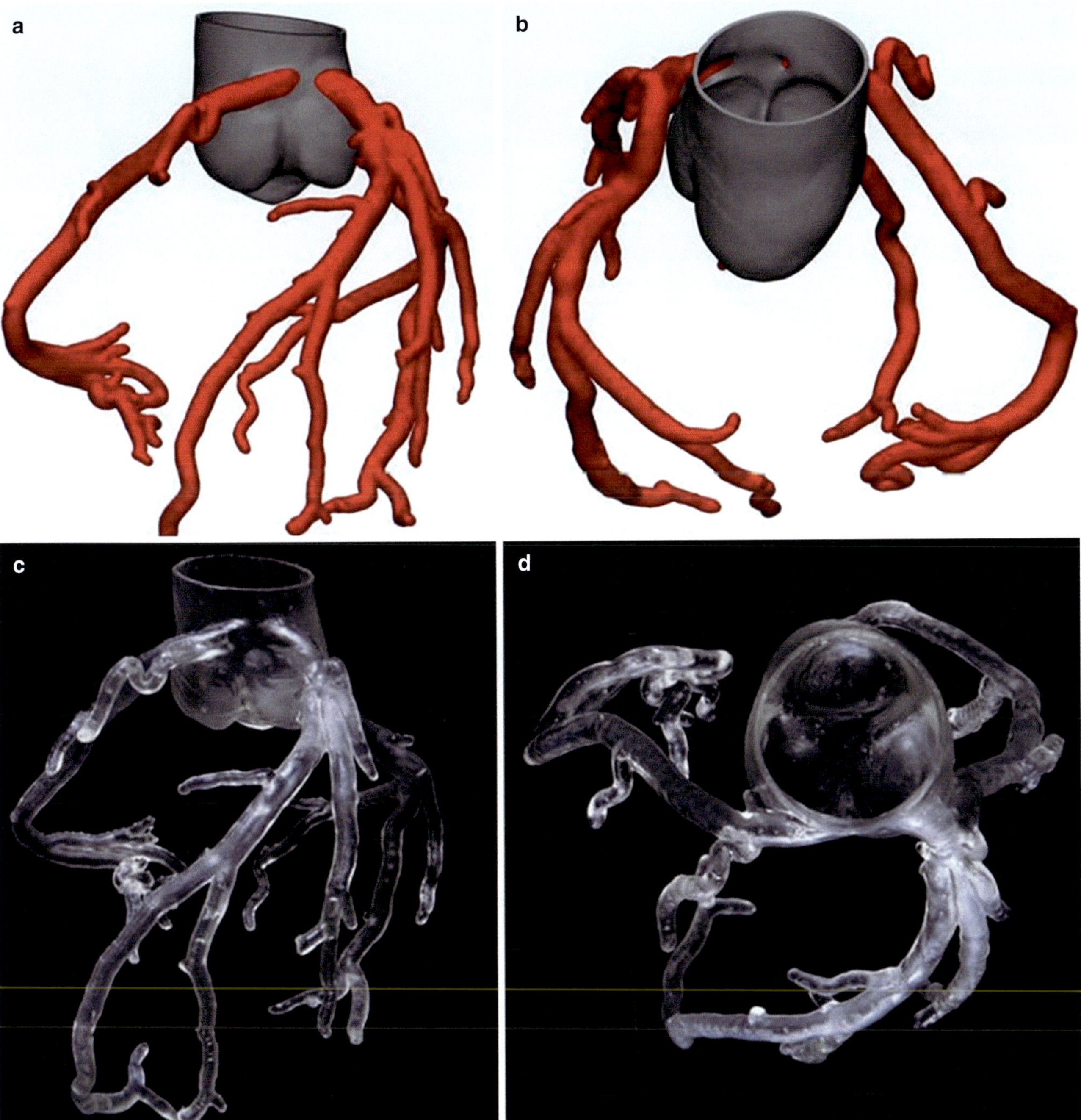

Fig. 8.4 3D printing of the left and right coronary artery openings at the sinus junction. (**a**) The left and right coronary artery openings at the sinus junction can be seen on the outer wall of the computer three-dimensional reconstruction aortic root model; (**b**) The left and right coronary artery openings at the sinus junction can be seen on the inner wall of the computer three-dimensional reconstruction aortic root model; (**c**) 3D printing of the outer wall of the aortic root model can show that both the left and right coronary artery open at the sinus junction; (**d**) 3D printing of the inner wall of the aortic root model can show both left and right coronary artery opening at the sinus junction. The image data, computer three-dimensional reconstruction, and 3D-printed model were obtained from Zhongshan Hospital affiliated with Fudan University

Department of Cardiovascular Surgery of Xijing Hospital by using medical reconstruction software such as Mimics based on CTA image data of the patients with coronary atherosclerosis. Using the corresponding printer, the author produced a 3D-printed model close to the aortic root with coronary artery structure, which can help better recognize the anatomical structure of the aortic root in advance, better observe the distribution of coronary

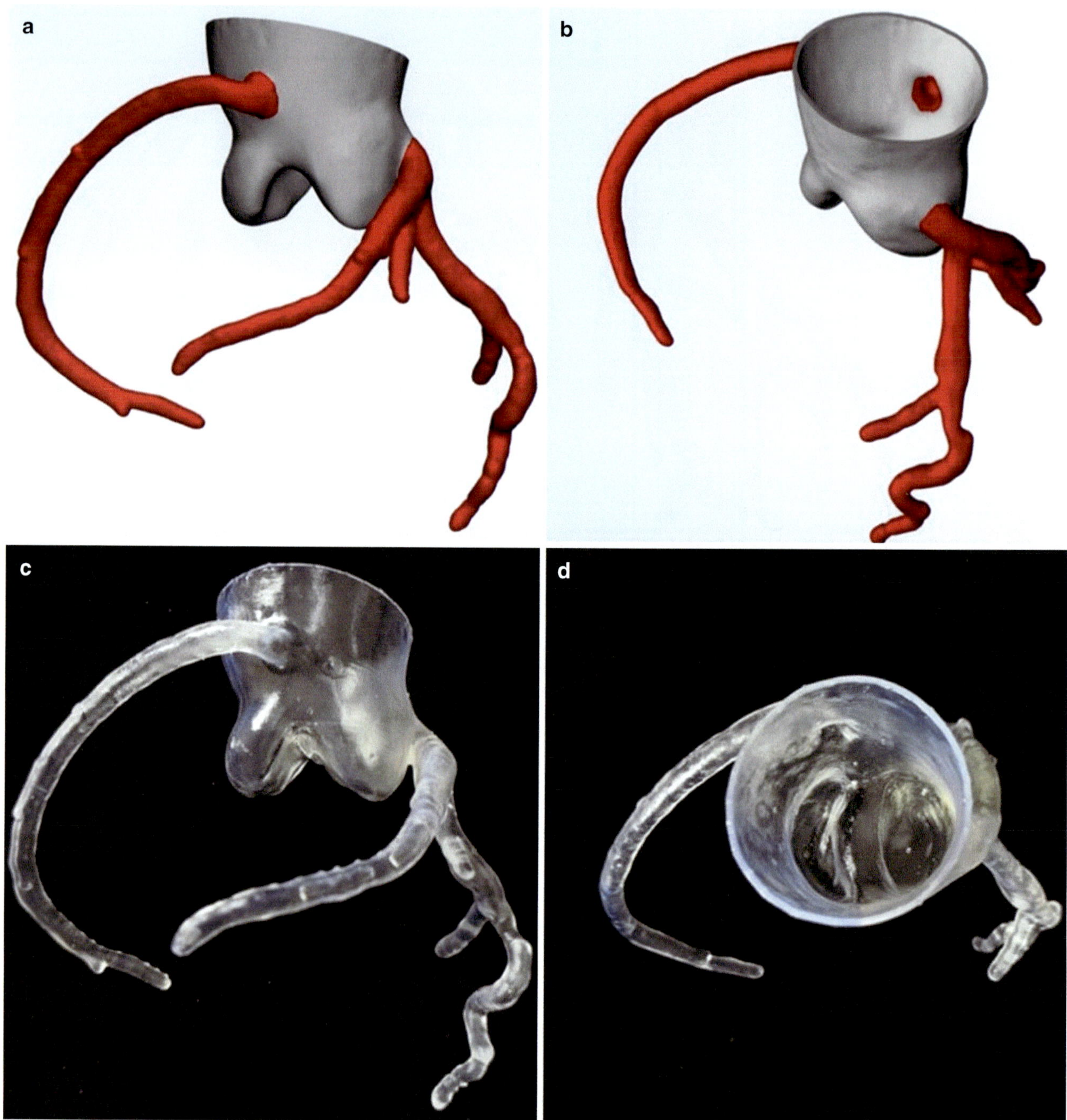

Fig. 8.5 3D printing of the opening of one side of the coronary artery in the ascending aorta. (**a**) The right coronary artery opens at the ascending aorta in the outer wall of the computer three-dimensional reconstruction aortic root model; (**b**) The right coronary artery opens at the ascending aorta in the inner wall of the three-dimensional computer reconstruction aortic root model; (**c**) The right coronary artery opens at the ascending aorta in the outer wall of the 3D-printed aortic root model; (**d**) The right coronary artery opens at the ascending aorta in the inner wall of the 3D-printed aortic root model. The image data, three-dimensional computer reconstruction, and three-dimensional printing model were obtained from the Department of Cardiovascular Surgery of Xijing Hospital

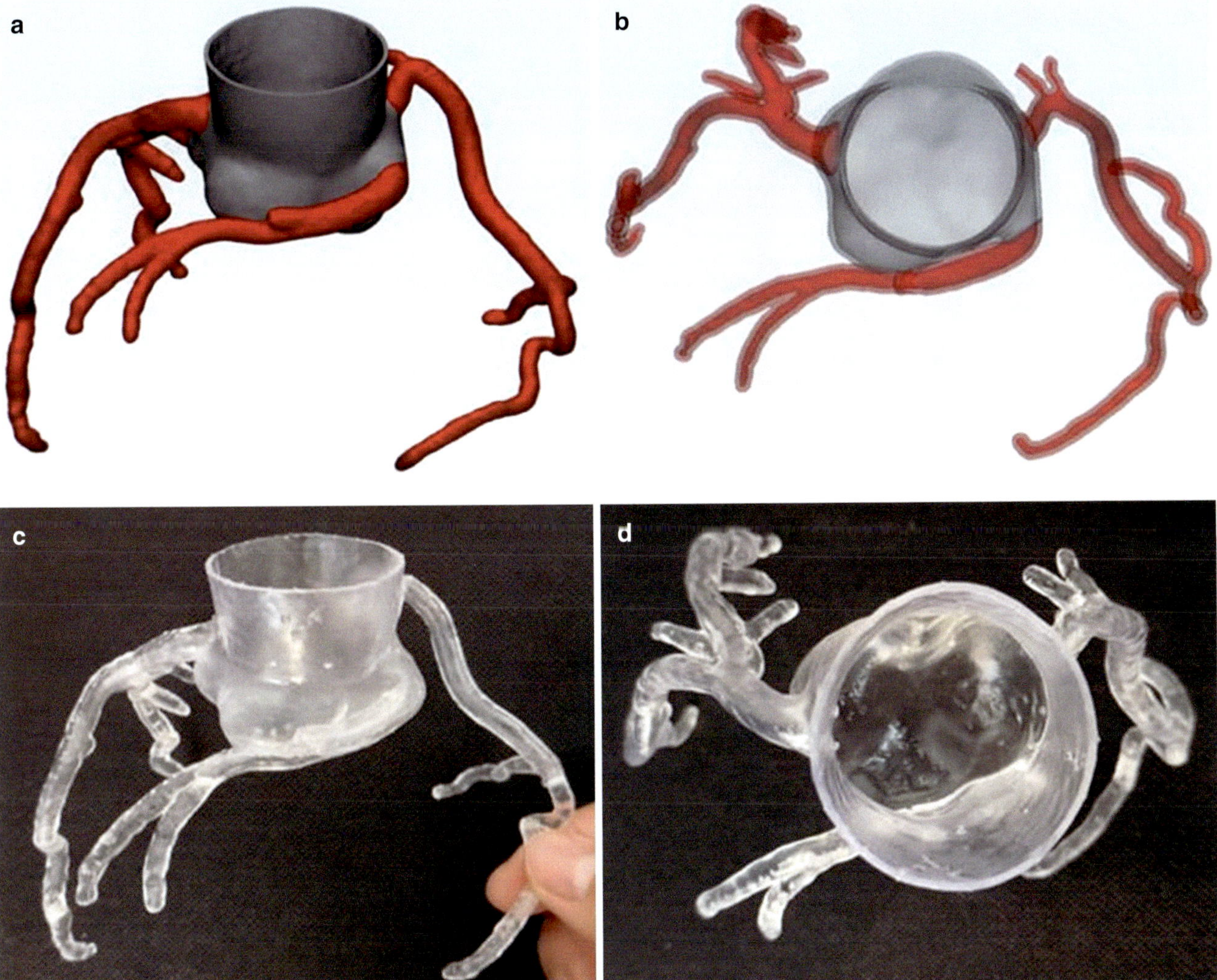

Fig. 8.6 3D printing of the coronary artery with three openings (**a**) The three openings of the coronary artery can be seen on the inner wall of the computer three-dimensional reconstruction aortic root model; (**b**) The three openings of the coronary artery can be seen on the inner wall of the digital aortic root model; (**c**) The three openings of the coronary artery can be seen on the outer wall of the 3D-printed aortic root model; (**d**) The three openings of the coronary artery can be seen on the inner wall of the 3D-printed aortic root model. The image data, three-dimensional computer reconstruction, and 3D-printed model were obtained from the Department of Cardiovascular Surgery of Xijing Hospital

atherosclerotic plaques, and to more intuitively see the location, degree, and calcification of coronary artery stenosis [9] (Fig. 8.7).

The application of 3D medical printing of coronary artery at the aortic root is especially beneficial for patients who have already had their transcatheter aortic valve replaced (see Chap. 6 of this book). According to the CTA images of patients undergoing TAVR, the author's Cardiovascular Surgery Department of Xijing Hospital prints 3D models of patients' aortic roots with coronary arteries, which can be used to judge the relationship among the patient's coronary artery opening, sinus, and stent in a more intuitive way. The patency of the approach during coronary artery stenting (Figs. 8.8 and 8.9) will be of great help to patients after TAVR.

8.4 Application of 3D Printing in Coronary Artery Fistula Disease

Coronary artery fistula (CAF) is one of the most common congenital coronary artery malformations and has a hemodynamic significance [10]. The coronary artery originates from abnormal communication between the aortic root and the heart cavity, pulmonary artery, coronary sinus, and superior and inferior vena cava. Abnormal blood flow leads to marked dilation of the coronary artery, sometimes causing spindle-shaped dilatation or cystic aneurysms [11]. Coronary artery fistula was first proposed by Krause in 1865 and first diagnosed by Biovck in 1947. Sakarupara classified congenital coronary artery fistula into five types

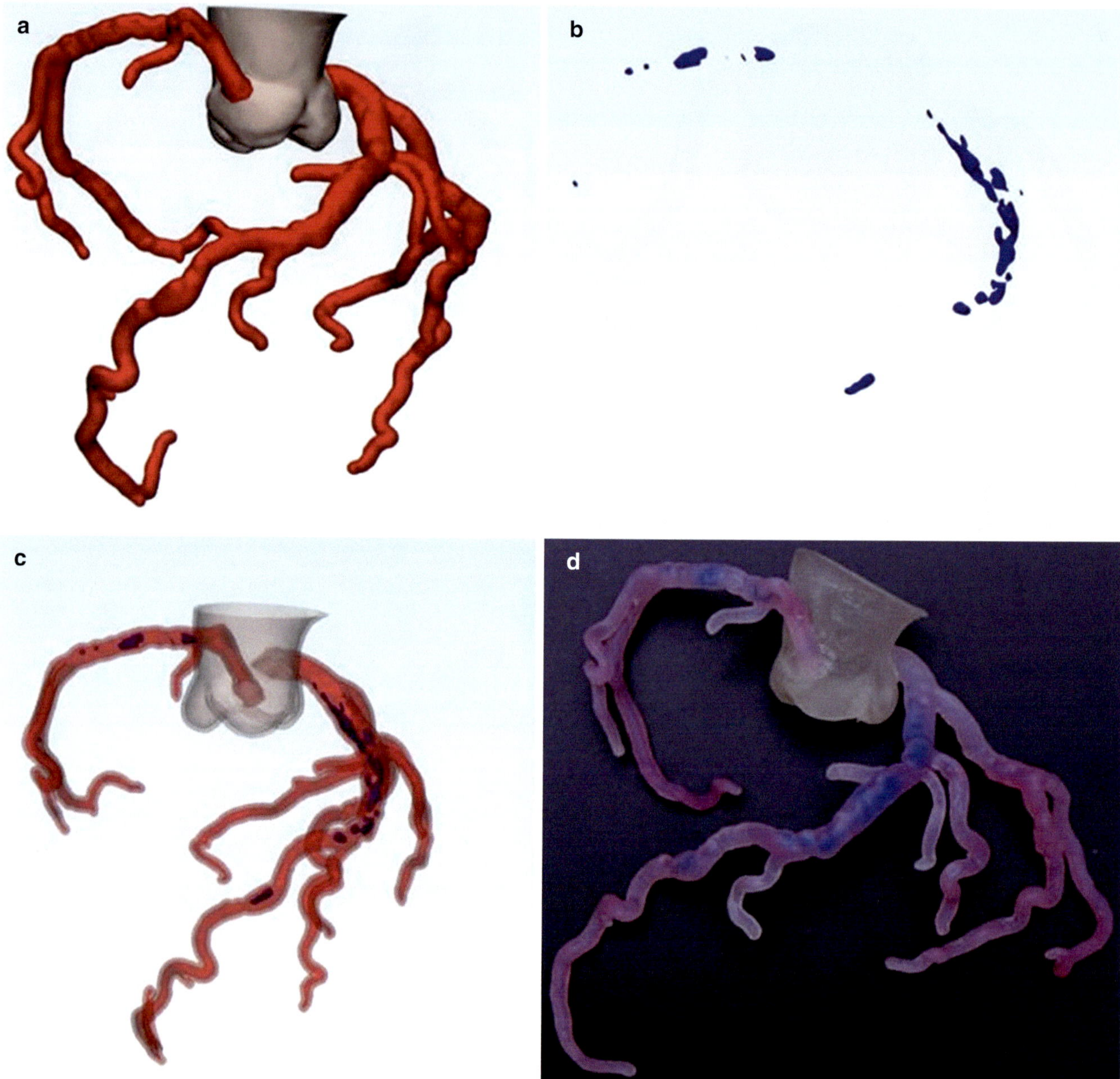

Fig. 8.7 3D-printed coronary atherosclerosis model. (**a**) Computer three-dimensional reconstruction aortic root model; (**b**) Computer three-dimensional reconstruction of the coronary atherosclerosis part; (**c**) Computer three-dimensional reconstruction of the aortic root with coronary atherosclerosis; (**d**) 3D printing of the aortic root with coronary atherosclerosis model; the red indicates the coronary artery, and the blue indicates the atherosclerotic part. The image data, three-dimensional computer reconstruction, and three-dimensional printing model were obtained from the Department of Cardiovascular Surgery of Xijing Hospital

according to the opening position of the coronary artery fistula: drainage into the right atrium, drainage into the right ventricle, drainage into the pulmonary artery, drainage into the left atrium, and drainage into the left ventricle. Right coronary artery fistula is the most common type, while right coronary artery-right ventricular fistula is also common. In the case of large fistula, if the shunt enters the right ventricular cavity, the increase of the right heart load and the pulmonary blood flow will lead to pulmonary hypertension; if the shunt enters the left ventricular cavity, the systemic circulation pressure will affect the coronary flow, and the left ventricular load will increase, which will lead to myocardial infarction, left ventricular enlargement, heart failure, and other pathological changes. Most patients with

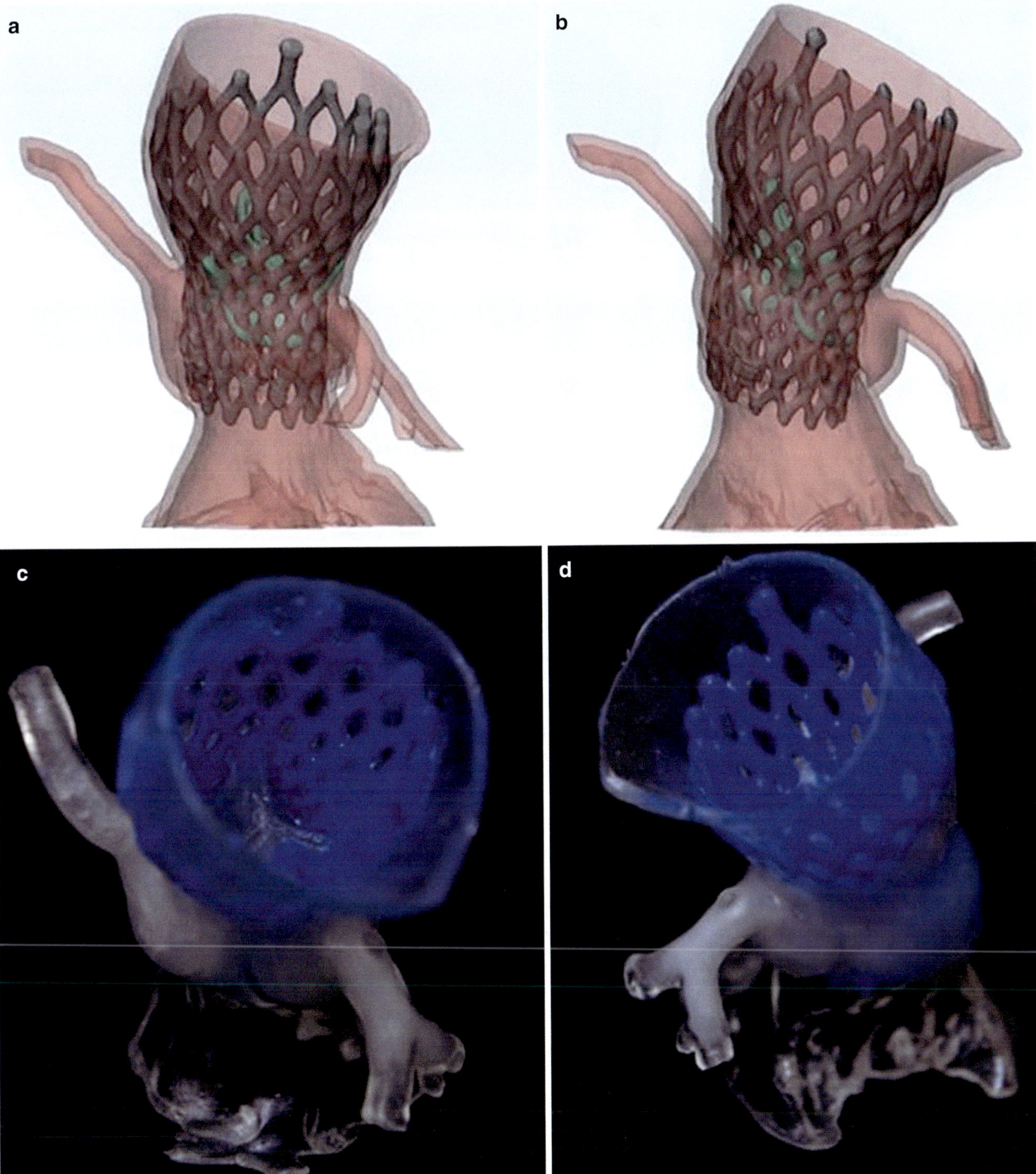

Fig. 8.8 A 3D-printed aortic root model after TAVR of the venous valve. (**a**) Computer three-dimensional reconstruction model showing right coronary artery patency after TAVR; (**b**) Computer three-dimensional reconstruction model showing left coronary artery patency after TAVR; (**c**) The 3D-printed model showing right coronary artery patency after TAVR; (**d**) The 3D-printed model showing left coronary artery patency after TAVR. The image data, three-dimensional computer reconstruction, and three-dimensional printing model were obtained from the Department of Cardiovascular Surgery of Xijing Hospital

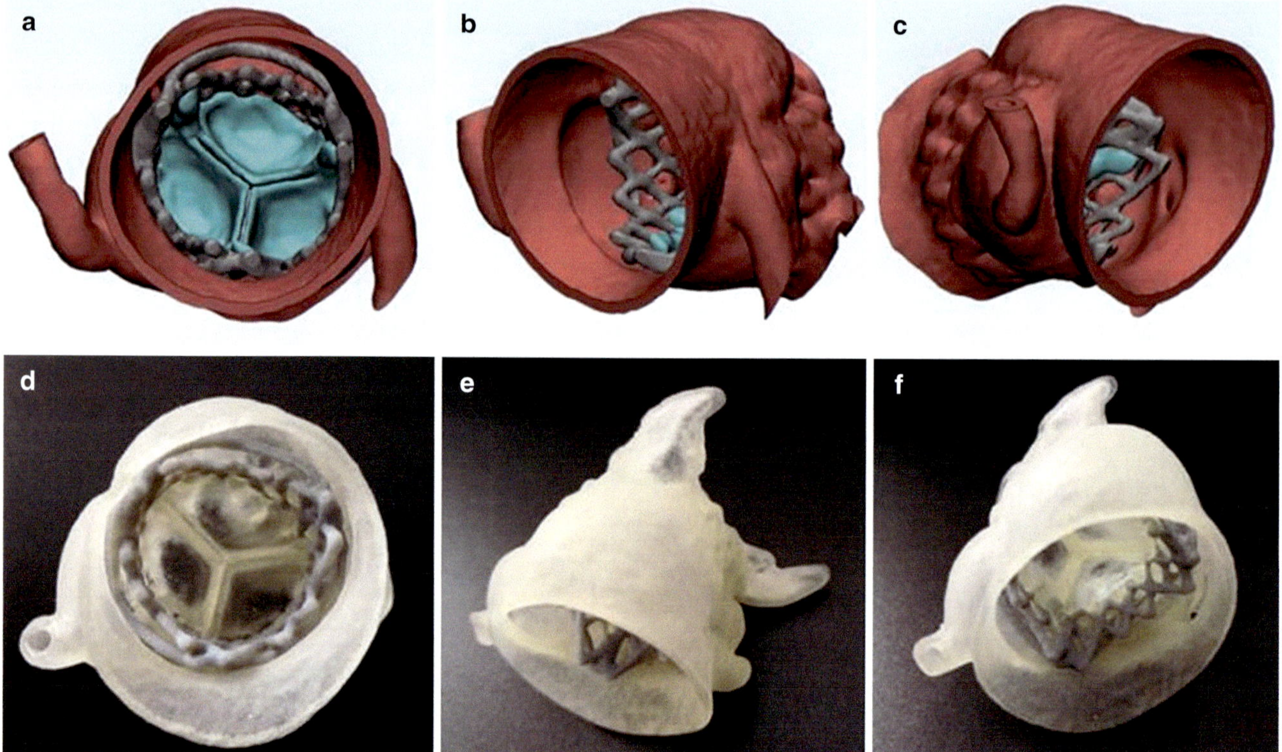

Fig. 8.9 3D-printed aortic root model after TAVR of the J-valve. (**a**) The position of the stent and the coronary artery can be seen by the computer three-dimensional reconstruction model; (**b**) The right coronary artery was obvious in the three-dimensional reconstruction model; (**c**) The left coronary artery was obvious in the three-dimensional reconstruction model; (**d**) The positions of the stent and the coronary artery can be seen in the 3D-printed model; (**e**) The 3D-printed model showed patency of the right coronary artery after surgery; (**f**) The computer three-dimensional reconstruction model showed left coronary artery patency after surgery. The image data, three-dimensional computer reconstruction, and 3D-printed model were obtained from the Department of Cardiovascular Surgery of Xijing Hospital

coronary artery fistula have a shunt through the fistula, which will result in decreased distal coronary artery blood flow and cause coronary artery "stealing" phenomenon (diastolic phase is the most obvious), and thus reduce myocardial blood flow perfusion and lead to myocardial ischemia in the corresponding areas. Patients usually suffer from panic, shortness of breath, and fatigue after exercise. The characteristic symptoms are typical or atypical angina pectoris, and most symptoms are similar to those of coronary heart disease and angina pectoris.

Coronary artery fistula is often confused with other congenital heart diseases that produce continuous cardiac murmurs and can be confirmed through coronary angiography. After examination, 3D reconstruction and printing of a physical model from the patient's preoperative CTA image data can be employed. Thus, the visualization of the direction, location, and size of the fistula can help doctors to develop the operation plan, select the type, size, and location of the occluder, and choose the most reasonable surgical approach [12]. According to CTA images of patients with coronary artery fistula, the author's Department of Cardiovascular Surgery of Xijing Hospital built and printed three-dimensional models in vitro. These models were used for surgical planning and postoperative evaluation and achieved favorable results (Fig. 8.10).

Interventional procedures for coronary artery fistula usually require a tail catheter from the femoral artery to the ascending aorta to show the location, shape, and size of fistula. Then the compressed occluder passes through the fistula into the right ventricle via conveying system. After the occluder is released, the coronary artery fistula will be blocked in the ascending aorta or coronary artery opening, and the operation is completed (Fig. 8.11).

8.5 Application of 3D Printing Coronary Artery in Preoperative In Vitro Simulated Tests

Coronary artery blood flow maintains the normal activity of myocardial cells. When coronary artery stenosis occurs, the blood flow decreases, which is likely to lead to myocardial ischemia or even myocardial infarction or coronary heart disease in severe cases, and coronary stent implantation will be required in the intervention. The number of stents implanted differs among patients. Lauren Shepard

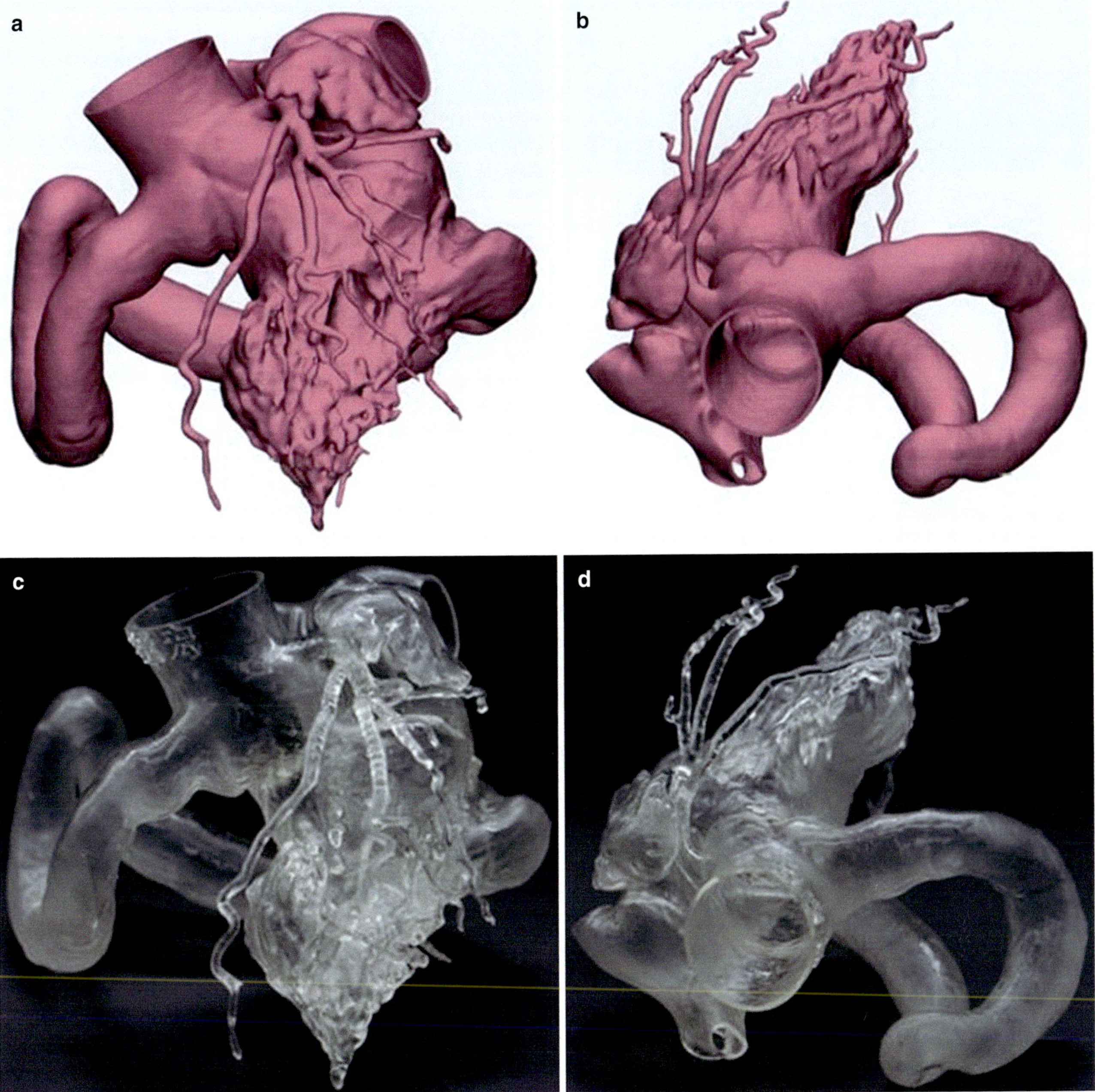

Fig. 8.10 3D printing of coronary artery fistula. (**a**) Fistula from the right sinus to the left ventricle in the computer three-dimensional reconstruction model; (**b**) A different view of the computer three-dimensional reconstruction model; (**c**) 3D-printed fistula model from the right sinus to the left ventricle; (**d**) The 3D-printed model shown from a different angle than in (**c**). The image data, three-dimensional computer reconstruction, and 3D-printed model were obtained from the Department of Cardiovascular Surgery of Xijing Hospital

et al. [13]. used CTA and MRI images of patients to establish heart models in order to minimize the number of the stents. The coronary artery was extracted and simulated in vitro to evaluate the changes in stress in different parts of the coronary artery implanted with different stents to guide clinical understanding of the biomechanics of the coronary artery and to solve the related problems of arterial stenosis. Bhavik N [14] and other British scholars used a 3D-printed model to test the coronary flow reserve fraction (FFR) in vitro. Based on the results, an approach for predicting FFR, which improves the accuracy of FFR measurements and that of coronary artery stenosis assessments, was developed. In addition, Susann Beier et al. [15]. overcame deficiencies in spatial resolution/signal noise and artifacts during PC-MIR examination in vivo by using 3D-printed models, which assisted in the measure-

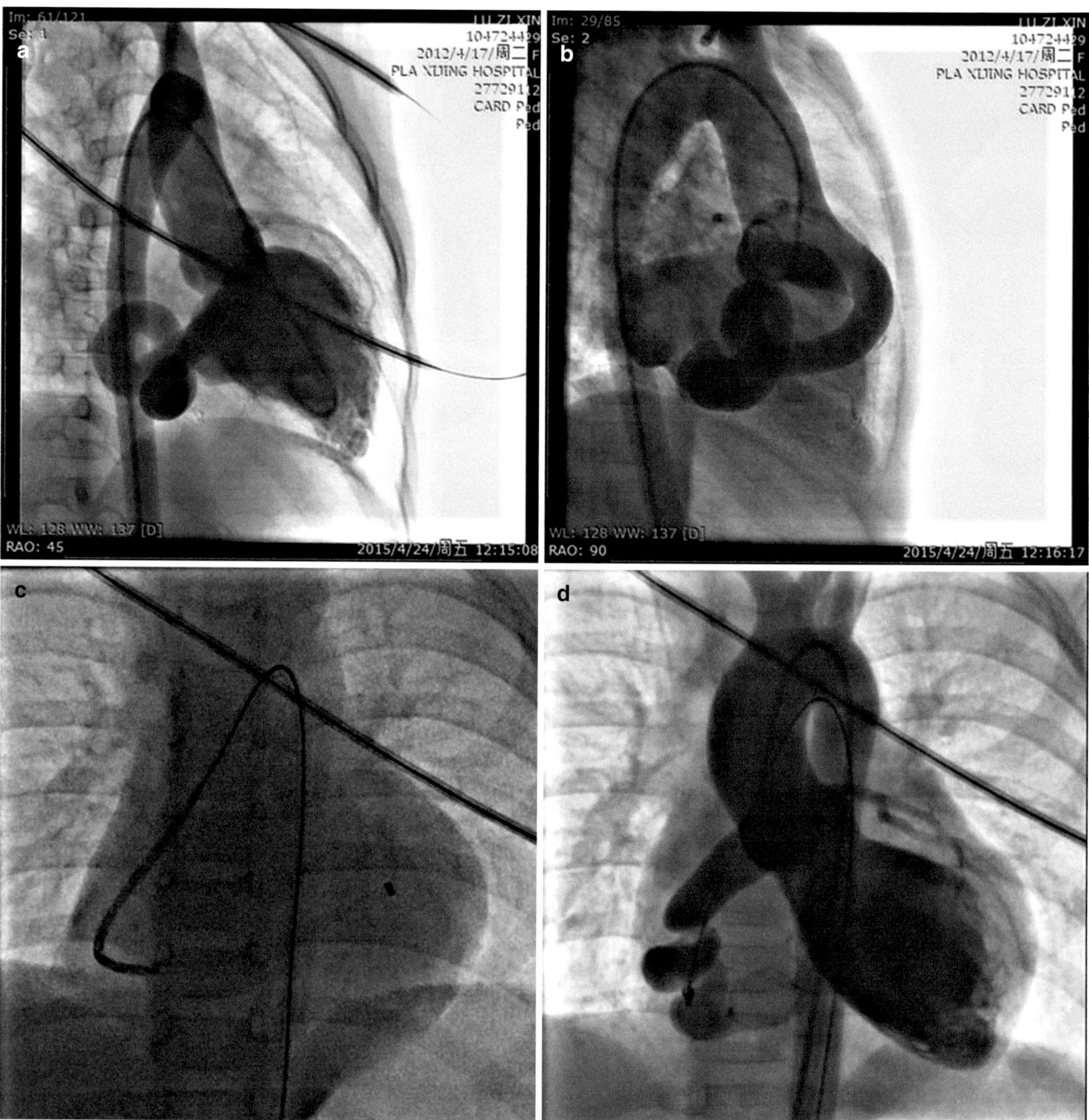

Fig. 8.11 Procedure of coronary artery fistula intervention. (**a**) The position, shape, and size of the coronary artery fistula are shown by angiography from the pigtail catheter in the left ventricle. (**b**) The position, shape, and size of the coronary artery fistula were revealed by the tail catheter from the femoral artery to the right anterior oblique angiography of the ascending aorta. (**c**) A compressed occluder was introduced into the right ventricle via the coronary artery fistula via a delivery system. (**d**) Reangiography of the ascending aorta showing occlusion of coronary artery fistula. Images were obtained from the Department of Cardiovascular Surgery of Xijing Hospital

ment of left coronary artery blood flow. More ideal results were obtained compared with the results of computer-simulated hemodynamics.

The wide application of 3D printing of the coronary artery provides reliable and intuitive guidance for the diagnosis, treatment, and clinical teaching of coronary artery disease [16]. With the development of medical 3D printing technology and the continual updating of printers, medical 3D printing will continue to rapidly develop in the field of coronary artery intervention [17].

References

1. Rowe SP, Zimmerman SL, Johnson PT, Fishman EK. Evaluation of Kawasaki's disease-associated coronary artery aneurysms with 3D CT cinematic rendering. Emerg Radiol. 2018;25:449–53.
2. Li L, Hao J, Qu S, Fang Y. The diagnostic value of three-dimensional CT angiography for patients with acute coronary artery disease. Exp Ther Med. 2018;16:945–9.
3. Giannopoulos AAM, Steigner MLM, George EM, Barile MM, Hunsaker ARM, Rybicki FJM, Mitsouras DP. Cardiothoracic applications of 3-dimensional printing. J Thorac Imaging. 2016;31:253–72.
4. Ciannopoulos AA, Mitsouras D, Yoo S-J, Liu PP, Chatzizisis YS, Rybicki FJ, Giannopoulos AA, Yoo S-J. Applications of 3D printing in cardiovascular diseases. Nat Rev Cardiol. 2016;13:701–18.
5. Chad M, Dugas MA, Jeffrey M, Schussler M. Advanced technology in interventional cardiology: a roadmap for the future of precision coronary interventions. Trends Cardiovasc Med. 2016;26:466–73.
6. Kandaswamy E, Zuo L. Recent advances in treatment of coronary artery disease: role of science and technology. Int J Mol Sci. 2018;19:424.
7. Vagberg W, Persson J, Szekely L. Cellular-resolution 3D virtual histology of human coronary arteries using x-ray phase tomography. Sci Rep. 2018;8:1–7.
8. Sodian R, Schmauss D, Markert M, Weber S, Nikolaou K, Haeberle S, Vogt F, Vicol C, Lueth T, Reichart B, Schmitz C. Three-dimensional printing creates models for surgical planning of aortic valve replacement after previous coronary bypass grafting. Ann Thorac Surg. 2008;85:2105–8.
9. Javan R, Herrin D, Tangestanipoor A. Understanding spatially complex segmental and branch anatomy using 3D printing: liver, lung, prostate, coronary arteries, and circle of Willis. Acad Radiol. 2016;23:1183–9.
10. Jian S, Xianxian Z. Recent progress in diagnosis and therapy of coronary artery fistulae. Adv Cardiovasc Dis. 2017;38:25–8.
11. Hailong Q, Jian Z, Jianzheng C, Meiping H, Qiang G, Jimei C, Shusheng W, Gang X, Hujun C, Xiaowei C. The application value of virtual reality technology in the surgical treatment of coronary artery fistula and abnormal origin of coronary artery. Chin J Clin Thorac Cardiovasc Surg. 2019:217–21. https://doi.org/10.25039/x46.2019.OP63.
12. Ganguli A, Pagan-Diaz GJ, Grant L, Cvetkovic C, Bramlet M, Vozenilek J, Kesavadas T, Bashir R. 3D printing for preoperative planning and surgical training: a review. Biomed Microdevices. 2018;20:1.
13. Shepard L, Sommer K, Izzo R, Podgorsak A, Wilson M, Said Z, Rybicki FJ, Mitsouras D, Rudin S, Angel E, Ionita CN. Initial simulated FFR investigation using flow measurements in patient-specific 3D printed coronary phantoms. Proceedings of SPIE--the International Society for Optical Engineering. 2017:10138.
14. Modi BN, Ryan M, Chattersingh A, Eruslanova K, Ellis H, Gaddum N, Lee J, Clapp B, Chowienczyk P, Perera D. Optimal application of fractional flow reserve to assess serial coronary artery disease: a 3D-printed experimental study with clinical validation. J Am Heart Assoc. 2018;7:e010279.
15. Beier S, Ormiston J, Webster M, Cater J, Norris S, Medrano-Gracia P, Young A, Gilbert K, Cowan B. Overcoming spatio-temporal limitations using dynamically scaled in vitro PC-MRI – a flow field comparison to true-scale computer simulations of idealized, stented and patient-specific left main bifurcations. Conf Proc IEEE Eng Med Biol Soc. 2016;2016:1220–3.
16. Oliveira-Santos M, Oliveira Santos E, Marinho AV, Leite L, Guardado J, Matos V, Pego GM, Marques JS. Patient-specific 3D printing simulation to guide complex coronary intervention. Rev Port Cardiol. 2018;37:541 e541–4.
17. Vukicevic M, Mosadegh B, Min JK, Little SH. Cardiac 3D printing and its future directions. JACC Cardiovascular Imaging. 2017;10:171–84.

3D Printing of Cardiac Tumors

9

Lanlan Li, Zhenxiao Jin, Yanyan Ma, and Vladimiro L. Vida

Cardiac tumors, which are rare cardiac diseases, can be classified into primary cardiac tumors and secondary cardiac tumors. In 2004, the WHO classified cardiac tumors into benign tumors, tumor-like lesions, and malignant tumors [1]. 75% of primary cardiac tumors are benign, and the other 25% are malignant tumors. According to previous reports, three-fourths of all cardiac tumors are benign tumors, nearly half of which are myxomas, with the other half being lipomas, papillary fibroelastoma, and rhabdomyomas; most malignant tumors were undifferentiated sarcomas, followed by angiosarcoma, rhabdomyosarcoma, lymphoma, and so on [2].

Cardiac tumors may cause various symptoms, such as heart obstruction, arrhythmia, abnormal valve function, pulmonary embolism, etc., and are easily confused with other heart diseases. The location, size, shape, activity, and the relationship of the tumors with the surrounding tissues can significantly affect the hemodynamics of the heart. Therefore, early accurate diagnosis and effective treatment of heart tumors are very important for the prognosis of patients [2, 3].

9.1 Diagnosis of Cardiac Tumors

Cardiac magnetic resonance (CMR) is the main diagnostic method for cardiac tumors [4], which can define the multiparameter tissue features of cardiac tumors, as well as the location and extent of the tumors through different sequences can be used. Computed tomography angiography (CTA) can also help determine the location and extent of tumors. Echocardiography is used for routine screening for heart masses and tumors, and 3D echocardiography can provide some details associated with tumors [5]. In addition, the three types of image data can also be used to construct 3D heart models, which may contribute to a better understanding of the influence of the tumors on the cardiac anatomy and aid in determining the operation plan (Fig. 9.1).

L. Li · Z. Jin · Y. Ma
Xijing Hospital, Xi'an, China

V. L. Vida (✉)
University of Padua, Padua, Italy

9.2 Surgical Procedures for Heart Tumors

Surgical resection of cardiac tumors is currently the first choice of clinical treatments, and a good prognosis and low recurrence rate can be expected in the case of benign cardiac tumors. While surgical treatment of malignant cardiac tumors can relieve symptoms, almost all cardiac malignancies have a poor prognosis. Surgical treatment is usually palliative and the tumor is prone to recur (Fig. 9.2).

Surgeons may also face with the following difficulties: (1) some benign heart tumors are found to have grown to a large size with a wide base or be located at a special position, causing a high risk and great difficulties of surgical resection [6]; (2) malignant tumors are difficult to completely resect, with a recurrence rate, and once the recurrence occurs, it is difficult for patients to undergo a second thoracotomy; (3) some patients cannot tolerate the severe trauma of thoracotomy because of their poor physical condition, or some patients are unwilling to undergo thoracotomy. With the wide application of minimally invasive technology in cardiovascular surgery, a growing number of heart operations are being performed through various types of minimally invasive incisions, including ultrasound-guided percutaneous radiofrequency ablation of intramyocardial cardiac tumors, which has also brought about new methods and new techniques for the treatment of cardiac tumors.

9.3 Application of 3D Printing in the Diagnosis and Treatment of Cardiac Tumors

In recent years, significant advances have been made in several imaging techniques, including CTA, MRI [7], and echocardiography. However, the limitation of these technologies

J. Yang et al. (eds.), *Cardiovascular 3D Printing*, https://doi.org/10.1007/978-981-15-6957-9_9

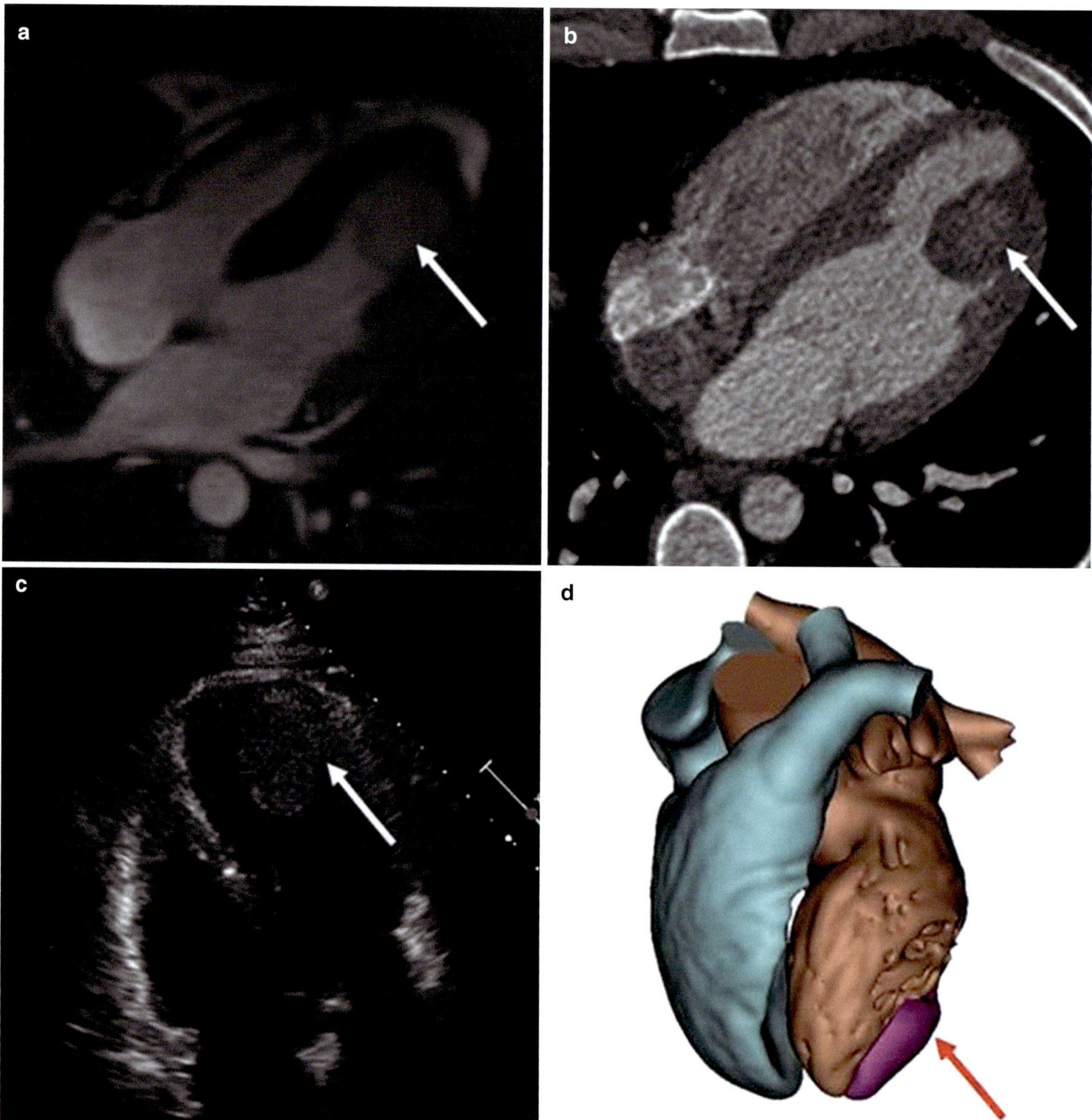

Fig. 9.1 Preoperative multimodality imaging in patients with cardiac tumors. (**a**) Preoperative magnetic resonance imaging; (**b**) Preoperative CTA imaging; (**c**) Preoperative echocardiography; (**d**) Computer 3D model. The image data and computer-based 3D reconstruction were obtained from the Department of Cardiovascular Surgery in Xijing Hospital

sometimes demonstrates inadequacy in diagnosis and treatment. 3D printing can provide a precise model of the patient's anatomical structure [8, 9]. In addition, the distinction between single anatomical structures and printing substructures with different colors can enable surgeons to clearly determine the optimal resection plane, the scope of the procedure, and the relationship with adjacent important tissues before surgery [10]. The insight into the potential risks of surgery can help physicians recognize possible complications before entering the surgical site and, thus, design individualized treatment strategies [11, 12].

Because cardiac tumors often have complex 3D structures which would change the normal cardiac anatomy, it is important to identify the size of the tumor and its location relative to the heart structure so that the surgery will be successfully conducted. It is also important to know the changes in cardiac anatomy after tumor resection [13]. In addition, for rare malignant tumors requiring surgical resection, 3D printing

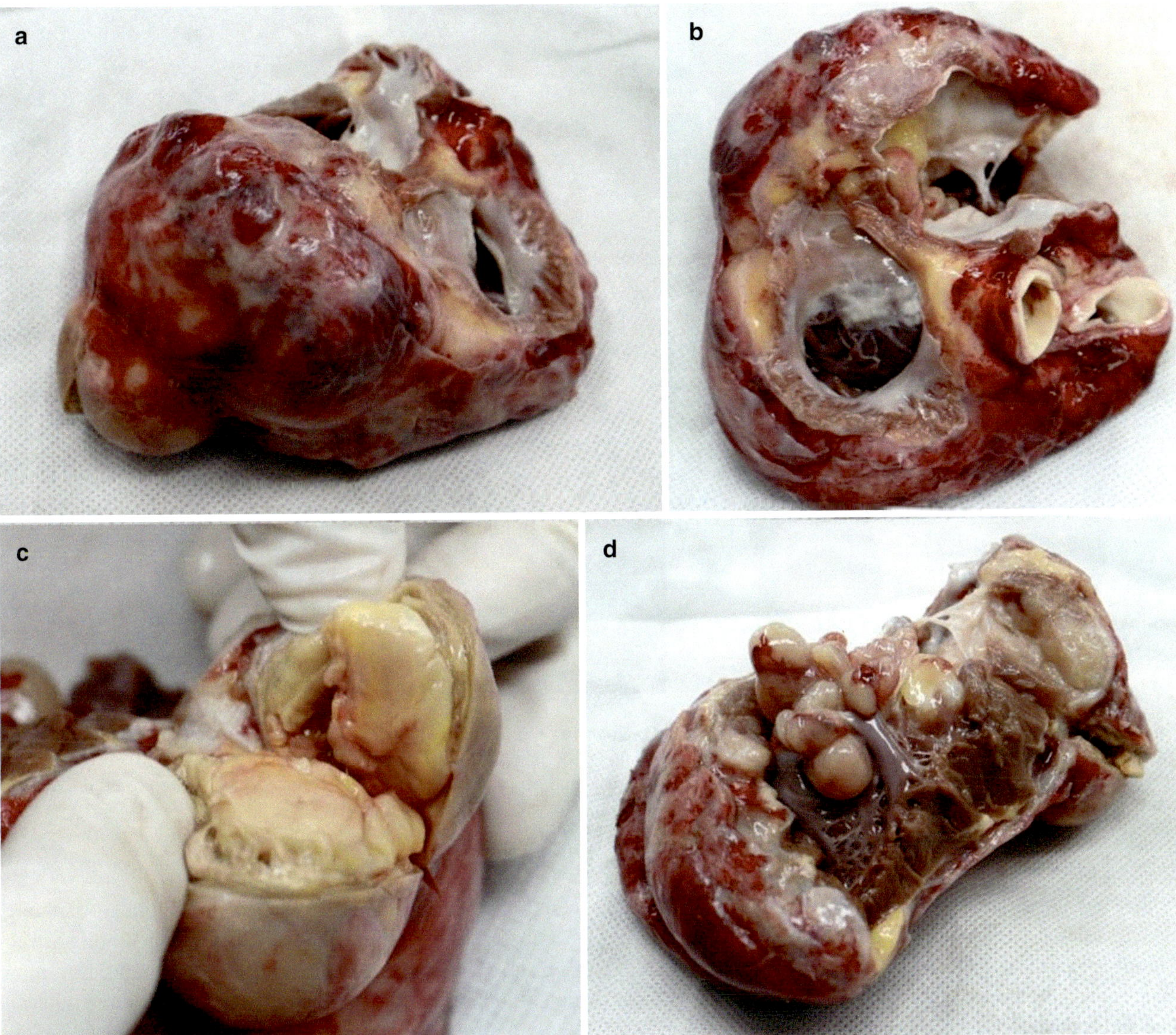

Fig. 9.2 Images of cardiac transplantation in patients with cardiac malignancies. (**a**) Large tumor on the surface of the left ventricle; (**b**) The tumor had invaded the bilateral ventricles and the septum. (**c**) Cystic necrosis and fat liquefaction were observed upon incision of the tumors. (**d**) Cardiac dissection revealed the tumor protruding into the left ventricle with infiltrating growth. The photographs are from the Department of Cardiovascular Surgery, Xijing Hospital

can help the surgeon determine the tumor boundaries during surgical planning [14]. Based on CTA images of patients with cardiac tumors, American scholar R.A. Moore [15] and his colleagues constructed 3D models of different regions of the heart and distinguished them by a variety of colors. The model showed that the heart tumor was located in the right atrium. By hiding the heart tumor module, the compression degree of the right heart system and the coronary artery circulation near the heart tumor were observed to provide an effective basis for the establishment of the surgeon's operation plan.

In 2016, Odeaa Al Jabbari's team [11] printed a 3D model of a patient's complex cardiac tumor that appeared at the junction of the right atrium and the inferior vena cava. Surgeons need to accurately determine the extent to which the tumor extends behind the diaphragm to the inferior vena cava and whether the tumor can be resected from the sternotomy alone or in combination with a laparotomy. Considering the patient's previous history of right nephrectomy, it was difficult to conduct the surgery. Accurate 3D models of the patient's heart and tumor can help the surgeon plan a feasible surgical procedure.

The left ventricular CTA images of patients with left ventricular tumors in Fig. 9.1 were 3D printed in the Cardiovascular Surgery Department of Xijing Hospital. It can be clearly seen that the tumors are located in the left

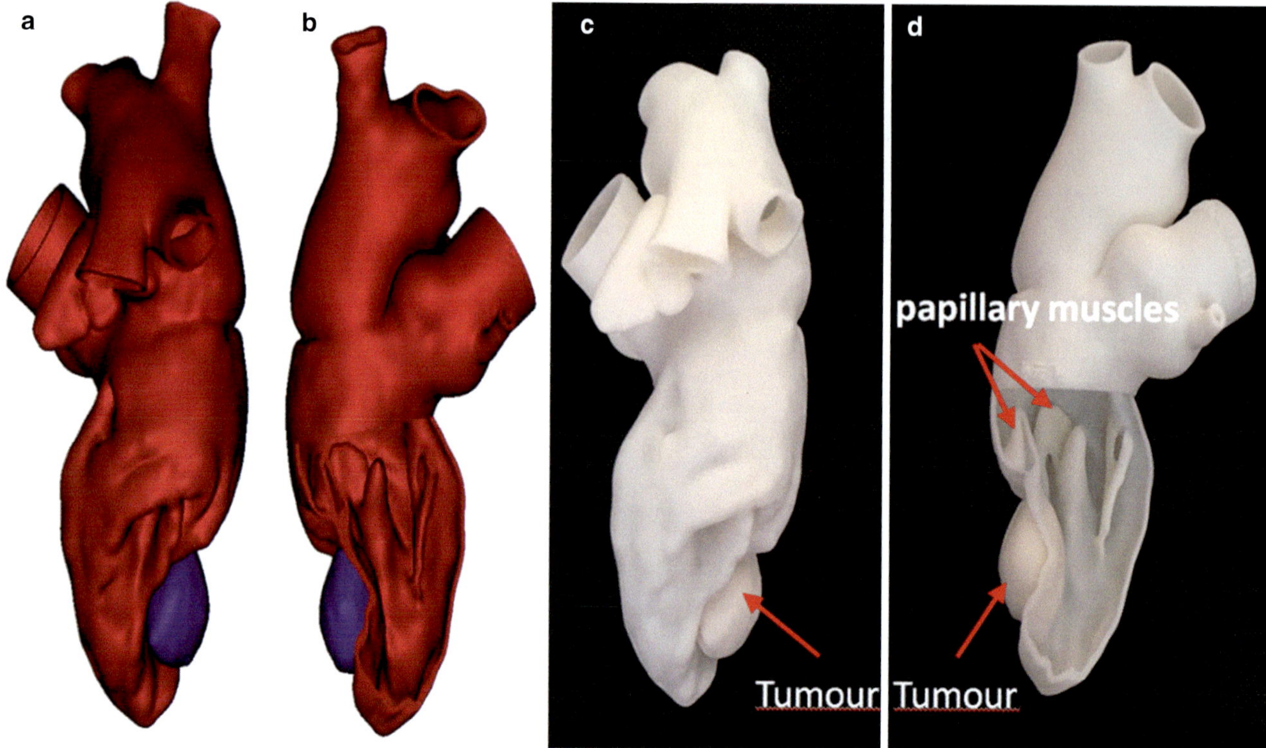

Fig. 9.3 3D-printed model of a left ventricular tumor. (**a**) The left ventricle is red, and the tumor is purple. (**b**) The relationship between the tumor and the local anatomy can be seen from the section of the left ventricle. (**c**) A 3D-printed model of the patient's left cardiac system; (**d**) The 3D-printed model showed the tumor located just below one of the papillary muscles. The image data, computer 3D reconstruction, and 3D printing models were obtained from the Cardiovascular Surgery Department of Xijing Hospital

ventricular lumen, and the basal part of which is wide and closely related to the surrounding normal cardiac tissues. Complete resection is difficult to achieve by surgery, and the other end of the tumor involves the mitral papillary muscle. The surgery would involve the mitral valve, which is related to a high risk of postoperative cardiac insufficiency. Therefore, this patient is not suitable for surgery. The technique of ultrasound-guided radiofrequency ablation was conducted, and good results were achieved (Fig. 9.3).

9.4 Summary

The type, size, and location of heart tumors vary greatly, which has a significant impact on cardiac hemodynamics. Cardiac tumors can be easily diagnosed by echocardiography and other imaging methods. However, surgical resection remains the main treatment for patients with surgical indications because of the different management strategies of cardiac tumors. Therefore, multimodal methods based on echocardiography, CTA, CMR, and other types of imaging data are of great significance for surgical indications and surgical planning. For difficult cardiac tumor cases, image data should be obtained prior to surgery so that 3D reconstruction can be performed during subsequent surgical planning. Compared with 2D imaging data, computer 3D reconstruction and 3D-printed models of cardiac tumors can show more potential interactions between tumor structures and adjacent cardiac structures. Thus, the relationship between cardiac tumor and other anatomic structures of the heart can be more directly evaluated by the surgeon, and these models can allow in vitro simulation of the surgical process or interventional surgery and facilitate the development of individualized surgical schemes to ensure the effectiveness and safety of surgical treatment.

References

1. Bruckner BA, Reardon MJ. Benign cardiac tumors: a review. Methodist Debakey Cardiovasc J. 2010;6:20–6.
2. Simpson L, Kumar SK, Okuno SH, Schaff HV, Porrata LF, Buckner JC, Moynihan TJ. Malignant primary cardiac tumors: review of a single institution experience. Cancer. 2008;112:2440–6.
3. Ekmektzoglou KA, Samelis GF, Xanthos T. Heart and tumors: location, metastasis, clinical manifestations, diagnostic approaches and therapeutic considerations. J Cardiovasc Med (Hagerstown). 2008;9:769–77.
4. Beroukhim RS, Prakash A, Buechel ER, Cava JR, Dorfman AL, Festa P, Hlavacek AM, Johnson TR, Keller MS, Krishnamurthy R,

Misra N, Moniotte S, Parks WJ, Powell AJ, Soriano BD, Srichai MB, Yoo SJ, Zhou J, Geva T. Characterization of cardiac tumors in children by cardiovascular magnetic resonance imaging: a multicenter experience. J Am Coll Cardiol. 2011;58:1044–54.
5. Xuemei C. The application of echocardiography in clinical diagnosis of primary cardiac tumors. Image Technology. 2017;29:67–9.
6. Pineda AM, Santana O, Cortes-Bergoderi M, Lamelas J. Is a minimally invasive approach for resection of benign cardiac masses superior to standard full sternotomy? Interact Cardiovasc Thorac Surg. 2013;16:875–9.
7. Hartung MP, Grist TM, Francois CJ. Magnetic resonance angiography: current status and future directions. J Cardiovasc Magn Reson. 2011;13:19.
8. Mahmood F, Owais K, Taylor C, Montealegre-Gallegos M, Manning W, Matyal R, Khabbaz KR. Three-dimensional printing of mitral valve using echocardiographic data. J Am Coll Cardiol Img. 2015;8:227–9.
9. Lulu R. The application progress of three dimensional printing in the field of cardiothoracic surgery in children. Int J Pediatr. 2018;45:251–5.
10. Shan Yibo WY, Hongcan S. Research progress of 3d printing in cardiothoracic surgery. Chin J Thorac Cardiovasc Surg Clin. 2016;32:692–4.
11. Al Jabbari O, Abu Saleh WK, Patel AP, Igo SR, Reardon MJ. Use of three-dimensional models to assist in the resection of malignant cardiac tumors. J Card Surg. 2016;31:581–3.
12. Schmauss D, Gerber N, Sodian R. Three-dimensional printing of models for surgical planning in patients with primary cardiac tumors. J Thorac Cardiovasc Surg. 2013;145:1407–8.
13. Padalino MA, Reffo E, Cerutti A, Favero V, Biffanti R, Vida V, Stellin G, Milanesi O. Medical and surgical management of primary cardiac tumours in infants and children. Cardiol Young. 2014;24:268–74.
14. Son KH, Kim KW, Ahn CB, Choi CH, Park KY, Park CH, Lee JI, Jeon YB. Surgical planning by 3d printing for primary cardiac schwannoma resection. Yonsei Med J. 2015;56:1735–7.
15. Riggs KW, Dsouza G, Broderick JT, Moore RA, Morales DLS. 3d-printed models optimize preoperative planning for pediatric cardiac tumor debulking. Transl Pediatr. 2018;7:196–202.

3D Printing of Cardiomyopathy

10

Yanyan Ma, Liwen Liu, Lijun Yuan, and Alex Pui-Wai Lee

Cardiomyopathy is a disease which involves heart tissue and is characterized by abnormal heart structure, heart failure, and arrhythmia, with great heterogeneity and diversity [1]. Cardiomyopathy can be classified into primary cardiomyopathy and secondary cardiomyopathy, and primary cardiomyopathy can be further classified into three types according to the etiology and pathology: dilated cardiomyopathy (DCM), hypertrophic cardiomyopathy (HCM), and restrictive cardiomyopathy (RCM). DCM and HCM are the two most common clinical phenotypes of primary cardiomyopathy, which are important causes of chronic heart failure and sudden cardiac death (SCD) in young patients. Dilated cardiomyopathy is the most common type of cardiomyopathy, accounting for approximately 60% of all the cases, and is more common in men than women, similar in adults and children. The incidence of dilated cardiomyopathy is approximately 7/100,000 per year, and it is most common among the 20-to-60-year-old age group. Obstructive hypertrophic cardiomyopathy accounts for approximately two-thirds of all hypertrophic cardiomyopathy cases. Epidemiological studies show that the incidence of hypertrophic cardiomyopathy in the normal population is approximately 0.2% and has a clear family history, but a considerable number of patients have no obvious clinical symptoms.

Electrocardiograms, echocardiography, CTA, cardiac magnetic resonance imaging (MRI), cardiac catheterization, and cardiac angiography are commonly used in auxiliary examinations for cardiomyopathy [2, 3]. Echocardiography is the standard diagnostic method for assessing ventricular function, which can accurately measure the size of cardiac chambers and ventricular systolic function and can be used to observe abnormal valve closure and pericardial lesions. Echocardiography, by measuring regional or global ventricular wall motion, can be used to accurately assess ventricular systolic dysfunction. Using CMR, the enlarged heart can be distinguished from ischemic dilated cardiomyopathy, which develops relatively slowly with subendocardial contrast agents. For hypertrophic cardiomyopathy, CMR provides more accurate measurements of interventricular septum and wall thickness, range of lesions, and systolic function [4, 5].

10.1 Treatment of Cardiomyopathy

Hypertrophic cardiomyopathy (HCM) is a type of hereditary cardiomyopathy characterized by asymmetric left ventricular hypertrophy. Current treatment methods mainly include drug therapy [6], surgical treatment, and alcohol septal ablation (ASA) [7–9]. For patients with outflow obstruction secondary to septal hypertrophy, symptoms persist despite optimal drug treatment. Myocardial septal myectomy (MM) and alcohol septal ablation can be performed at this stage [10] Surgical treatment requires thoracotomy, which may result in a left bundle branch block, while alcohol ablation is less invasive but does not relieve obstruction of the left ventricular outflow tract in some patients. The newly developed minimally invasive interventional therapy (the Liwen Procedure), which can effectively improve the thickness of the ventricular septum and relieve obstruction of the left ventricular outflow tract, has been widely studied. Cardiac transplantation may be considered for patients with dilated cardiomyopathy who do not respond to medical treatment.

Y. Ma · L. Liu
Xijing Hospital, Xi'an, China

L. Yuan
Tangdu Hospital, Xi'an, China

A. P.-W. Lee (✉)
Laboratory of Cardiac Imaging and 3D Printing, Li Ka Shing Institute of Health Science; Department of Medicine and Therapeutics, Faculty of Medicine, The Chinese University of Hong Kong, Hong Kong, China

Division of Cardiology, Department of Medicine and Therapeutics, The Chinese University of Hong Kong, Hong Kong, China
e-mail: alexpwlee@cuhk.edu.hk

J. Yang et al. (eds.), *Cardiovascular 3D Printing*, https://doi.org/10.1007/978-981-15-6957-9_10

10.2 Application of 3D Printing in Hypertrophic Cardiomyopathy

The symptom improvement rate after septal myocardial resection was 70%. Compared with drug therapy, septal myocardial resection can effectively improve the prognosis of successful patients. However, the complex anatomy of the left ventricular outflow tract and the limited visual range of the left ventricle may make surgery more risky and difficult. A previous study found that approximately 5% of patients with complete atrioventricular block required permanent pacemaker implantation. Other complications include ventricular septal perforation, aortic valve insufficiency, arrhythmia, and deterioration of left ventricular function. The complexity of surgical intervention makes the outcomes highly dependent on the operator's surgical skills and experience. Therefore, by using 3D printing technology to create the patient's individualized 3D model, the operator can determine the left ventricular geometry and observe the unique view of the outflow tract, and preoperative simulation of myectomy can effectively guide surgery. Surgical septal resection (morrow procedure) is the preferred treatment for patients with severe hypertrophic cardiomyopathy. However, the complex anatomy of the left ventricular outflow tract and the limited intraoperative visibility of the left ventricle increase the risks and technical challenges of surgery. In 2015, Yang Dh [11] and others used multicolor 3D printing technology to construct the hypertrophic left ventricular myocardium and the papillary muscle. The 3D-printed model provided surgeons with visual information about the left ventricular system, including the extent of septal hypertrophy and the position and length of the papillary muscle. The model was disassembled to understand the internal structure of the ventricle, simulate the operation, and determine the operation plan. The patient's individualized 3D-printed model provided the surgeon with very clear information about the geometry of the left ventricle, and the medical team was able to perform preoperative simulations that effectively guided ventricular septal resection in obstructive hypertrophic cardiomyopathy. Due to the extensive involvement of the hypertrophic myocardium in this patient, complete removal of the hypertrophic myocardium below the aortic valve was not possible, and an incision was made at the apex of the heart in addition to the routine procedure. The hypertrophic myocardium near the lower part of the interventricular septum and involving the anterior papillary muscle of the mitral valve was resected with this approach, and the outflow tract obstruction was completely relieved. The serious complications of mitral regurgitation were prevented, and satisfactory clinical results were obtained.

The American scholar Hermsen [12] used a cardiomyopathy model to compare the sample volume after surgical resection with the sample volume of the in vitro model. It was found that there is a good consistency between them, which indicates that the use of cardiomyopathy models represents a new method for surgical training.

Surgeons can use patient-specific 3D-printed models for preoperative visualization of actual operations. Combined with the growing experience of surgical simulation and related data, 3D-printed models are of great significance for improving surgeons' skills and experience. In addition, 3D printing can provide more educational opportunities, especially those of patients with a small left ventricle, a small surgical field, or a high surgical risk (Fig. 10.1).

Liu Liwen, professor of the Ultrasound Department of Xijing Hospital, developed a new type of Liwen Procedure for hypertrophic obstructive cardiomyopathy, that is, percutaneous transmyocardial radiofrequency ablation under the guidance of ultrasound for hypertrophic obstructive cardiomyopathy [13]. The procedure is guided by ultrasound through a percutaneous transepicardial puncture through the tip of the heart to the ventricular septal hypertrophy. High-frequency waves can induce local hypertrophy for myocardial coagulation necrosis to achieve the goal of widening the left ventricular outflow tract [14, 15]. 3D printing can be used to observe the cardiac anatomy, especially the coronary artery distribution, and to guide surgical planning and risk assessment in the Liwen Procedure. A real 3D model of heart was constructed with preoperative CTA or MRI data of patients with obstructive hypertrophic cardiomyopathy. The coronary artery was displayed in a computer 3D model or a 3D-printed model to prevent the electrode from damaging the coronary artery and the conduction bundle and to ensure the safety of the operation. The anatomic structure of the patient's heart could be fully understood, the optimal puncture site could be determined, and the proper electrode needle path could be set (Fig. 10.2). A 3D model corresponding to the 2D CTA image and ultrasound image also could effectively guide the operation and shorten the operation time.

The Liwen Procedure has been performed in over 100 patients and achieved excellent early clinical results. It was highly endorsed by TCT President Martin B Leon and CSI Conference President Horst Silvert. The results have been published in J Am Coll Cardiol. 2018; 72 (16):1898–1909 [16].

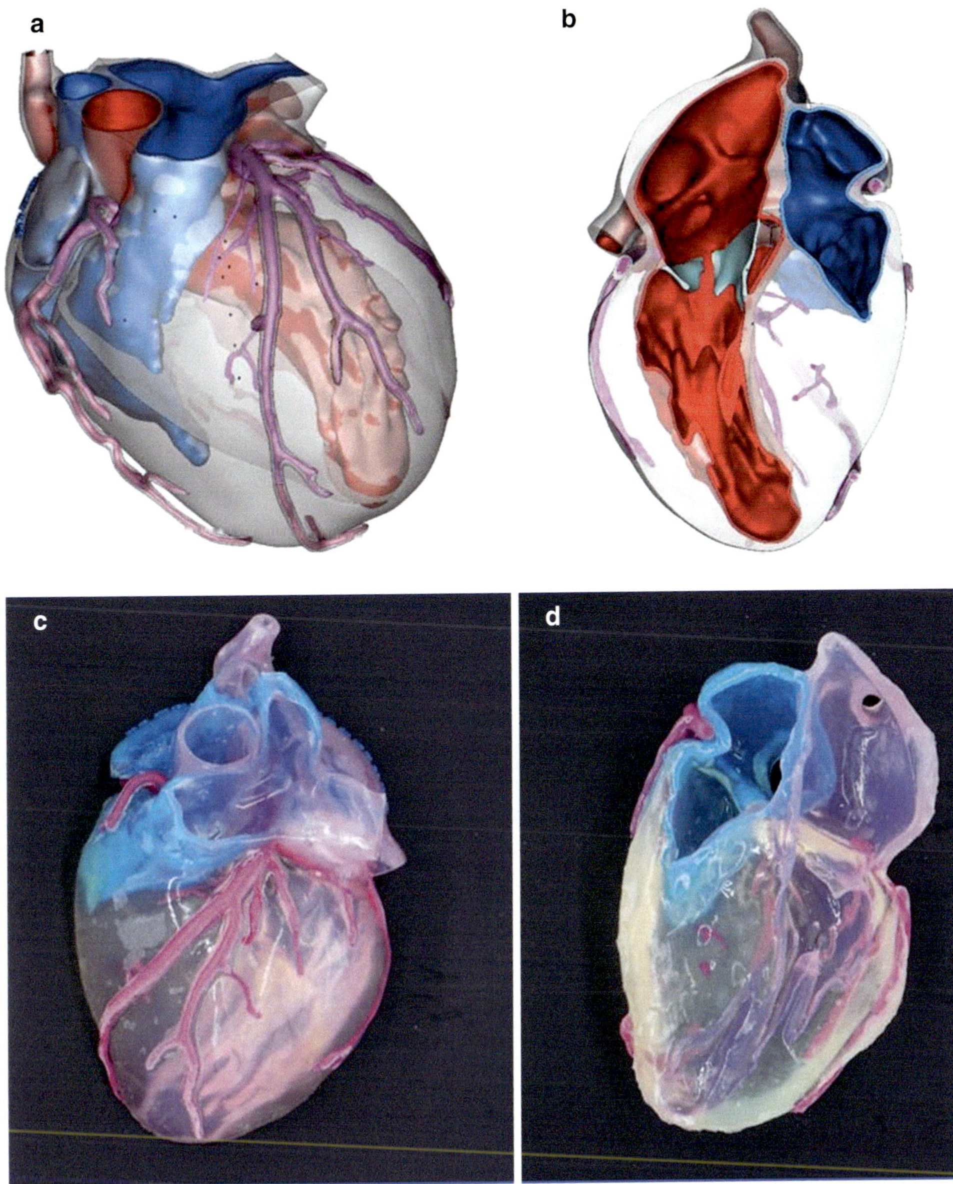

Fig. 10.1 3D-printed model of hypertrophic cardiomyopathy. (**a**) Computer modeling revealed the external structure of hypertrophic cardiomyopathy; (**b**) Computer modeling showed the internal structure of hypertrophic cardiomyopathy; (**c**) The 3D-printed model showed the external structure of hypertrophic cardiomyopathy. (**d**) The 3D-printed model showed the internal structure of hypertrophic cardiomyopathy. The image data, computer 3D reconstruction, and 3D-printed model were obtained from the Cardiovascular Surgery Department of Xijing Hospital

10.3 Summary

With the development of imaging technology, cardiomyopathy can now be easily diagnosed. However, determining the optimal treatment strategy remains a difficult problem because of the great differences in the range and classification of cardiomyopathy. Surgical excision remains the preferred treatment for cardiomyopathy in patients who meet the indications. However, determining the extent of resection, avoiding too much or too little resection, and complications such as ventricular septal perforation and atrioventricular block after operation are key to ensuring the surgical effect and long-term survival. Therefore, multimodal methods based on echocardiography, CTA, CMR, and other imaging data are of great significance for surgical indication and surgical planning [17]. For difficult cases of cardiomyopathy, image data should be obtained prior to surgery so that 3D reconstruction can be performed during subsequent surgical planning. The 3D-printed model can directly display the degree, range, and adjacent relationship of hypertrophic myocardium. New techniques for the treatment of cardiomyopathy, such as the Liwen Procedure, require even more intensive 3D printing modeling. In addition to similar surgical guidance, 3D-printed models can also assist in providing angulation of the heart, and the direction, depth, and range of radiofrequency ablation are important to improve safety and effectiveness.

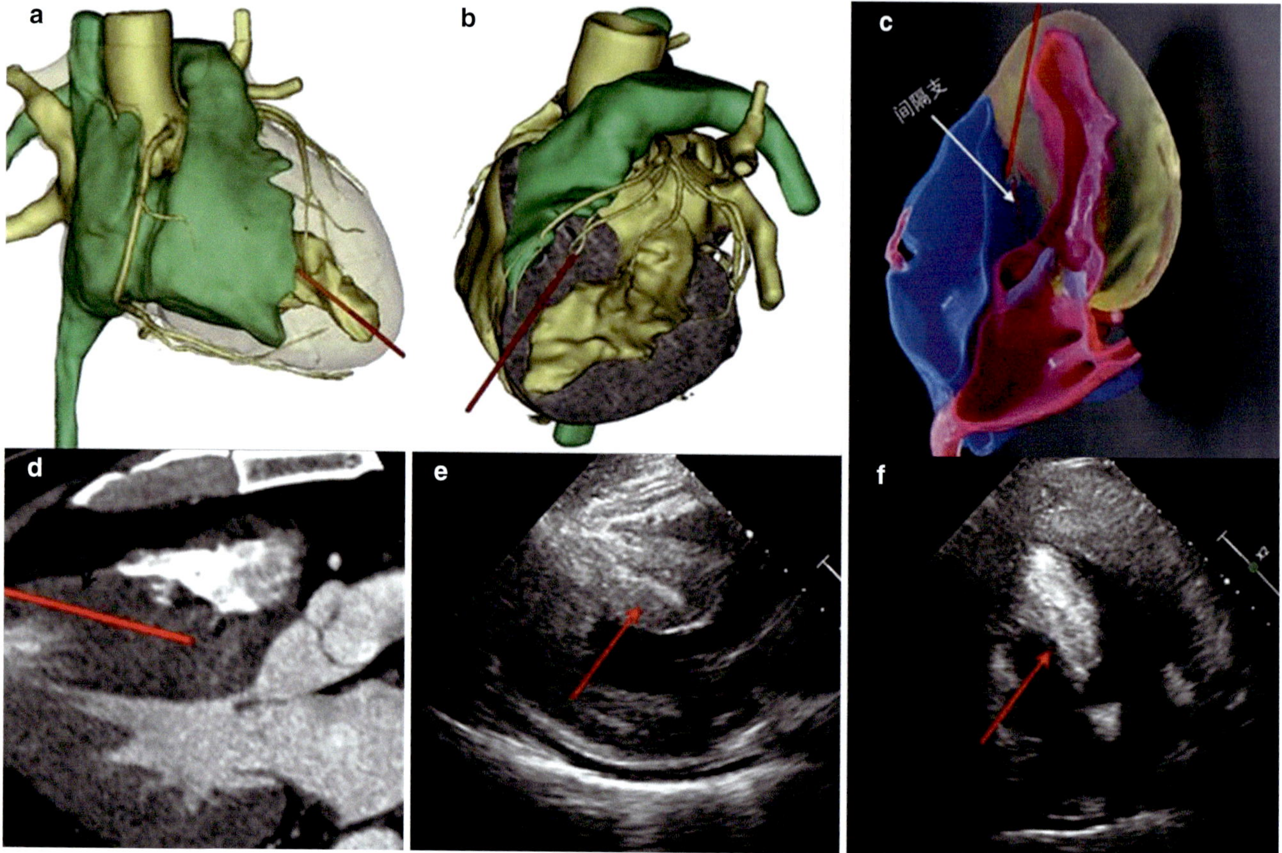

Fig. 10.2 Ultrasound-guided percutaneous transluminal myocardial septal radiofrequency ablation for the treatment of obstructive hypertrophic cardiomyopathy. (**a**) A 3D model based on CTA images: The myocardium is translucent, the right heart is green, and the left heart is yellow. (**b**) The computer section shows the myocardium. The red line is a simulated electroacupuncture approach. The approach is shown to avoid the surface coronary artery and to ablate the septal branches during operation. (**c**) A 3D cardiac printing model based on CTA images; (**d**) CTA 2D imaging display of the surgical path of radiofrequency ablation; (**e**, **f**) Usltrasound images in radiofrequency ablation. The image data for the computer 3D reconstruction and the 3D-printed models were from the National Innovation Center for Additive Materials Manufacturing and the Cardiovascular Surgery Department of Xijing Hospital

References

1. Crossen K, Jones M, Erikson C. Radiofrequency septal reduction in symptomatic hypertrophic obstructive cardiomyopathy. Heart Rhythm. 2016;13:1885–90.
2. Honghu W, Dawei W. Coronary CTA in the hypertrophic heart disease patients with angina pectoris in application value. Chin J CT and MRI. 2016;14:64–8.
3. Tian L, Shihua Z, Minjie L. Contrast-enhanced cardiovascular magnetic resonance imaging for differentiating the patients with ischemic heart disease and primary dilated cardiomyopathy. Chin Circ J. 2014;(29):284–7.
4. Elliott PM, Anastasakis A, Borger MA, Borggrefe M, Cecchi F, Charron P, Hagege AA, Lafont A, Limongelli G, Mahrholdt H, McKenna WJ, Mogensen J, Nihoyannopoulos P, Nistri S, Pieper PG, Pieske B, Rapezzi C, Rutten FH, Tillmanns C, Watkins H. ESC guidelines on diagnosis and management of hypertrophic cardiomyopathy: the task force for the diagnosis and management of hypertrophic cardiomyopathy of the European society of cardiology (esc). Eur Heart J. 2014;35:2733–79.
5. American College of Cardiology Foundation/American Heart Association Task Force on Practice G, American Association for Thoracic S, American Society of E, American Society of Nuclear C, Heart Failure Society of A, Heart Rhythm S, Society for Cardiovascular A, Interventions, Society of Thoracic S, Gersh BJ, Maron BJ, Bonow RO, Dearani JA, Fifer MA, Link MS, Naidu SS, Nishimura RA, Ommen SR, Rakowski H, Seidman CE, Towbin JA, Udelson JE, Yancy CW. ACCF/AHA guideline for the diagnosis and treatment of hypertrophic cardiomyopathy: executive summary: a report of the American college of cardiology foundation/American heart association task force on practice guidelines. J Thorac Cardiovasc Surg. 2011;142:1303–38.
6. Sherrid MV, Shetty A, Winson G, Kim B, Musat D, Alviar CL, Homel P, Balaram SK, Swistel DG. Treatment of obstructive hypertrophic cardiomyopathy symptoms and gradient resistant to first-line therapy with beta-blockade or verapamil. Circ Heart Fail. 2013;6:694–702.
7. Cooper RM, Shahzad A, Hasleton J, Digiovanni J, Hall MC, Todd DM, Modi S, Stables RH. Radiofrequency ablation of the interventricular septum to treat outflow tract gradients in hypertrophic obstructive cardiomyopathy: a novel use of cartosound® technology to guide ablation. Europace. 2016;18:113–20.

8. Maron BJ, Rowin EJ, Casey SA, Maron MS. How hypertrophic cardiomyopathy became a contemporary treatable genetic disease with low mortality: shaped by 50 years of clinical research and practice. JAMA Cardiol. 2016;1:98–105.
9. Leonardi RA, Kransdorf EP, Simel DL, Wang A. Meta-analyses of septal reduction therapies for obstructive hypertrophic cardiomyopathy: comparative rates of overall mortality and sudden cardiac death after treatment. Circ Cardiovasc Interv. 2010;3:97–104.
10. Kim LK, Swaminathan RV, Looser P, Feldman DN. Incorrect icd-9 codes and percentages. JAMA Cardiol. 2017;2:230.
11. Yang DH, Kang JW, Kim N, Song JK, Lee JW, Lim TH. Myocardial 3-dimensional printing for septal myectomy guidance in a patient with obstructive hypertrophic cardiomyopathy. Circulation. 2015;132:300–1.
12. Hermsen JL, Burke TM, Seslar SP, Owens DS, Ripley BA, Mokadam NA, Verrier ED. Scan, plan, print, practice, perform: development and use of a patient-specific 3-dimensional printed model in adult cardiac surgery. J Thorac Cardiovasc Surg. 2017;153:132–40.
13. Liu L, Liu B, Li J, Zhang Y. Percutaneous intramyocardial septal radiofrequency ablation of hypertrophic obstructive cardiomyopathy: a novel minimally invasive treatment for reduction of outflow tract obstruction. EuroIntervention. 2018;13:e2112–3.
14. Zuo L, Sun C, Yang J, Liu B, Zhou M, Guo R, Yu S, Ge J, Xiong L, Liu L. Percutaneous trans-apex intra-septal radiofrequency ablation of hypertrophic cardiomyopathy. Minim Invasive Ther Allied Technol. 2018;27:97–100.
15. Liu L, Zhou M, Zuo L, Li J, Chen W, Xu B, Hsi DH. Echocardiography guided Liwen procedure() for the treatment of obstructive hypertrophic cardiomyopathy in a patient with prior aortic valve replacement surgery: Liwen procedure for intra-myocardial radiofrequency ablation. Echocardiography. 2018;35:1230–2.
16. Liu L, Li J, Zuo L, Zhang J, Zhou M, Xu B, Hahn RT, Leon MB, Hsi DH, Ge J, Zhou X, Zhang J, Ge S, Xiong L. Percutaneous intramyocardial septal radiofrequency ablation for hypertrophic obstructive cardiomyopathy. J Am Coll Cardiol. 2018;72:1898–909.
17. Hongning S, Ruiqiang G. Application and research progress of three-dimensional printing based on medical imaging in diagnosis and treatment of cardiovascular diseases. Chin J Med Imaging Technol. 2017;33:375–80.

3D Printing of Vascular Disease

11

Jincheng Liu, Jian Yang, Guangyuan Song, Vladimiro L. Vida, Wei Yi, Tiesheng Cao, Yang Liu, Alessandro Fiocco, Alvise Guariento, Claudia Cattapan, Weixun Duan, Shiqiang Yu, Francesco Bertelli, and Matteo Andolfatto

11.1 Coarctation of Aortic Arch and 3-Dimensional Printing

Wei Yi, Tiesheng Cao, Yang Liu

Coarctation of the aorta (CoA) refers to congenital vascular narrowing in the initial segment of the descending aorta, which accounts for 5%–8% of the cases of congenital heart disease (CHD). It is reported that the majority of CoA patients will develop secondary symptoms to various degrees (such as hypertension, stroke, collateral formation, aortic dissection, and ventricular hypertrophy) and even death if left untreated [1].

Surgery is the main treatment for CoA [2, 3]. The surgical indications are a gradient of systolic arterial pressure of the upper and lower limbs of > 50 mmHg and a vascular diameter at the CoA site of <50% inner aortic diameter at normal segment. The body growth and development of infants and children will lead to relative stenosis of the aortic stent segment, so stent implantation is not recommended, and surgery remains the major treatment. For adult patients, balloon angioplasty combined with NuMED Cheatham Platinum (CP) stent (BCMED, USA) implantation has become the common minimally invasive surgical approach for CoA [4, 5]. During the surgical procedure, the patient is in the supine position. Then, the left radial artery and the right femoral artery are punctured under local anesthesia, and the arterial sheath catheter is placed. Afterward, angiography is carried out to determine the coarctation site, length, degree, proximal and dismal inner aortic diameters, relationship with surrounding blood vessels, and presence of other vascular disease. The guide wire catheter is then passed through the coarctation lesion to the ascending aorta, the appropriately sized covered stent (CP stent) and balloon in balloon (BIB) catheter are selected, the balloon is dilated, and the stent is released after maneuvering to the predetermined position along the guide wire (Fig. 11.1) [6, 7]. The CP-covered stent has the advantages that the stent has potent radial support force for the vascular wall, which can avoid stent displacement; at the same time, it allows for late expansion, thus laying the foundation for a second operation (especially in young patients) [8, 9].

CoA is mainly diagnosed through ultrasound and CTA, and the CTA-based 3D printing technology can provide beneficial guidance for planning the surgical procedure for CoA.

11.1.1 3D Modeling of CoA

The 3D printing of CoA is similar to other cardiovascular 3D printing approaches. In brief, it can be summarized as image preparation → modeling → DICOM file conversion to an STL file → 3D printing using the printer → model postprocessing.

1. Image preparation
   - To prepare the specific 3D model for CoA patients, clinical image data should be first collected. The image data should meet the requirement of being capable of determining the cavity volume; as a result, only three imaging technologies are practical, namely, electrocardiograph (ECG)-gating computed tomography (CTA),

J. Liu · J. Yang · W. Yi · Y. Liu · W. Duan · S. Yu
Xijing Hospital, Xi'an, China

G. Song
Fuwai Hospital, Chinese Academy of Medical Sciences, Beijing, China

V. L. Vida (✉)
University of Padua, Padua, Italy

T. Cao
Tangdu Hospital, Xi'an, China

A. Fiocco · A. Guariento · C. Cattapan · M. Andolfatto
Paediatric and Congenital Cardiac Surgery Unit, Department of Cardiac, Thoracic and Vascular Sciences and Public Health, University of Padua, Padua, Italy

F. Bertelli
Unit of Maternal Fetal Medicine, Department of Child and Woman's Health, University of Padua, Padua, Italy

J. Yang et al. (eds.), *Cardiovascular 3D Printing*, https://doi.org/10.1007/978-981-15-6957-9_11

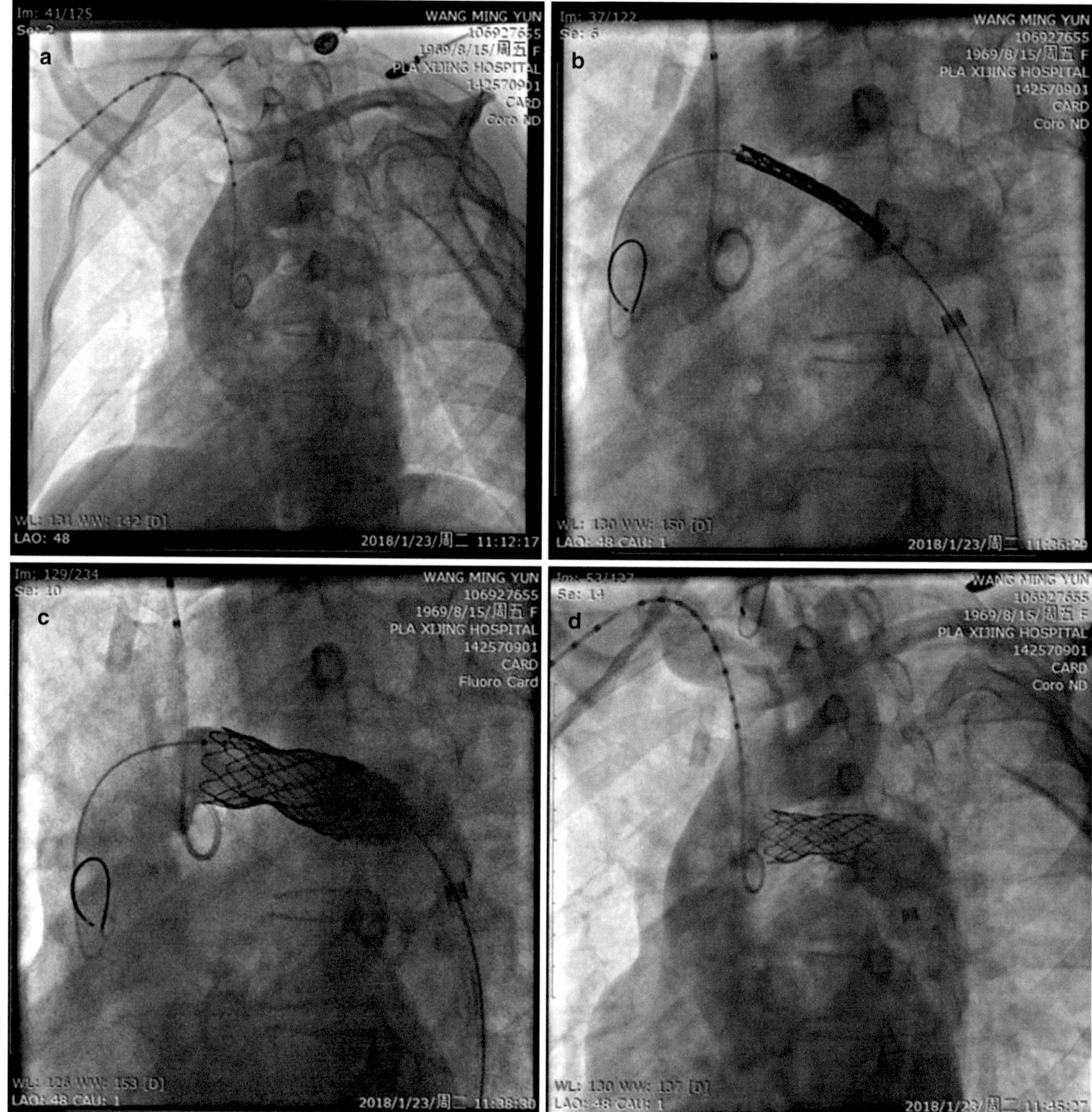

Fig. 11.1 Graphs displaying the steps for interventional therapy in CoA. (**a**) the swine tail catheter is sent to the ascending aorta through the right radial artery, and the imaging displays the coarctation position, morphology, and diameter of the narrowest site; (**b**) the stent compressed through the femoral artery approach crosses the coarctation site to enter the aortic arch; (**c**) the balloon is sufficiently dilated at the coarctation site; (**d**) ascending aorta angiography displays the blood flow within the stent. Image data are provided by the Department of Cardiovascular Surgery of Xijing Hospital

volume three-dimensional echocardiography, and cardiac magnetic resonance (CMR). Ultrasound-based imaging is restricted by manual operation and technical limitations; for instance, the loss of anatomical data in ultrasound images will make ultrasound unsuitable for preparing 3D models for CoA patients. CTA can provide favorable (0.3–0.7 mm) tissue resolution, which contributes to clearly identifying skeleton and pathological calcium deposition. Apart from the excellent spatial resolution, CTA can also be adopted for patients with a CMR-incompatible pacemaker, pacemaker guide wire, and metal implant. Thus far, CTA has become a major image source of preoperative and postoperative 3D printing in CoA patients.

2. Modeling
   (a) Preoperative modeling
   ① The patient medical images (DICOM file) are opened with the computer-assisted design software Mimics, and the coronary plane, cross-section plane, and sagittal plane are displayed. The coarctation position is observed and confirmed, and the diameter of the coarctation can be precisely measured through preliminary threshold segmentation (Fig. 11.2).
   ② Region growing. Exclude images and floating pixels that are not connected with the selected point in the current mask.
   ③ Image segmentation. Use the independent split mask function to isolate the cardiac region image.

Generally, it is necessary to perform multiple independent mask operations on three planes until the ascending aorta, arterial duct, brachiocephalic trunk, left common carotid artery, left subclavian artery, and coarctation segment of descending aorta are separated to form the preliminary preoperative model (Fig. 11.3).

   (b) Postoperative modeling (the unmentioned steps are the same as those mentioned above)
   ① Postoperative modeling consists of two parts: postoperative lumen and stent modeling. First, the stent image is separated through threshold segmentation, which will be then preserved separately. Next, the threshold segmentation scope is increased to separate the stent and the lumen and observe the images, and the diameter of the narrowest postoperative coarctation in the same patient is increased from 2.05 mm to 8.44 mm (Fig. 11.4).
   ② After repeated image segmentation, the Edit Masks tool is used to outline the lumen at the postoperative coarctation and to wipe the stent part layer by layer to obtain the outlined postoperative model (Fig. 11.4).

3. The Conversion of DICOM Files into STL files

The DICOM files of the original 3D model are imported into 3-Matic software for postprocessing, including the excision of the additional parts, beautifying details, and remedying defects. Finally, the hollow function is used to mold the model, and then the STL files are exported for printing (Fig. 11.5).

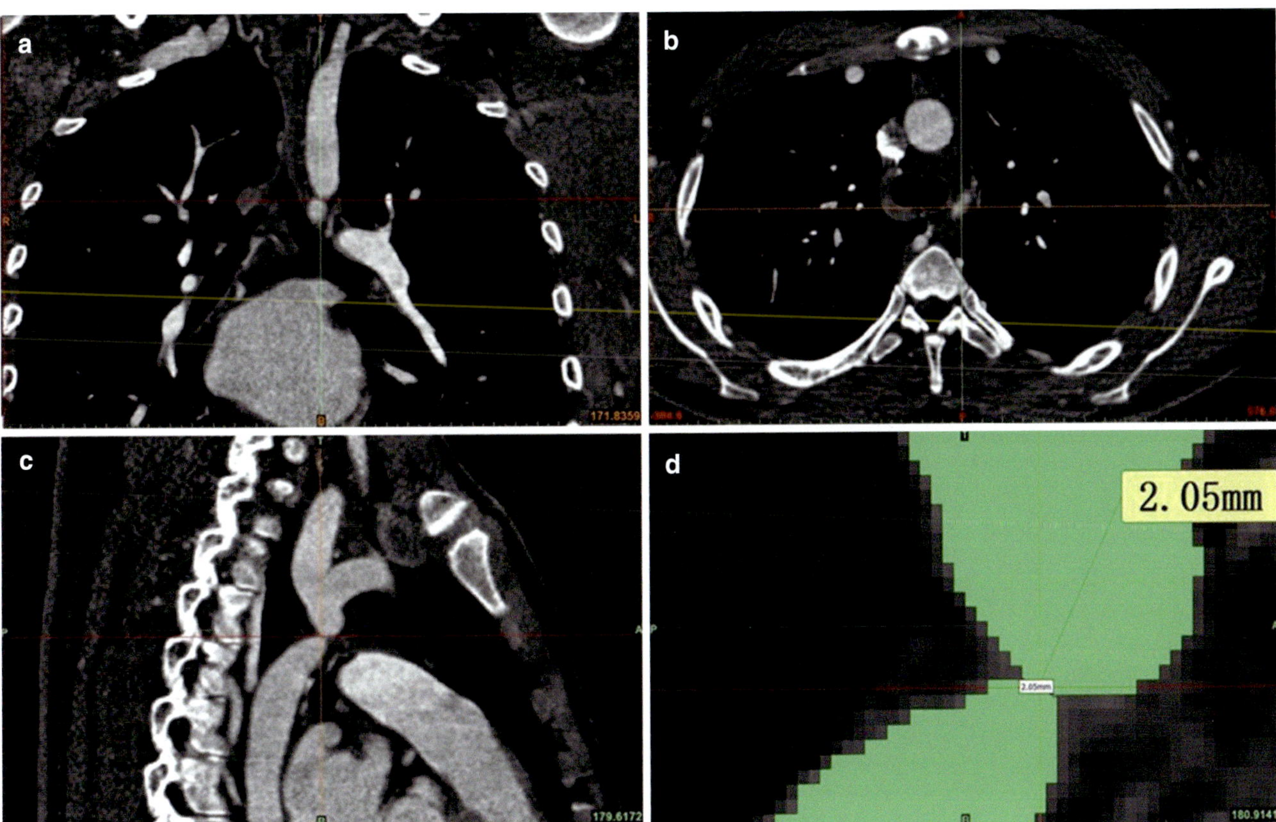

Fig. 11.2 Determine coarctation in the patient and measure its diameter. (**a**) coronary plane; (**b**) cross-section plane; (**c**) sagittal plane; (**d**) the coarctation diameter is 2.05 mm as measured after threshold segmentation. The image data are provided by the Department of Cardiovascular Surgery of Xijing Hospital

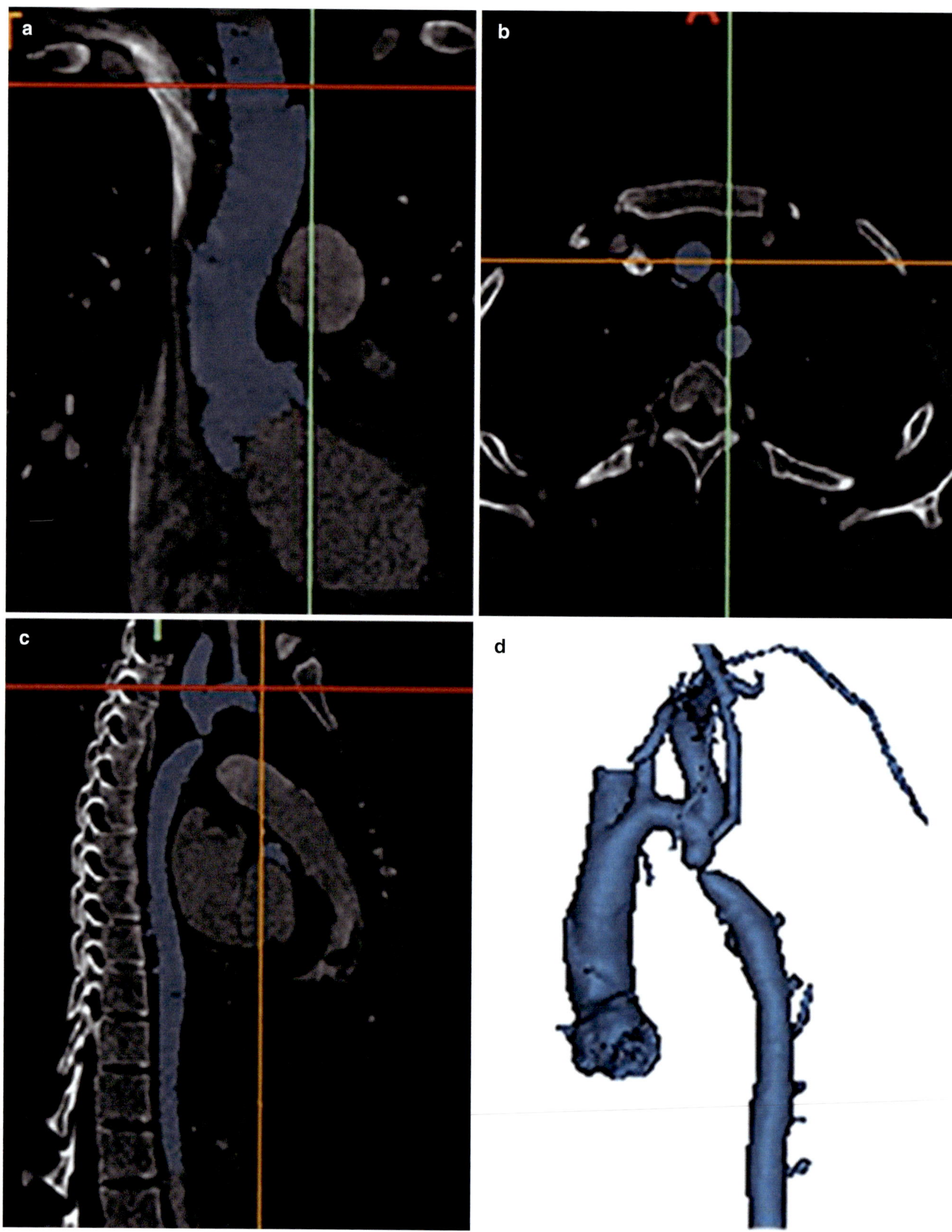

Fig. 11.3 Independent mask operation on multiple planes and construction of the preliminary preoperative model. (**a**) independent mask on the coronary plane; (**b**) independent mask on a cross section; (**c**) independent mask on the sagittal plane; (**d**) preoperative preliminary model after multiple independent mask operations. The image data and computer 3D reconstruction model are provided by the Department of Cardiovascular Surgery of Xijing Hospital

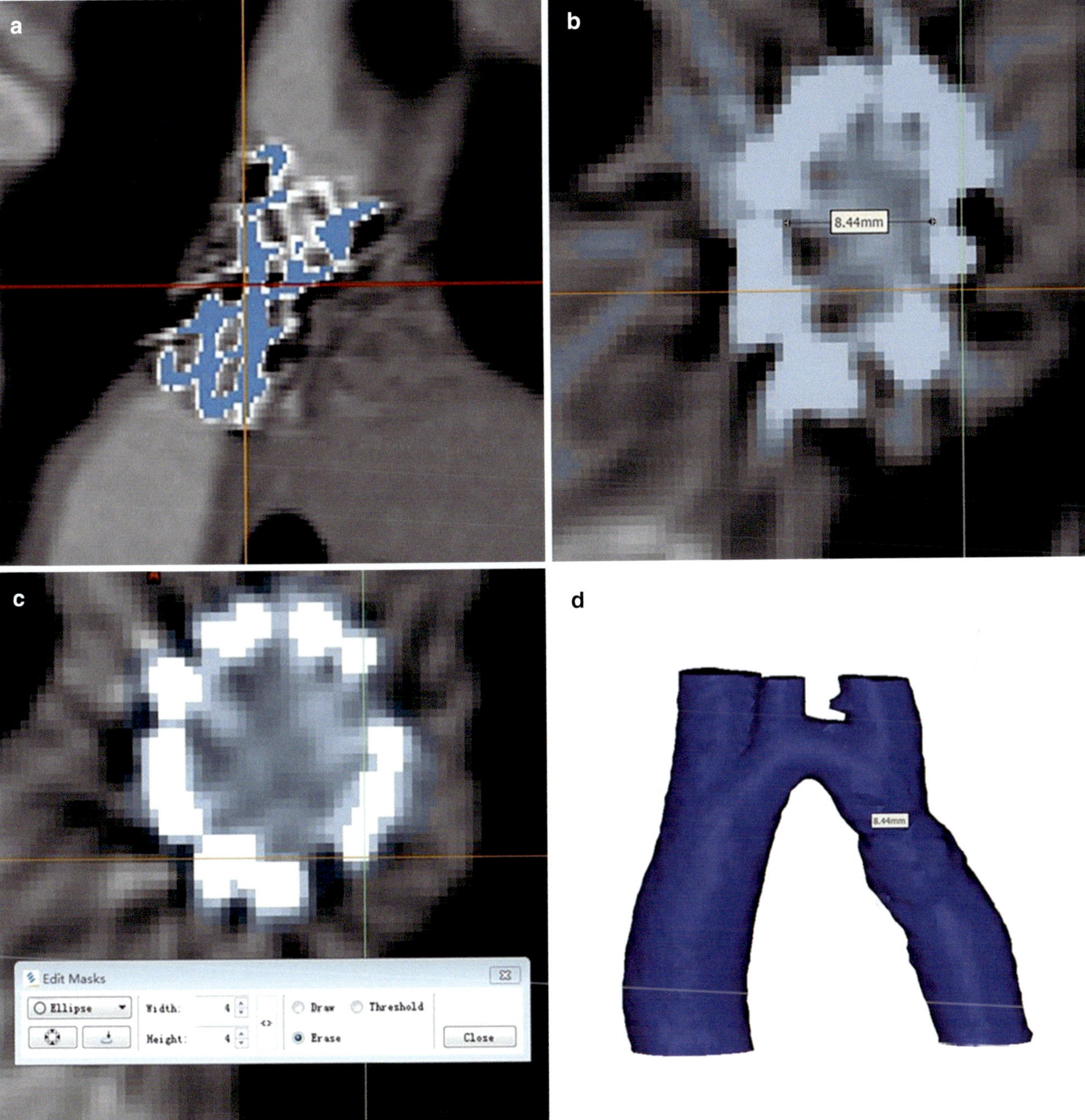

Fig. 11.4 Postoperative modeling steps for CoA patients. (**a**) the stent part is separated using the threshold segmentation function; (**b**) the narrowest diameter of the postoperative coarctation is measured as 8.4 mm; (**c**) the Edit Masks tool is used to wipe the stent part layer by layer, and the white region in the figure is the single-layer stent wiped; (**d**) the unrepaired postoperative model is constructed through multiple independent mask operations. The image data and computer 3D reconstruction model are provided by the Department of Cardiovascular Surgery of Xijing Hospital

4. 3D Printing

Finally, several factors should be considered when constructing the 3D model, including the material type and cost, resolution, construction rate and volume, and printer cost (Fig. 11.6). Common medical 3D printing methods are ① fused deposition modeling (FDM), ② selective laser sintering (SLS), ③ stereolithography apparatus (SLA), ④ direct writing (DW), and material jetting (MJ). Each method has its own merits and demerits, which should be selected according to different needs.

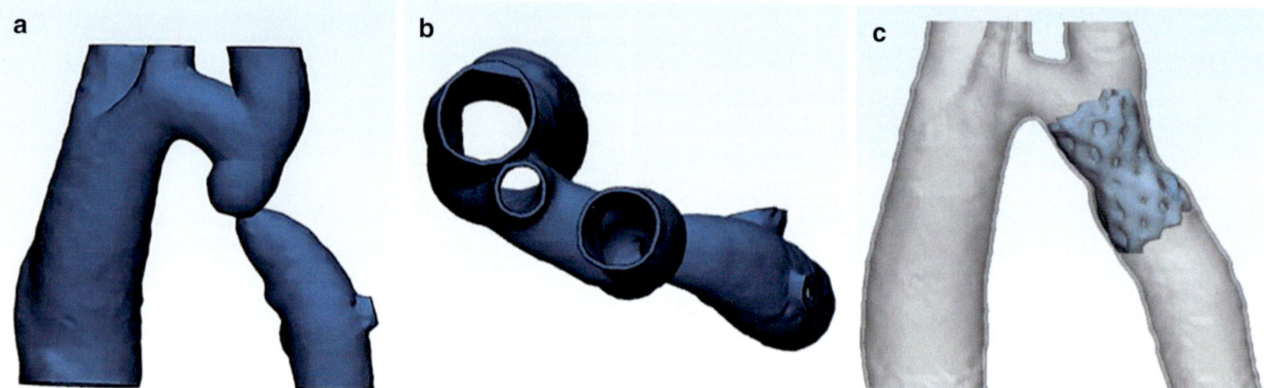

Fig. 11.5 The repaired model. (**a**) coronary plane presenting the preoperative model; (**b**) cross section displaying the preoperative model; (**c**) postoperative model of the patient, with changed luminal transparency. The image data and computer 3D reconstruction model are provided by the Department of Cardiovascular Surgery of Xijing Hospital

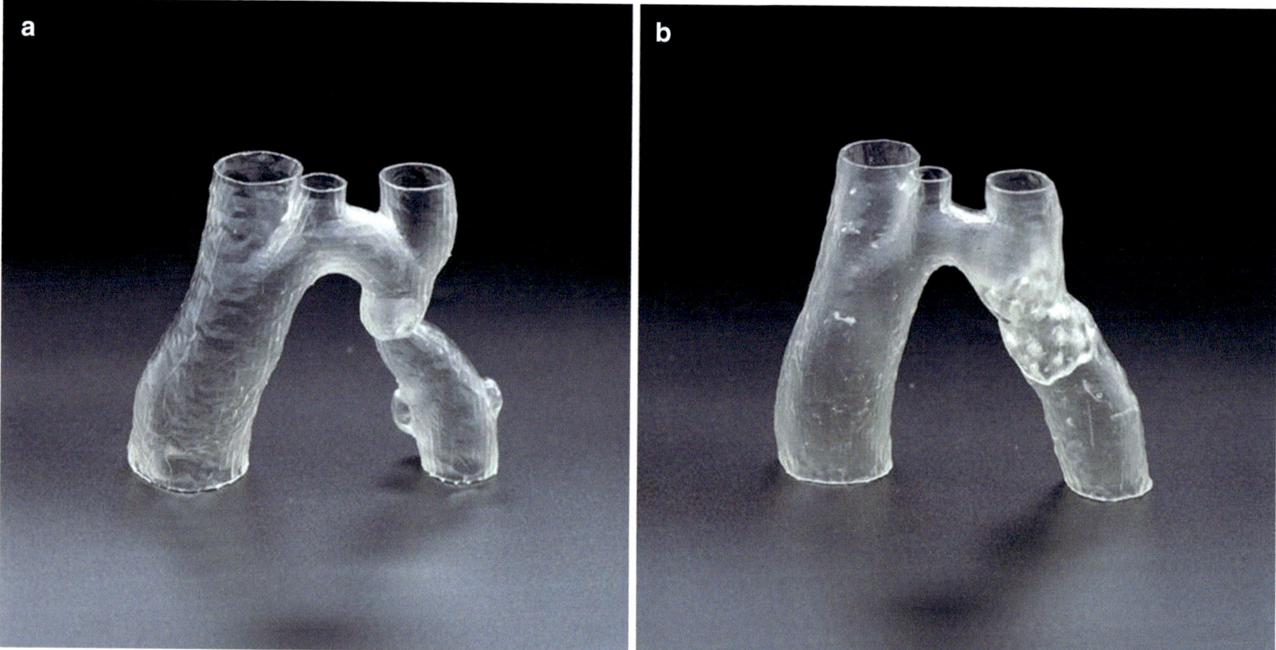

Fig. 11.6 SLA-printed physical CoA model. (**a**) preoperative model; (**b**) postoperative model. The 3D-printed model was developed at the College of Aeronautics of Xi'an Jiaotong University and Cardiovascular Surgery of Xijing Hospital

11.1.2 Application of 3D Printing in CoA

3D-printed patient-specific models can be applied in multiple aspects; for instance, they can be used as anatomical teaching tools and in the investigation of intracardiac blood flow function, model development, and preoperative planning of complicated diseases. Patient-specific models have been gradually utilized to assist in manufacturing or improving intracardiac consumable items [10].

11.1.2.1 Teaching Tools

Early 3D printing is used to manufacture the anatomical teaching model. A 3D-printed model can clearly display the complicated anatomical structure of the patient, present the relationship of normal and abnormal anatomical structures to the medical staff, and help the public better understand the status of the heart under special structures. The CoA patient-specific model has been utilized in the clinical training of resident physicians and nurses as well as for communication between physicians and patients [11].

11.1.2.2 Preoperative Planning

CoA usually causes other cardiac functional changes, such as left ventricular hypertrophy, ascending aorta thickening, and collateral vascular formation, and these changes cannot be precisely observed through 2D CTA, CMR, and echocardiography. Therefore, 3D-printed modeling can play a key role in assessing various CoA diseases with high preciseness. For example, surgery to infant patients of CoA is generally performed through left posterolateral thoracotomy. Their small chest and heart increases the difficulty of open surgery, but 3D models can help surgeons identify the patient's anatomical structure and allow a precise preoperative understanding of the complicated anatomical structure, which can greatly shorten the operation time and guarantee the operation safety [12].

For adolescents and adults, using a 3D-printed model for preoperative assessment can reduce the uncertainty of patient anatomical structure, decrease the operation and cardiopulmonary bypass time, and contribute to enhancing the surgical efficiency [13]. In 2007, Armillotta et al. [14] proposed the concept that 3D-printed models could be used in the preoperative planning of interventional surgery to test whether the device size and shape were suitable for the specific anatomical structure of the patient and to implement the predetermined surgery. In 2015, Valverde et al. [12] published a thesis suggesting that 3D-printed models could accurately replicate the patient's anatomical structure, which contributed to planning intravascular stent implantation for aortic arch hypoplasia. Francesca Romana Pluchinotta et al. [13] from Italy reported a rare case of severe coarctation at the original segment of the left common carotid artery in 2017 and indicated that a 3D model was conducive for preoperative planning and determination of the stent length and its optimal placement location.

11.1.3 Future Development of CoA 3D Printing

The CoA patient-specific 3D models can directly aid physicians in selecting the appropriate surgical approaches for different patients and predicting potential complications when used in combination with the high-resolution cardiac imaging, image processing software, and material science. In the near future, these models could also play a positive role in modifying consumables used in heart surgery.

However, there are some problems to be urgently solved regarding the 3D printing of CoA. The first is error, such as the manual error made during modeling and the error resulting from different printing methods. Therefore, to truly construct high-fidelity models, multiple imaging modes and different 3D printing methods should be used to verify the accuracy of the geometric structure of the heart. The second problem is about materials. The use of TangoPlus family materials (Stratasys) to print the realistic heart anatomical models through the PJ printing technique is currently the best method, but there are still huge differences in these materials compared with real cardiac tissue. For example, the three-layer structure of the aortic vascular wall in a patient cannot be recreated, and thus, 3D models cannot be used to accurately measure and describe the hemodynamic changes at the site of CoA. Finally, the different material characteristics between normal and pathological aortic vessels should also be considered, which has put forward higher requirements for 3D printing of CoA.

In the future, 3D printing of CoA will develop toward transplantable and individualized treatments. 3D-printed titanium alloy, for example, is currently utilized in maxillofacial and orthopedic repair surgery. For heart 3D printing, individualized custom production of therapeutic devices, stents, catheters, and plugging devices may be realized in the near future. These applications hold promising and broad prospects, although additional research is still needed.

11.2 Aortic Dissection and 3-Dimensional Printing

Alessandro Fiocco, Alvise Guariento, Claudia Cattapan

Aortic dissection is the rupture of the intima and part of the middle layer of the aorta caused by hypertension, cystic necrosis in the middle layer of the aortic wall, atheromatous plaque formation, and trauma [15]. The dissection spreads to differing degrees in the middle layer by peeling, thereby forming a false lumen. Aortic dissection is a dangerous, rapidly developing cardiovascular disease with a high mortality rate [15]. The incidence of aortic dissection is about 0.2–0.8 per 100,000 people; it is more common in men than in women. There are two classical clinical classifications of aortic dissections: the Stanford classification and the DeBakey classification. According to the Stanford system, aortic dissections are classified into Stanford type A and type B, based on whether the rupture is superior or inferior to the subclavian artery. In a Stanford type A dissection, rupture is superior to the subclavian artery and occurs in the ascending aorta [16], While in type B, the rupture is inferior to the subclavian artery and occurs in the descending aorta. The DeBakey system classifies the aortic dissections into types I, II, and III. Type I dissection involves the ascending aorta, the aortic arch, and the descending aorta; type II involves the ascending aorta. Types I and II are equivalent to the Stanford type A dissection. Type III dissection involves the descending aorta and is equivalent to the Stanford type B dissection [17]. The most common symptoms of acute aortic dissection are severe pain in the chest, back, and abdomen with tearing. Patients often experience severe pain without relief even after rest or nitroglycerin injection. Most patients with aortic dissection have hypertension. Some patients have severe chest pain accompanied by transient hypotension or common transient syncope. Rupture of the dissection or pericardial tamponade should be considered immediately if the patient exhibits symptoms of hypotensive shock, such as paleness, rapid heart rate, and low blood pressure.

One can usually detect aortic root dissection with transthoracic echocardiography [18]. The more common diagnostic methods for identifying aortic dissection are multislice spiral computed tomography (CT) and CT angiography (CTA). CTA can be used not only to make a definite diagnosis of aortic dissection but also to determine the scope of the aortic dissection, the location of the rupture, and the perfusion of the branch vessels. CTA can be used to distinguish the true lumen and the false lumen of the ascending aorta, the aortic arch, and the descending aorta, thereby contributing to classifying the aortic dissection and to planning the therapeutic strategy. For example, DeBakey type I aortic dissection involves dissection of the ascending aorta, the aortic arch, and the descending aorta. The aortic vessels are divided into the true and the false lumens, with the true lumen obviously compressed and the systemic vessels involved as well (Fig. 11.7). CTA images of a DeBakey II aortic dissection showed that the ascending aorta was divided into a true and a false lumen and that the descending aorta was normal (Fig. 11.8). CTA images of a DeBakey III aortic dissection showed that the descending aorta was divided into a true and a false lumen, whereas the ascending aorta was normal (Fig. 11.9). CTA plays an important role in planning the therapeutic strategy for different types of aortic dissections. Rapid diagnosis is usually required because aortic dissection is acute and potentially lethal. One can also use magnetic resonance imaging (MRI) to make a definite diagnosis. However, it is not commonly used because it is time-consuming and has other downsides. At present, aortography is the gold standard of diagnosis. Endovascular repair and other interventional procedures are usually performed simultaneously.

Once diagnosed, patients with acute aortic dissection should be operated on as soon as possible despite the high

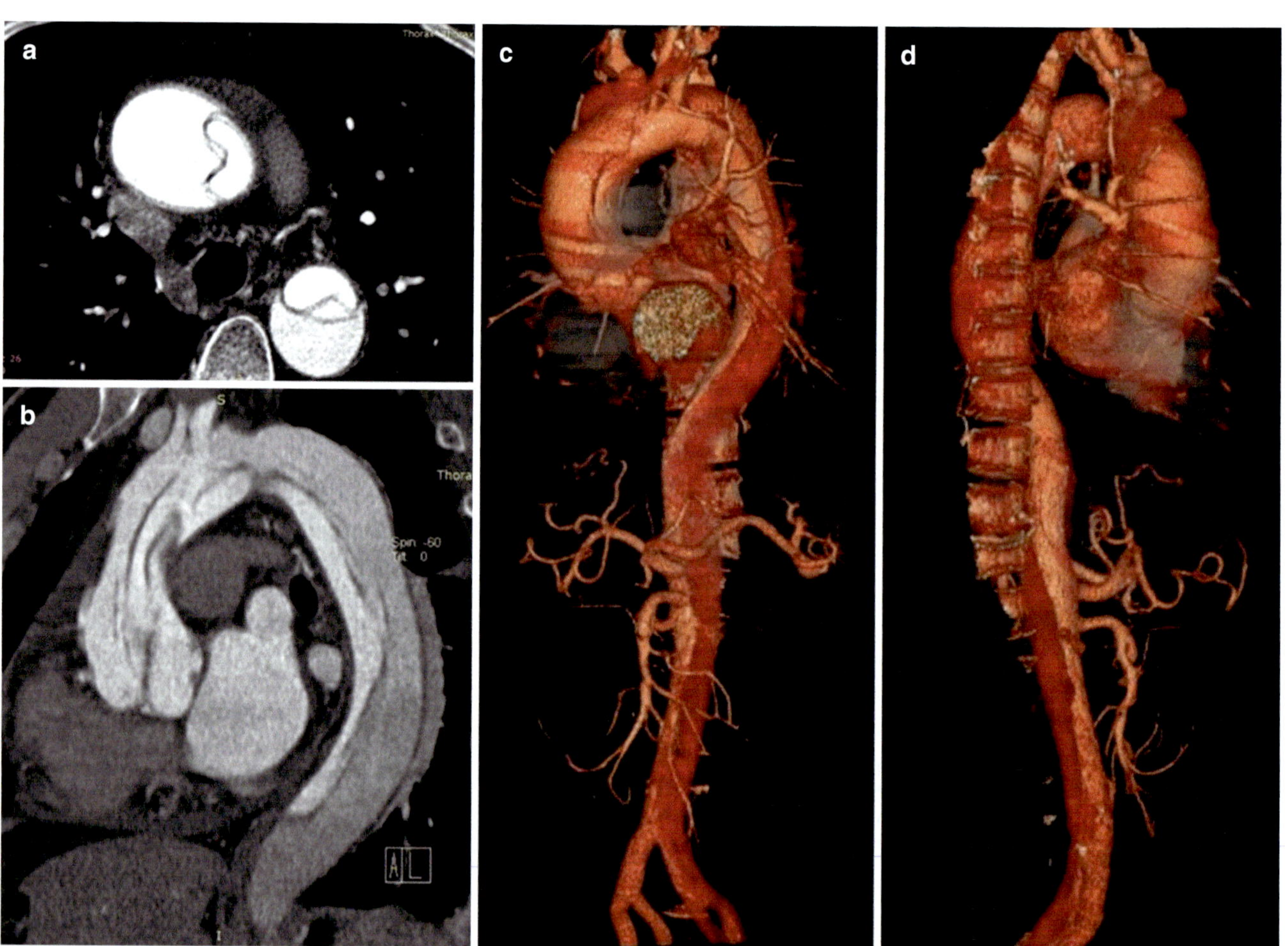

Fig. 11.7 Computed tomography angiographic image of a DeBakey type I aortic dissection. (**a**) Cross-sectional view shows that the ascending and descending aortas are divided into a true and a false lumen and that the true lumen is obviously compressed. (**b**) The ascending aorta, aortic arch, and descending aorta are involved in the dissection (sagittal view). (**c**) The left anterior oblique view of the computerized three-dimensional reconstructed image shows the systemic vascular involvement of a type I aortic dissection. (**d**) Computerized 3D reconstruction of the right anterior oblique view shows systemic vascular involvement in a type I aortic dissection. Images from the Department of Cardiovascular Surgery in Xijing Hospital

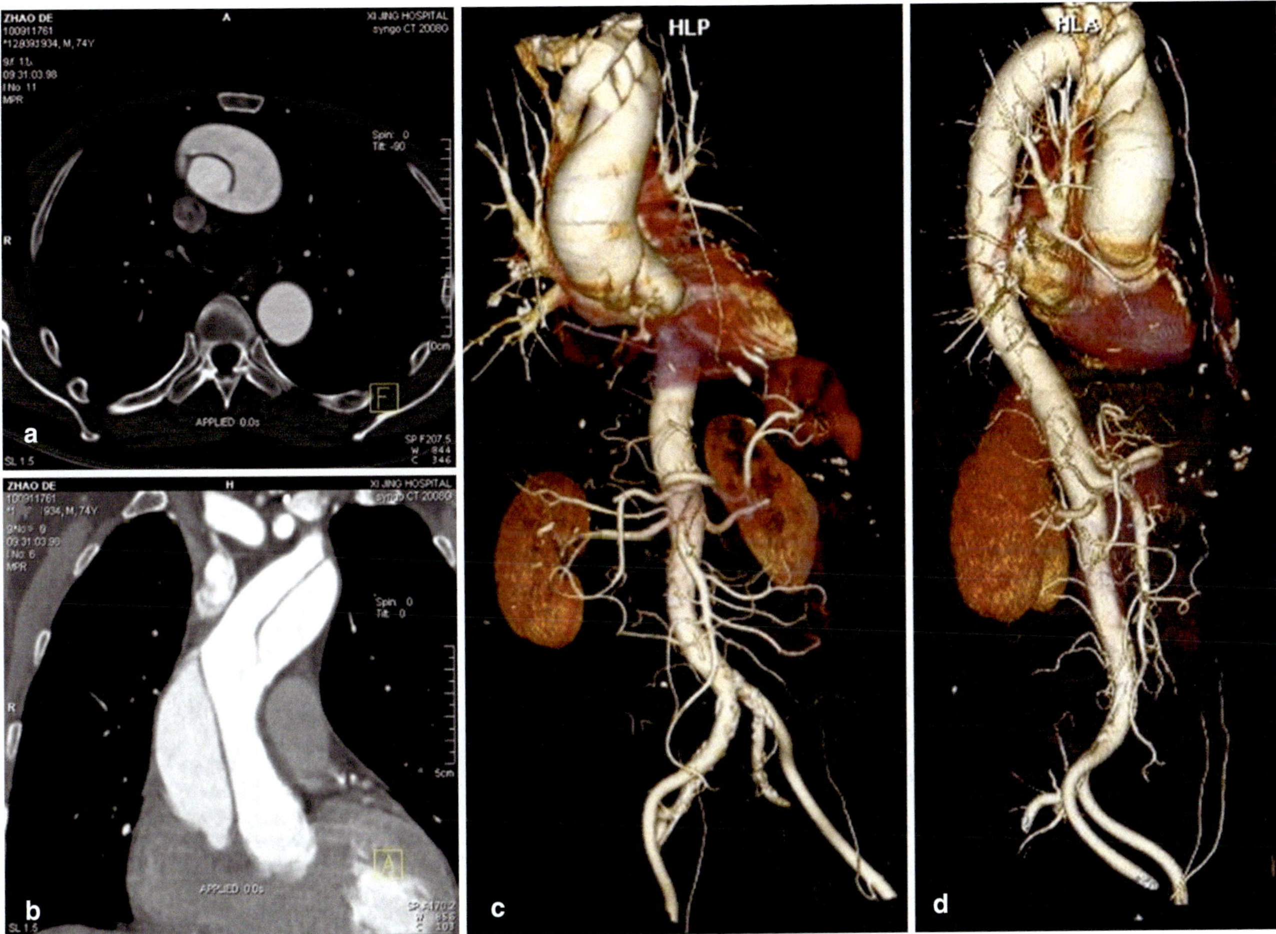

Fig. 11.8 Computed tomography angiographic images of a DeBakey type II aortic dissection. (**a**) The ascending aorta is divided into two lumens—a true lumen and a false lumen. The descending aorta is normal. (**b**) The ascending aorta and aortic arch are involved in the dissection in the sagittal view. (**c**) The left anterior oblique view of the computer-aided 3-dimensional image shows the aorta. (**d**) Computerized 3-dimensional reconstruction of the right anterior oblique shows a normal aorta in a type II aortic dissection. Images from the Department of Cardiovascular Surgery in Xijing Hospital

risk of the operation, especially those with Stanford type A aortic dissection, who have a significantly higher mortality rate at the early stage [19] if not having surgery. Patients with type A aortic dissection need to undergo root and arch replacement or hybrid surgery for aortic arch revascularization under cardiopulmonary bypass and deep hypothermic circulatory arrest. With the rapid development of endovascular therapy, more and more cases of aortic dissection can be treated by minimally invasive interventional therapy. At present, most cases of type B aortic dissection can be treated with an endovascular stent. Type A dissection involving part of the arch and the ascending aorta can also be treated by endovascular intervention or minimally invasive hybrid surgery [20, 21] (Fig. 11.10). The development of minimally invasive endovascular treatment for aortic dissection is closely related to the advancement of imaging, especially the CTA-based 3D imaging of the aorta, which plays an important role in the diagnosis and treatment of aortic dissection.

In recent years, the application of 3D printing in the treatment of cardiovascular disease has developed gradually [22], mostly in the diagnosis and therapeutic preplanning of aortic dissection [23]. The 3D-printed model of an aortic dissection is currently based primarily on data from CTA scans, so the capturing of appropriate image data is very important for postprocessing image analysis, measurement, and 3D model printing. Patients who can cooperate should be trained to hold their breath to reduce the influence of the respiratory motion artifact in analysis of the images. The scans are usually performed of all layers from the top of the thoracic artery down to the femoral artery. To fully demonstrate the details of the aortic dissection, one must scan the entire lengths of the thoracic and abdominal aortas and the major branching vessels. Depending on the patient, the scan may extend to the blood vessels in the neck and legs. The scanning method can be selected according to the rhythm of the heart. At present, CTA examinations are mostly performed with nonionic con-

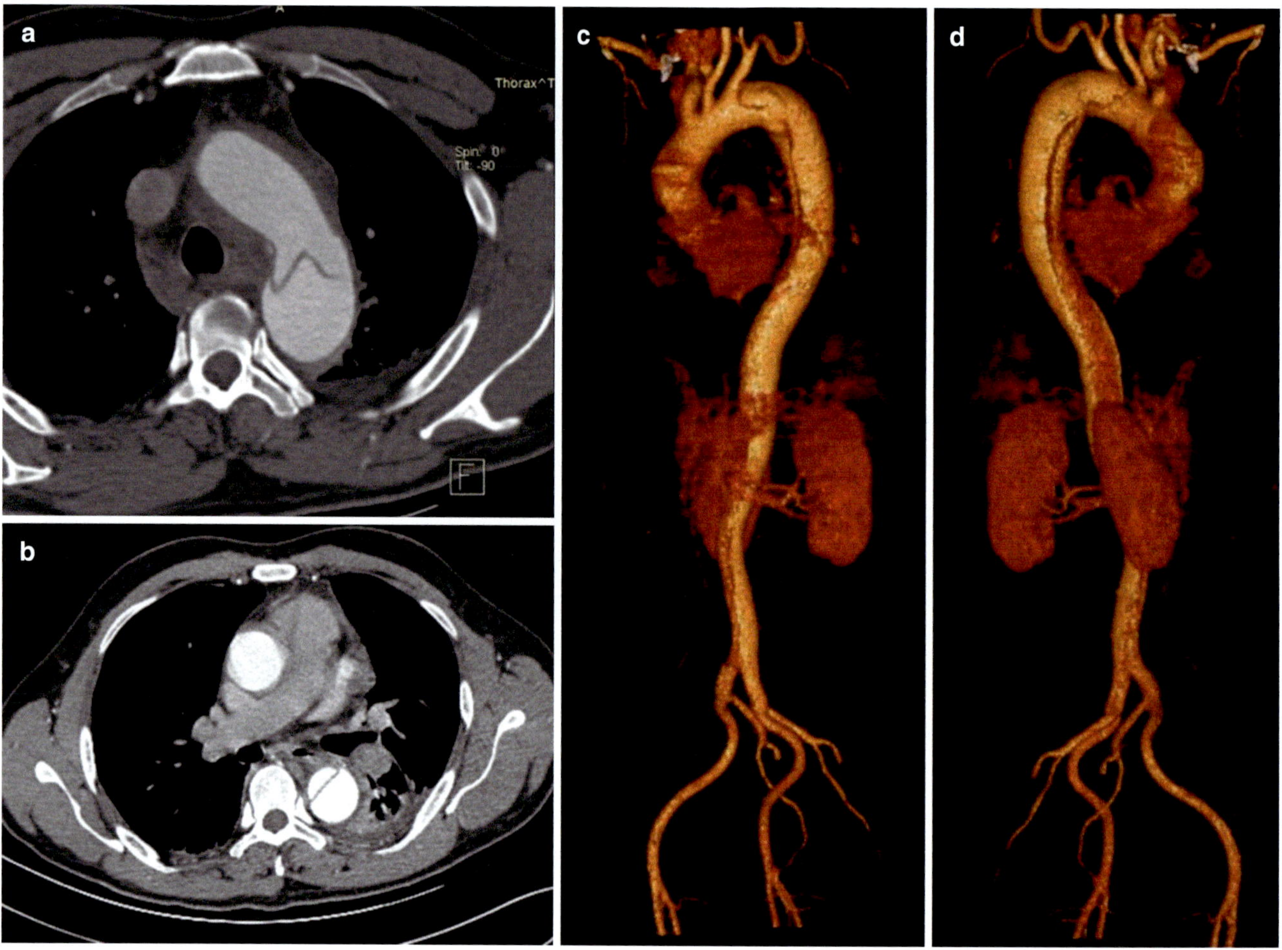

Fig. 11.9 Computed tomography angiographic image of a DeBakey type III aortic dissection. (**a**) The descending aorta is divided into 2 lumens, true and false, and the ascending aorta is normal. (**b**) Sagittal view of the descending aorta involved in the dissection. (**c**) The left anterior oblique view of the computerized 3-dimensional image shows the systemic vascular involvement of a type III aortic dissection. (**d**) Computerized 3-dimensional reconstruction of the right anterior oblique view shows systemic vascular involvement in a type III aortic dissection. Images from the Department of Cardiovascular Surgery in Xijing Hospital

trast medium. The injection dose is 1–2 ml/kg via an intravenous injection in the arm or the leg. The typical CTA images of an aortic dissection will show "double lumen sign." The true lumen and the false lumen have the same or different density. The false lumen is usually larger than the true one. However, for type A aortic dissection, it may be difficult to determine the location of the tears from the CTA images. Low-density imaging may occur in the false lumen in some cases due to different scanning time. For an aortic intramural hematoma, the aortic wall is thickened along the long axis without filling with the contrast medium. The image data obtained before and after the operation can be used for 3D printing. At present, there are many kinds of 3D printing technologies for aortic dissection. The accuracy, printing times, and material costs of different technologies have their own advantages and disadvantages. Therefore, a suitable printer should be selected for 3D printing.

Most patients with acute type A aortic dissection have operations in emergent situations, and most of the operations are open surgeries [24]. At present, the diagnosis and operation planning are usually based on CTA images; 3D printing has hardly been performed before operation. Nevertheless, if rapid printing is available, 3D printing before the operation can be helpful for developing the surgical strategy, selecting a suitable graft, communicating between doctors and patients, and teaching displays [25, 26]. A team led by Professor Hossien [27] from the University of Aachen, Germany, printed 3D models of patients with type A aortic dissection before the operation to guide the development of the surgical strategy and the measurement of the stent grafts. 3D printing can also be used for patient education and communication. At the same time, it is very helpful for clinical teaching, especially the 1:1 printing of detailed models. However, the team noted that for patients with acute type A

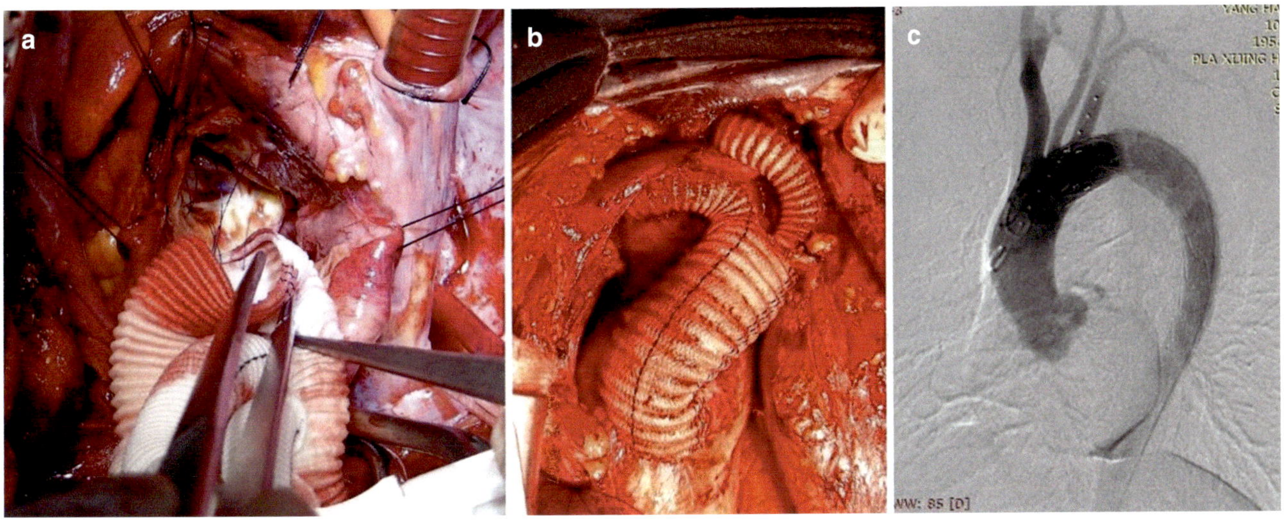

Fig. 11.10 Surgery for aortic dissection. (**a**) Aortic arch replacement by artificial vessels in type I aortic dissection. (**b**) The ascending aorta to the innominate artery and the common carotid artery reconstructed using artificial vessels. (**c**) Fluoroscopy of the endovascular repair of type III aortic dissection. Images from the Department of Cardiovascular Surgery in Xijing Hospital

dissection, the use of 3D printing depended on a new generation of rapid protoclassification technologies [27]. The traditional technology is time-consuming and is therefore not useful for such acute, dangerous cases before surgery.

In the Department of Cardiovascular Surgery in Xijing Hospital, the 3D printing technology is used to view the preoperative and postoperative images of a patient with DeBakey I dissection, which can clearly demonstrate the site of the aortic dissection, the true and false lumens, and the extent of the vascular involvement as well as the position and shape of the endovascular stent. These images are valuable for detecting an endoleak or other complications after the operation (Fig. 11.11).

In recent years, more and more cases of aortic dissection do not require open surgery, including most of type B dissections and some type A dissections involving part of the arch and the ascending aorta. These patients can be treated with minimally invasive endoluminal or hybrid surgery. In particular, more patients with DeBakey III aortic dissection can have endovascular repair. The procedure usually involves aortography with contrast to show the location of the tears of the aortic dissection and the true and false lumens. Then the stent graft system advances to the aorta mostly via the femoral artery. It is important to detect the location of the stent graft system in the true lumen and to stabilize it in the right landing zone. After the completion of the endovascular repair, the false lumen will disappear in the angiography and the superior aortic arch branch will have good blood perfusion (Fig. 11.12).

For minimally invasive interventional therapy, preoperative imaging is the main basis for diagnosis and surgical strategy preplanning. The clinical application of preoperative 3D printing has special advantages over conventional imaging in terms of the 3D structure of the aortic dissection and the characteristics of endovascular treatment. Based on the CT images, the 3D model of the aortic dissection can be printed to assess the disease before minimally invasive intervention. It can also provide intraoperative guidance and make communication with patients and their families more intuitive (Figs. 11.13 and 11.14)

Alice Finotello et al. [28] from the University of Genoa analyzed the 3D pathological anatomical images using 3D-printed models of patients with aortic dissection. The 3D-printed models are very useful for understanding the anatomical structure of the lesions and the accurate measurements. At the same time, surgical strategy design, in vitro preoperative simulation tests, and in vitro verification can be carried out on the basis of the 3D-printed model. According to the results, preplanning based on 3D-printed models improved the surgical accuracy and procedural success rates and significantly reduced the duration of their procedures.

In the cases of complex aortic dissection, distinct preoperative diagnosis and surgical strategy are critical. However, it is usually difficult to define the characteristics of the lesion by routine imaging examination. For these cases, 3D printing technology can help the operators to see the anatomical features of the lesion and the position of the tears directly with details. Operators can also confirm the proximal aneurysm neck and the anchorage area, which makes it easier for the operator to choose a reliable therapeutic strategy before the operation.

The Department of Cardiovascular Surgery in Xijing Hospital performed accurate CTA and 3D printing assessments of a patient who underwent endovascular repair for aortic dissection. In this case, based on the analysis of the

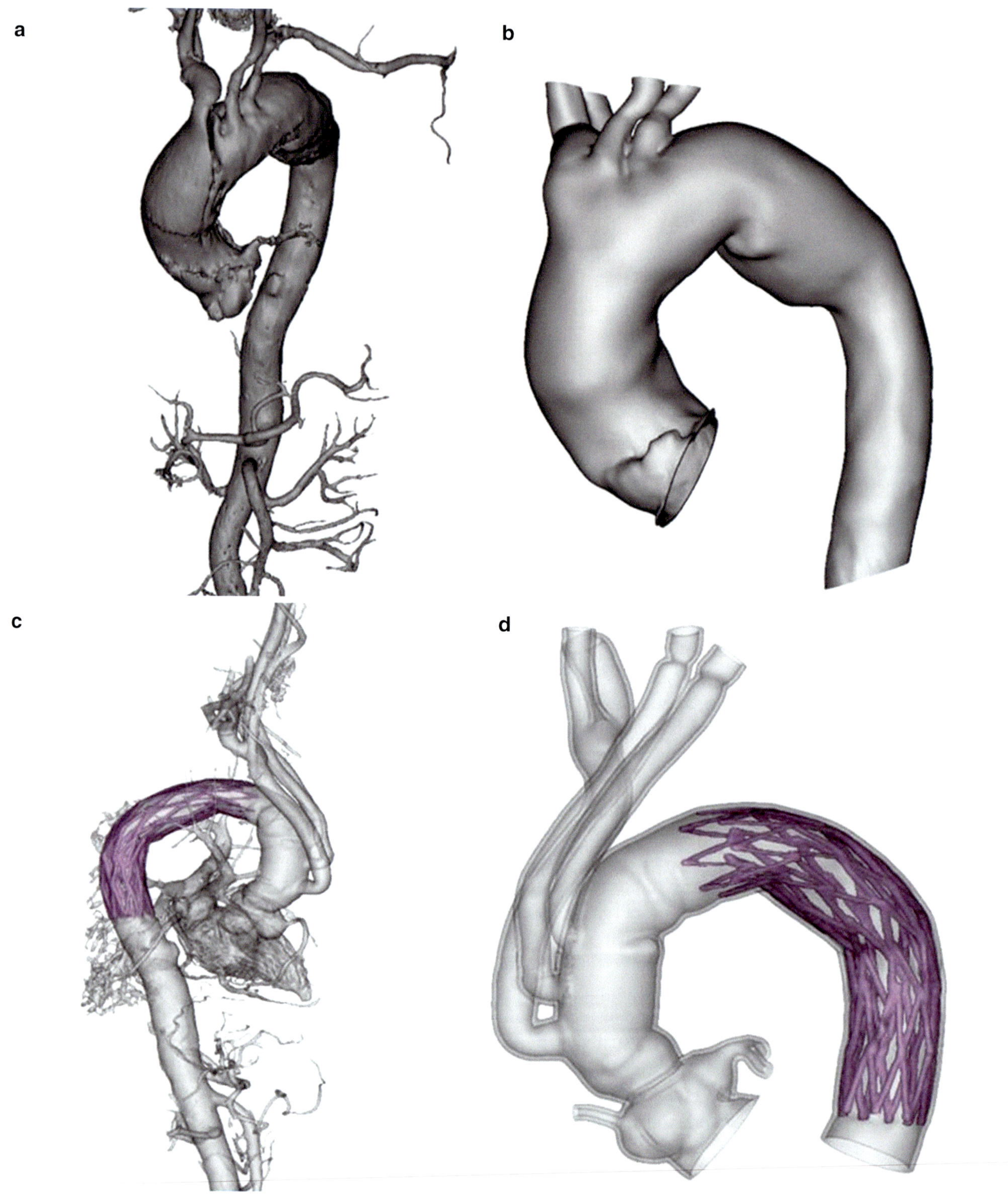

Fig. 11.11 3D printing of a DeBakey type 1 aortic dissection. (**a**) Computerized 3-dimensional (3D) reconstruction of the model shows the appearance of a type I aortic dissection. (**b**) A computer 3D reconstruction of the aortic arch and branches of the type I aortic dissection. (**c**) A 3D computer reconstruction of the arterial branches with the stent after surgery. (**d**) A computerized 3D reconstruction of the aortic dissection shows the location and shape of the stent after surgery Images from the Department of Cardiovascular Surgery at Xijing Hospital

3D-printed model, the occluder was selected to seal the pseudoaneurysm rupture with satisfactory results (Fig. 11.15).

For a Stanford type B aortic dissection with a proximal anchoring zone of insufficient length, the current surgical strategy for subclavian artery reconstruction includes hybrid surgery, the chimney technique, the branch stent technique, the sandwich technique, in situ fenestration, and so on. Preoperative 3D printing can further optimize the selection

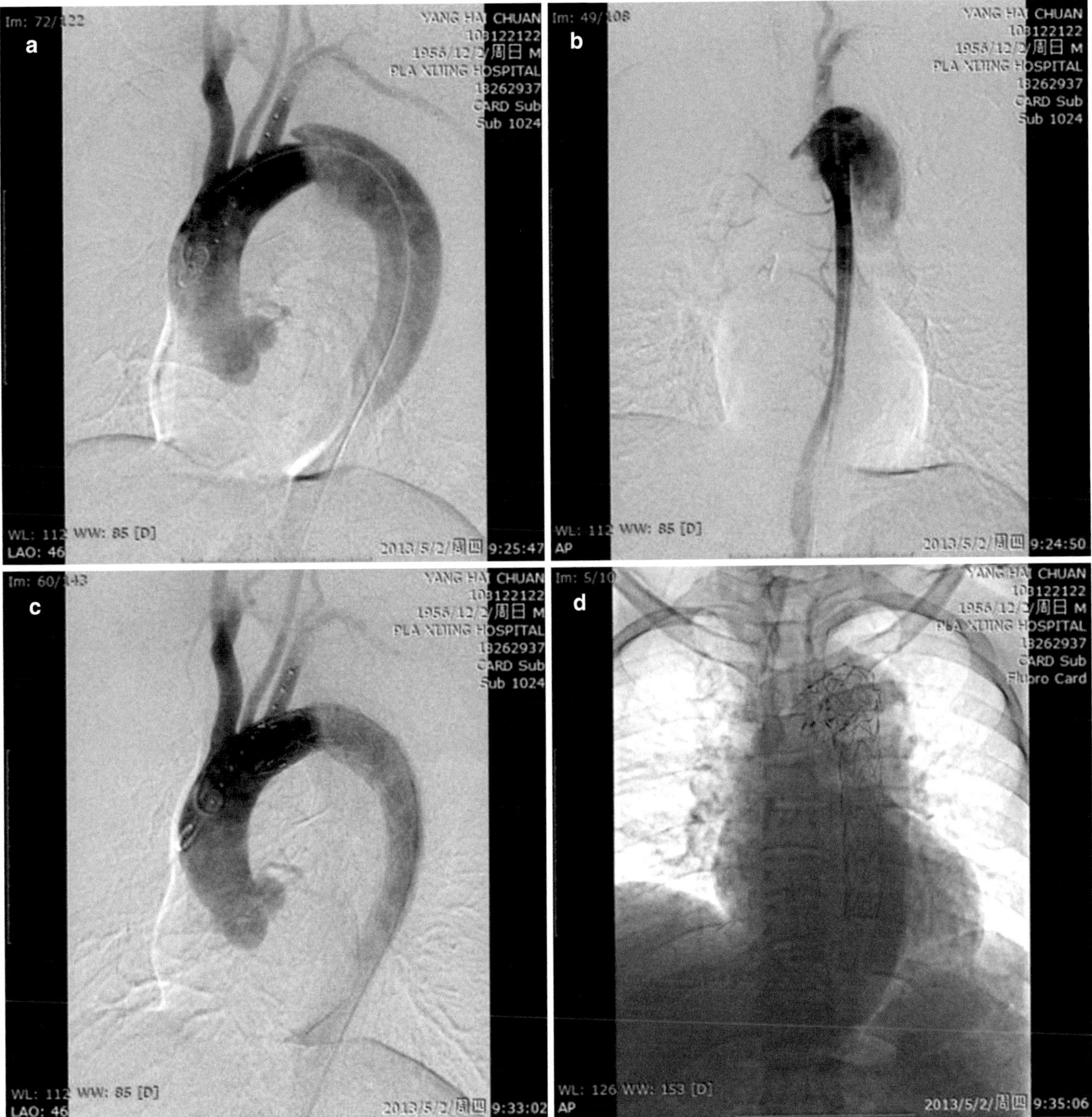

Fig. 11.12 Endovascular repair of type III aortic dissection. (**a**) Aortography with contrast medium in the ascending aorta shows the tears and the location of the aortic dissection with the true and false lumens. (**b**) Aortography with contrast medium in the aortic arch shows the tears and the descending branches. (**c**) The false lumen disappeared and the blood perfusion recovered after endovascular therapy. (**d**) Fluoroscopy shows the shape of the stent in the thoracic aorta after endovascular therapy. Images from the Department of Cardiovascular Surgery at Xijing Hospital

of these techniques. Especially for complicated cases with a difficult landing zone, preoperative 3D printing can contribute to more accurate intraoperative fenestration techniques and branch processing. For some special cases that need a custom-made stent, a 3D-printed model is necessary for in vitro measurement and personalized stent design and fabrication. 3D printing has also been used to assist in the in vitro fenestration design in cases of aortic dissection type B with a poor proximal anchoring zone. The difficulty of this procedure is related to the selection of the fenestration position. Only using the data from CTA to design the fenestration in vitro may lead to inaccurate measurement. The inaccurate alignment will lead to the failure of the procedures. In the past, the diameter of the external fenestration was much larger than that of the branch vessels in order to solve the problem of malalignment. This design could lead to a series

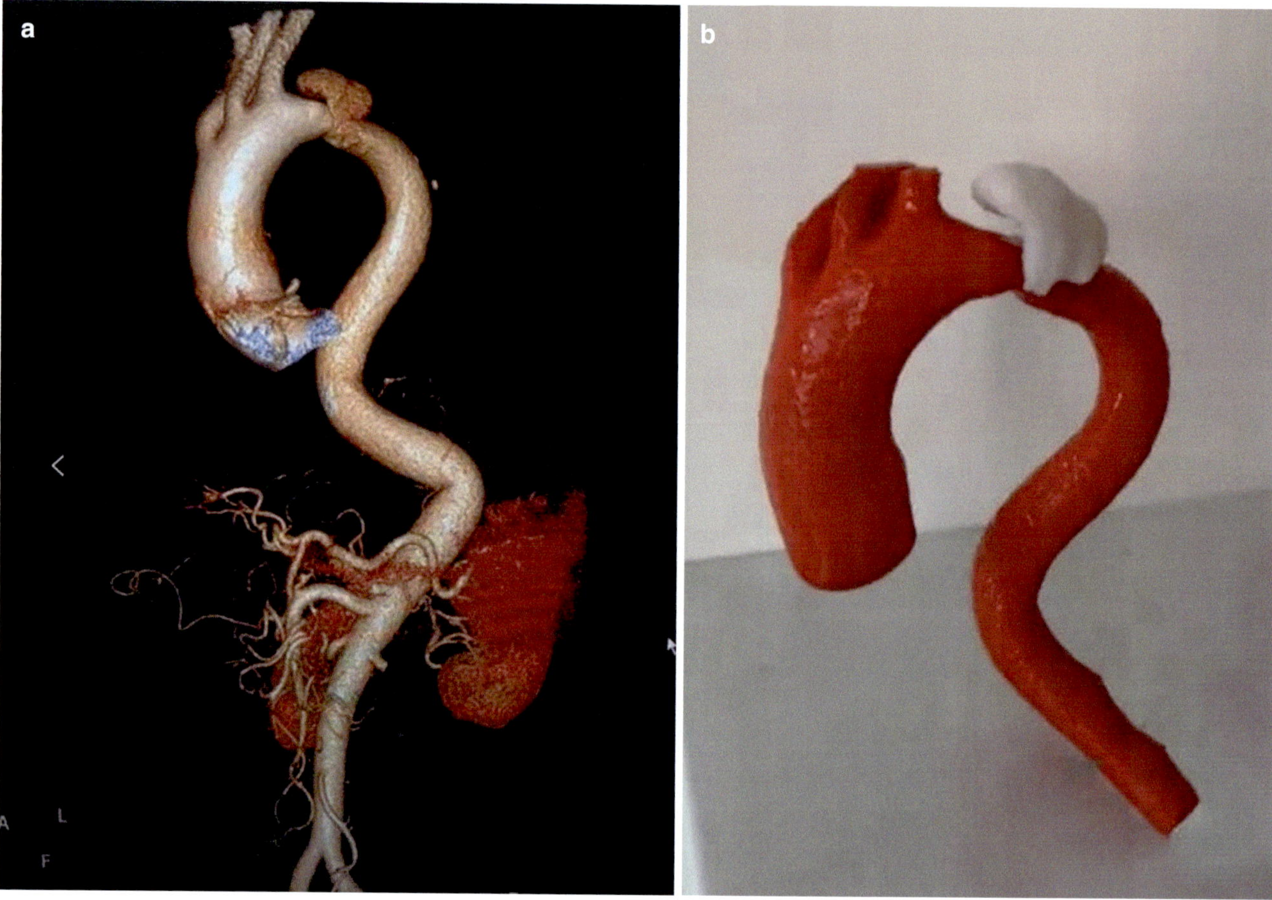

Fig. 11.13 Computed tomography angiographic image and 3-dimensional (3D)-printed model of a traumatic aortic dissection. (**a**) Computed tomography angiographic image. (**b**) 3D-printed image. Images and 3D-printed model from Tangdu Hospital at Air Force Military Medical University

of complications such as endoleak after the procedures. With 3D printing, the fenestration technique can be implemented more compatibly. The in vitro fenestration technique with 3D printing expands the indications for aortic dissection therapy.

Although endovascular therapy for aortic dissection has been widely used in the clinic, the long-term efficacy and complications remain controversial, especially the high rate of reoperation. Alice Finotello's team [28] from the University of Genoa use 3D printing for patient follow-up. On the one hand, 3D printing shows the anatomical problems and long-term prognosis of complications more accurately during the follow-up period. On the other hand, the 3D structure of the stent provides a more detailed basis for the next treatment strategy.

In addition, 3D printing contributes to effective clinical teaching, especially of complex aortic dissections that are difficult to teach and understand. The 3D printing technology based on the case model reflects the characteristics of the disease more accurately. For some complicated cases, in vitro simulation can be used to visualize the problems that may occur during the procedure, which is helpful to improve the preoperative strategy.

11.3 Aortic Aneurysm and 3-Dimensional Printing

Weixun Duan, Claudia Cattapan, Alvise Guariento

An aortic aneurysm is a localized or diffuse dilatation or bulging of the arterial wall caused by lesion or injury. It can occur anywhere in the arterial system, especially in the aorta and the carotid arteries. An aortic aneurysm is one of the most common aortic diseases which is mainly caused by arteriosclerosis, trauma, infections, immune system diseases, and Marfan syndrome. The morbidity shows a significant increase in men over 50 and the males have a higher morbidity than the females. The main clinical manifestations are a pulsatile mass on the body surface, severe pain when the aneurysm compresses the peripheral nerves or ruptures, and

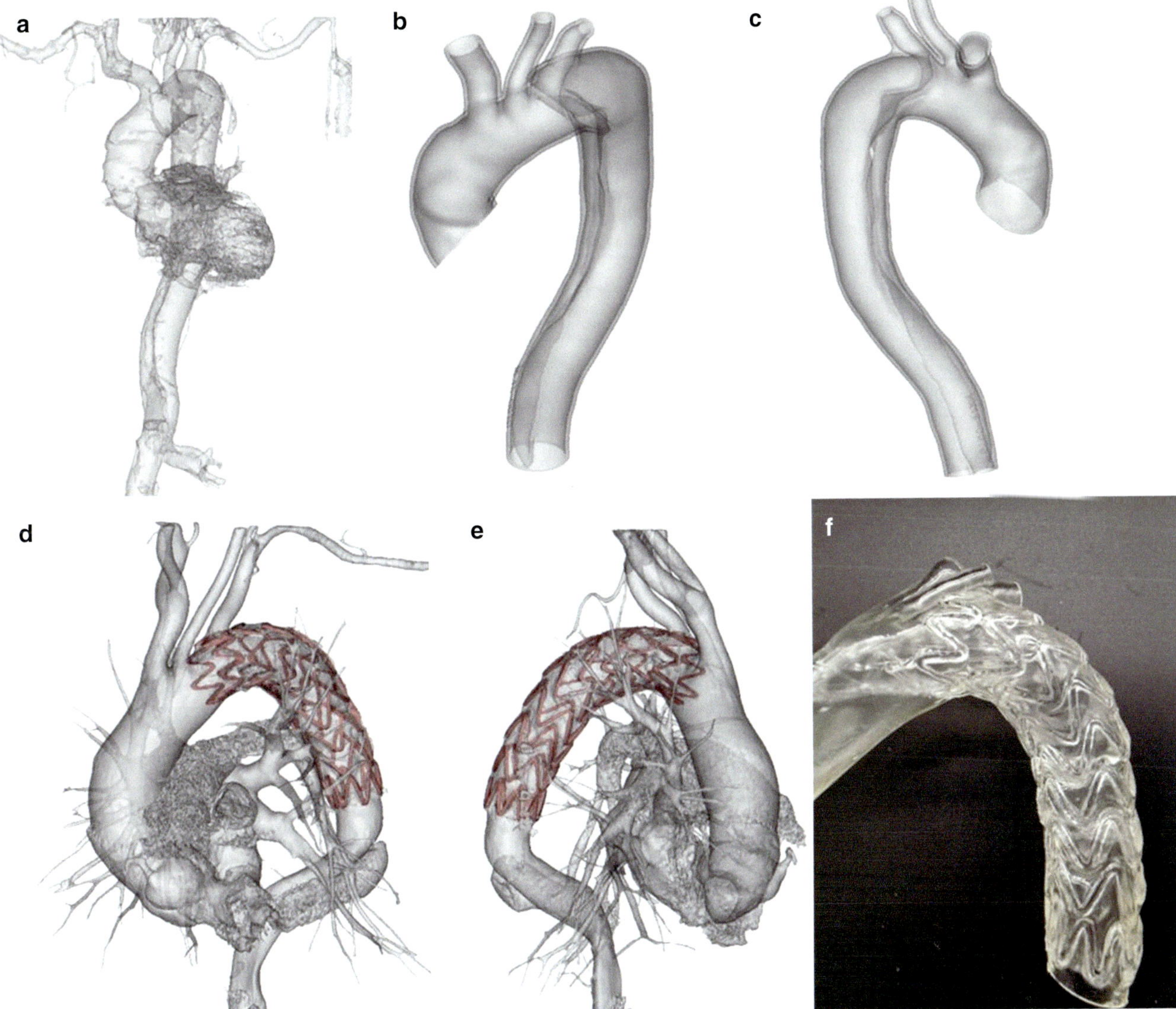

Fig. 11.14 3-Dimensional (3D) printing of a DeBakey type III aortic dissection. (**a**) Computer 3D reconstruction shows an aortic dissection with tears. (**b**) The left anterior oblique view of the 3D reconstruction model shows the location of the dissection and the tears. (**c**) The right anterior oblique view of the 3D reconstruction model shows the location of the dissection and the true and false lumens. (**d**) The left anterior oblique view of the 3D reconstruction model shows the relationship between the stent and the aortic arch after endovascular therapy. (**e**) The right anterior oblique view of the 3D reconstruction model shows the relationship between the stent and the aortic arch after the procedures. (**f**) A 3D-printed model of a type III aortic dissection after endovascular therapy with a stent graft. Images and 3D-printed model from the Department of Cardiovascular Surgery at Xijing Hospital

ischemia or necrosis of the limbs and organs due to distal arterial embolism caused by thrombus or plaque abscission in the lumen.

The location and size of an aortic aneurysm can be determined by a conventional color Doppler ultrasound examination [18]. The more frequently used diagnostic methods are multislice spiral CT and CTA, which are the most important methods for the diagnosis of an aortic aneurysm. These methods can clarify the size and location of the aneurysm, the relationship between the aneurysm and the surrounding tissues, the calcification of the artery wall, the thrombus in the aneurysm, and the hematoma formed after the rupture of the aneurysm. They can also provide more accurate reference for further treatment and are important basis for the planning of the surgical strategy. In addition, MRI can also perform similar CTA. MRI may be used without contrast injection in patients with renal insufficiency. Previously, aortography was the gold standard of diagnosis, but now it is mostly performed during the interventional procedures.

Treatment varies according to the location and characteristics of the aneurysm, including surgery, endovascular repair, and aneurysm embolization. The principles of surgi-

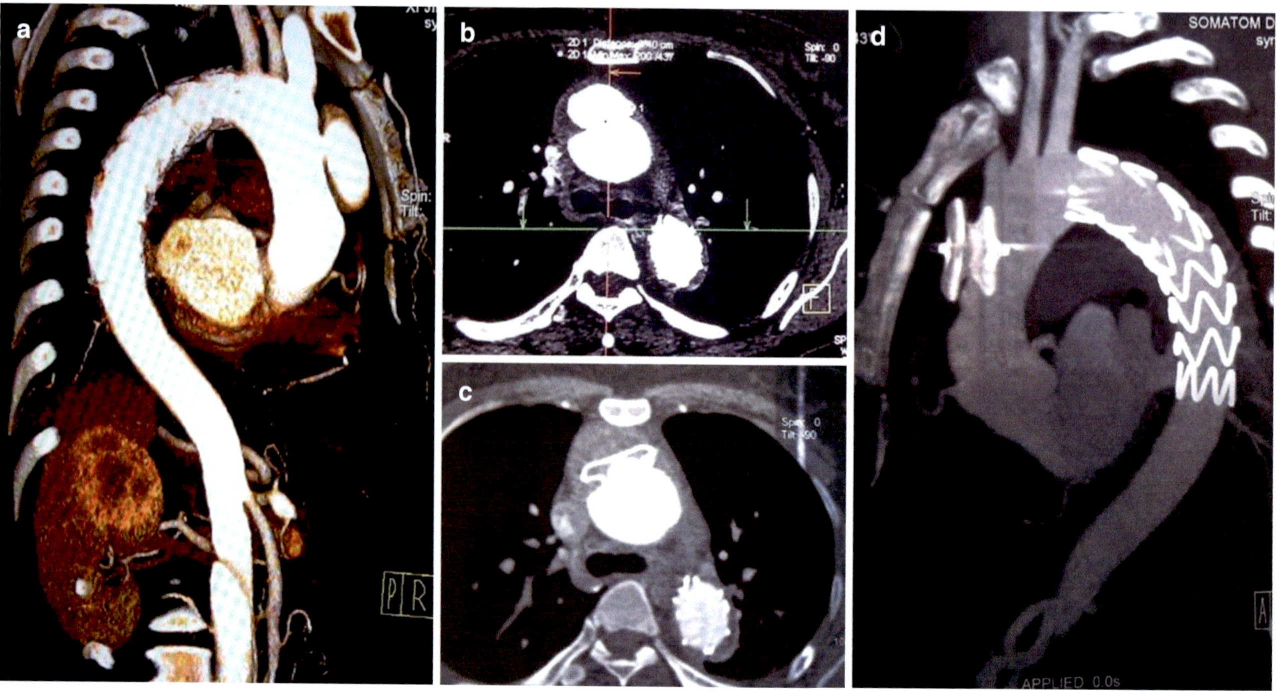

Fig. 11.15 Computed tomography angiographic images of patients with aortic dissection and pseudoaneurysm of the ascending aorta. (**a**) pseudoaneurysm of the ascending aorta occurred after endovascular repair of the aortic dissection. (**b**) The cross-sectional view showed a pseudoaneurysm in the ascending aorta. (**c**) The cross-sectional view showed that the pseudoaneurysm of the ascending aorta was occluded with an occluder. (**d**) Computer-assisted 3-dimensional reconstruction revealed an ascending pseudoaneurysm repaired with an occluder. Images from the Department of Cardiovascular Surgery at Xijing Hospital

cal treatment are resection of the aneurysm and arterial reconstruction. Reconstruction approaches include repair of arterial lacerations, artificial vessel graft, and end-to-end anastomosis, among others [29]. The Department of Cardiovascular Surgery of Xijing Hospital has performed 3D preoperative assessment of patients with an ascending aortic aneurysm to further understand the aneurysm and the branch vessels and determine further surgical plan (Fig. 11.16).

CTA, which clearly demonstrates aortic dilation, vascular tortuosity, and hematomas (Fig. 11.17), can provide a good display for diagnosing most thoracic aortic aneurysms and abdominal aneurysms.

At present, most aneurysms involving the aortic root require open surgery to replace the ascending aorta, such as in patients with Marfan syndrome. Most other thoracic aortic aneurysms and abdominal aneurysms can be repaired with endovascular therapy [30] (Fig. 11.18).

After the endovascular repair of an abdominal aneurysm, the shape and position of the stent can be shown clearly on CTA images (Fig. 11.19). Combined with 3D printing technology, the CTA images are extremely helpful for accurately delineating the size and the range of the abdominal aorta before and after the procedures (Fig. 11.20).

But the endovascular repair of an aneurysm has its limitations. In patients with insufficient proximal anchorage, large angulation, or lesions involving important branch vessels, the procedure can be difficult with a high rate of complications. In recent years, endovascular treatment of complex aortic diseases has been made possible by a series of branch reconstruction techniques, including the chimney and fenestration procedures and hybrid operations. The anchorage area of the main stent can be increased using these techniques. New technology can be used not only to treat the lesion completely but also to preserve the important branch vessels. The rapid development of 3D printing technology has become an important complement to traditional diagnostic imaging methods of abdominal aortic aneurysms [31, 32]. Compared with traditional CTA scanning, 3D printing is more intuitive and accurate. Through 3D printing technology, we can make a clear diagnosis. More importantly, physicians can observe the shape of the lesion in a 3D view and make decisions about the surgical strategy based on the 3D-printed model [33, 34]. In particular, the position, size, and angle of the stent and the procedural strategy can be determined more accurately [35]. Endovascular treatment of an aneurysm is different from an open operation. With the former, the operator cannot directly observe the true shape of the blood vessels; instead, he or she must combine fluoroscopy, angiography, and preoperative imaging data. Great challenges are encountered when dealing with complex anatomical structures, such as a complicated abdominal aortic aneurysm with a short, twisted neck, involving the renal

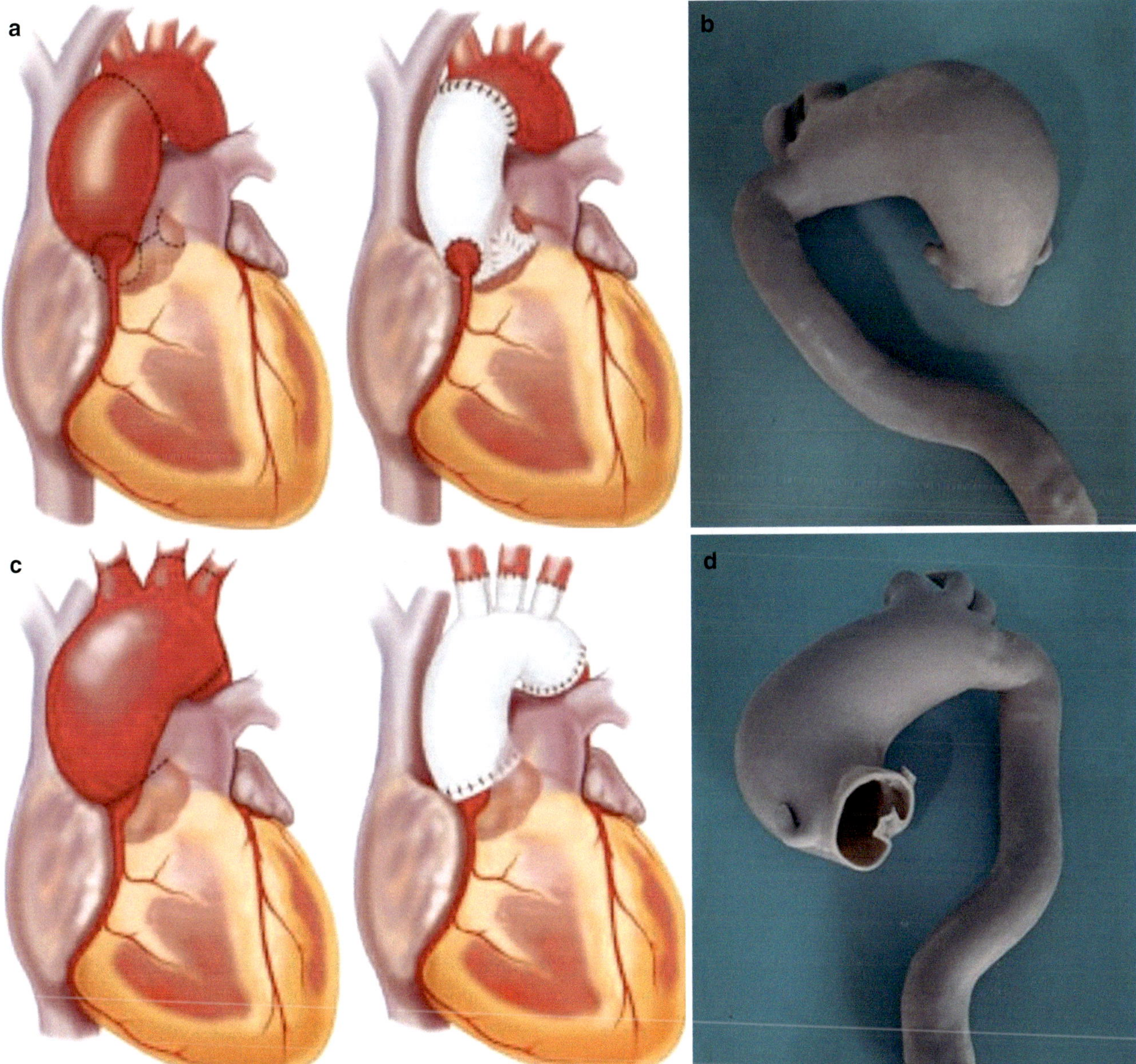

Fig. 11.16 A 3-dimensional-printed model of an ascending aortic aneurysm and possible surgical procedures. (**a**) Ascending aortic replacement with coronary artery bypass grafting for aneurysms involving the ascending aorta. (**b**) 3D-printed model of a patient with an ascending aortic aneurysm. (**c**) For aneurysms involving the ascending aorta and the aortic arch, the branches of the ascending aorta and aortic arch were reconstructed. (**d**) A 3D-printed model of ascending aortic aneurysm. The 3D-printed model is from the Xi'an Jiaotong University

artery or other important branches. It is difficult to display effectively the complex anatomical aspects of aortic aneurysms using only images obtained from CTA scans and computer 3D reconstructions. 3D printing shows the complex anatomical relationships in a 1:1 model. The precise measurements and surgical strategy can be recreated with the 3D-printed model [36, 37].

Dr. Tam's [38] team from St. Mary's Hospital in Hong Kong conducted a meta-analysis of 3D printing applications in the endovascular treatment of aortic aneurysms. Overall, 3D printing has been used primarily for the preoperative evaluation of abdominal aortic aneurysms and thoracic aortic aneurysms in order to preplan the surgical strategies. Based on previous studies, 3D printing technology can help the surgeon visualize the anatomical features of the lesion and judge the location and structure of the proximal neck and anchorage area. The rate of successful operations has increased, and the time of exposure to irradiation from digital subtraction angiography and the operating time were shortened with the use of 3D printing. 3D printing also contributes to effective doctor–patient communication and to teaching.

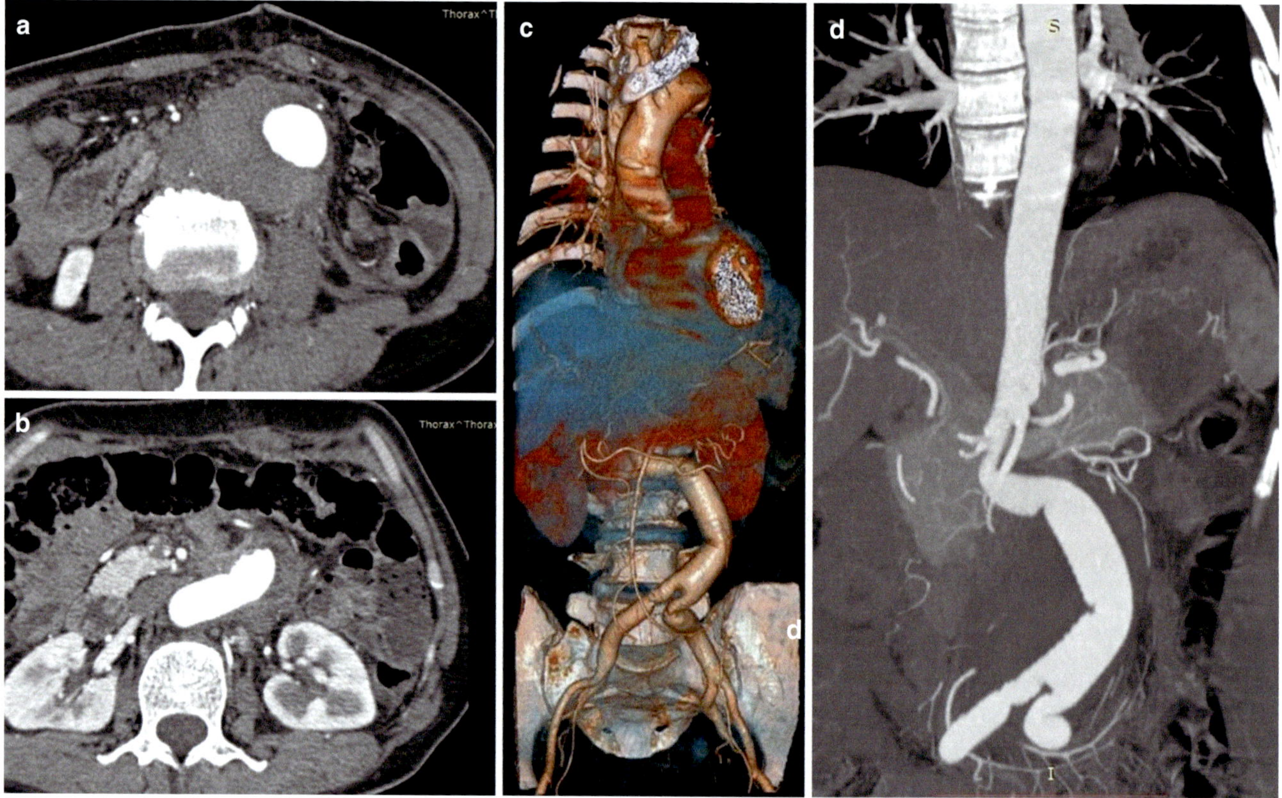

Fig. 11.17 Computed tomography angiographic images of the abdominal aneurysm. (**a**) cross-sectional view of the abdominal aorta shows distension and peripheral hematoma. (**b**) Abdominal aortic tortuosity shown in cross section. (**c**) A 3-dimensional (3D)-printed model of an abdominal aneurysm. (**d**) A 3D model display of a 3D abdominal aortic aneurysm and the surrounding hematoma. Images from the Department of Cardiovascular Surgery at Xijing Hospital

Torres's [37] team from the University of São Paulo created a transparent 3D-printed model of an abdominal aortic aneurysm. They simulated the procedure with this transparent model in vitro before the operation. This in vitro simulation helped strategy and stent selection and improved the efficiency of the operation by shortening the procedural time.

For the most common abdominal aortic aneurysm, a stent anchorage of at least 15–20 mm in the proximal portion of the lesion is generally required. However, the anchoring zone below the renal artery is less than 15 mm in some patients, and even the aortic aneurysm extends directly across the renal artery. For the endovascular treatment of this kind of complicated aneurysm, a series of fenestration techniques is often used. The fenestration is performed to preserve the important branches.

The key point of the fenestration technique is to carefully preplan the procedure according to the preoperative imaging data and determine the location and relative relationship of each branch artery. The inaccurate release of the stent may result in failure of fenestration or target organ ischemia. Accurate preoperative measurement and localization are essential. In the past, the fenestration procedure depended mainly on image measurements, which were the basis of a custom-made fenestration stent or a conventional stent. A custom-made stent graft is relatively accurate. But a custom-made stent is time-consuming and expensive. In emergency cases, i.e., patients with ruptured aortas, it is difficult to use a custom-made stent.

Traditional CTA can be used to reconstruct the anatomical performance of the aneurysm, but the measurements are not exact enough for strategic preplanning. The errors in measurement could lead to a mismatch between the aneurysm and the endovascular stent. Letta's team [18] from the University of Washington use 3D-printed models to perform the actual measurement of the aneurysm. Based on their models, the physicians can understand the morphological characteristics of all the branch vessels and directly and accurately measure the specific dimensions of the superior mesenteric artery, the bilateral renal artery, and the bilateral

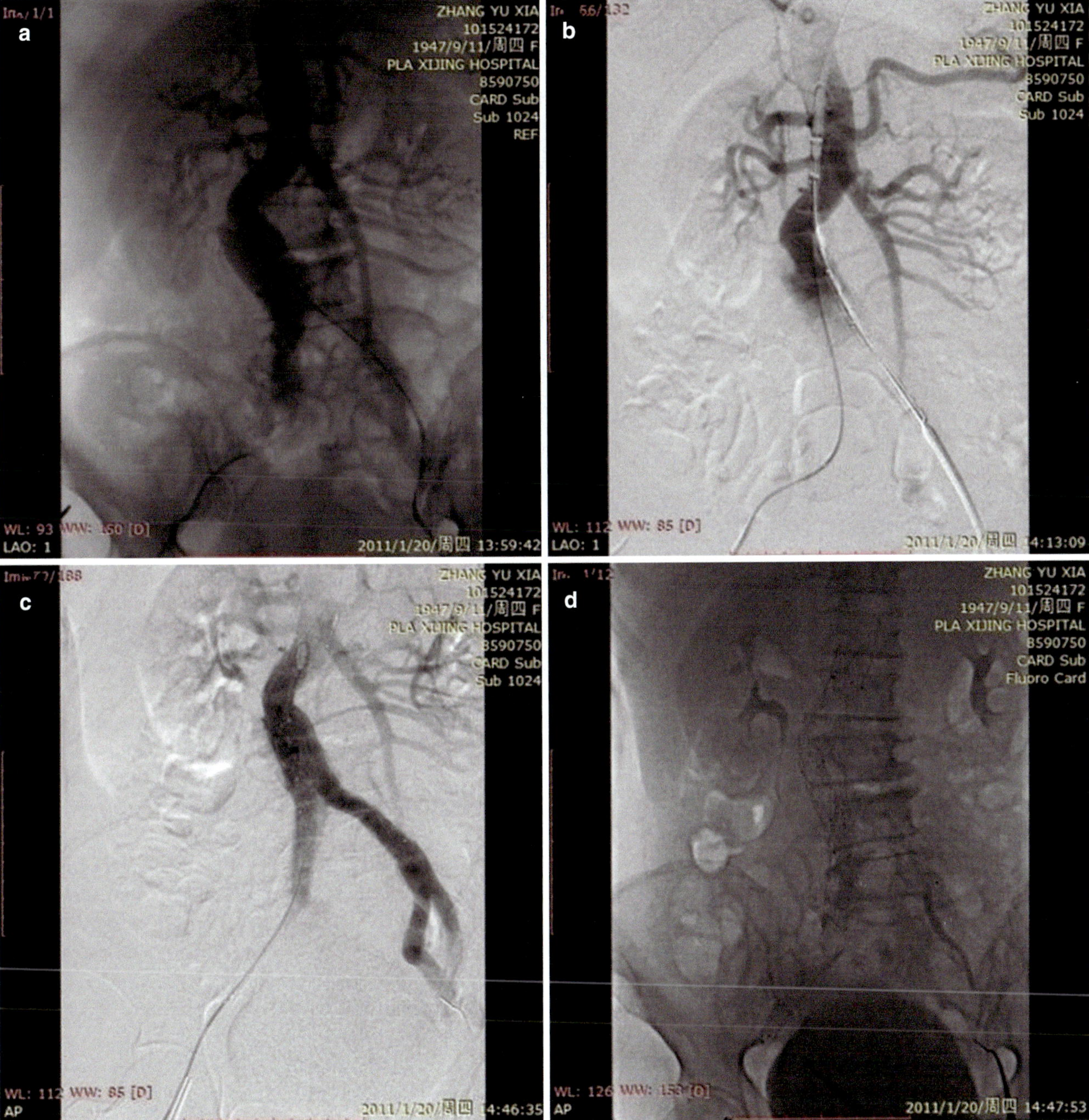

Fig. 11.18 Endovascular repair procedure for an abdominal aneurysm. (**a**) The location, shape, size, and involvement of the visceral branching vessels of the aneurysm were demonstrated by angiography. (**b**) A compressed stent graft delivery system was advanced by the femoral approach. (**c**) Angiography showed that the aneurysm was isolated and that the blood flow in the abdominal aorta was patent after release of the stent. (**d**) Fluoroscopy revealed the satisfactory shape of the stent in the abdominal aorta after endovascular therapy. Images from the Department of Cardiovascular Surgery at Xijing Hospital

iliac artery. For an abdominal aortic aneurysm with an angular neck, a 3D-printed model can accurately display the anatomical positions and directions of all the branches, which helps fenestration design in vitro before carrying out the procedures [39].

In addition, the design of custom-made stents can be verified with in vitro simulation based on the 3D-printed models [40]. It is helpful in preplanning the endovascular therapy [41]. This technique can improve the success rates of the procedures.

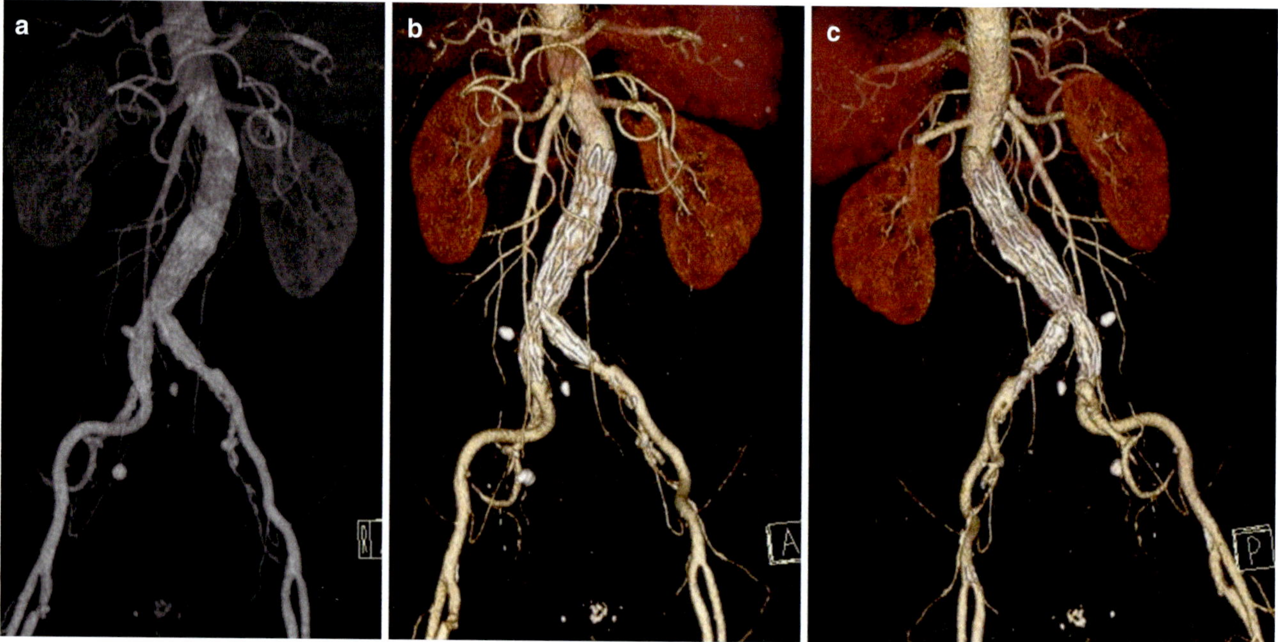

Fig. 11.19 Computed tomography angiographic images after endovascular repair of an abdominal aneurysm. (**a**) The coronary view shows the endovascular repair of the abdominal aorta below the level of the renal artery. (**b**) Endovascular repair of the abdominal aorta below the renal artery plane on computer-aided 3-dimensional images. (**c**) Endovascular repair of the abdominal aorta below the renal artery. Images from the Department of Cardiovascular Surgery at Xijing Hospital

11.4 Takayasu Arteritis and 3-Dimensional Printing

Shiqiang Yu, Francesco Bertelli, Matteo Andolfatto

Takayasu arteritis is a chronic nonspecific inflammatory disease of the aorta. It usually occurs in the brachiocephalic trunk, the renal artery, the thoracic and abdominal aorta, and the superior mesenteric artery [42] and may cause stenosis and occlusion in different parts of the arteries, and even aneurysm [43]. It is most common in young women.

The etiology of this disease is thought to be related to the autoimmune system. Based on the extent of involvement of the aorta, the patients were classified into four types: type I, brachiocephalic artery type; type II, aortic or renal artery type; type III, extensive type; and type IV, pulmonary artery type. Patients with Takayasu arteritis can have hypertension in the upper limbs and insufficient blood perfusion in the lower limbs because of aortic stenosis. The patients usually present with headache, dizziness, palpitations, cold lower limbs, and intermittent claudication. Some patients exhibit low skin temperature in the extremities and a decreased or no distal pulse [42]. Aortic stenosis can be detected if one hears a systolic vascular murmur. Laboratory tests show an erythrocyte sedimentation rate and high levels of high-sensitivity C-reactive protein in the active stage.

Takayasu arteritis is a systemic disease and is usually treated medically. Operative therapy may be considered for patients with severe symptoms due to partial aortic stenosis [44]. Surgical revascularization of the diseased vessels may be performed when the lesion is stable and when the body temperature and blood test results including the erythrocyte sedimentation rate, the white blood cell count, and immunoglobin G levels are normal [45]. Extracorporeal or intrathoracic revascularization and endarterectomy are feasible for patients with brachiocephalic artery stenosis [46, 47]. Serious stenosis of the thoracic or abdominal aorta can be reconstructed with an artificial graft. For patients with limited thoracoabdominal aortic stenosis, stenting of coarctation of the aorta is feasible [48].

In general, Takayasu arteritis with aortic stenosis or occlusion can be diagnosed with CTA [49, 50]. The CT scanning area should cover the whole body including the vessels in the neck, the main branches of the thoracic and abdominal arteries, the arteries of the lower limbs, and the coronary artery. Most patients with Takayasu arteritis have aortic stenosis who often have renal artery stenosis at the same time and usually have refractory hypertension and a large pressure difference between the upper and lower limbs. Takayasu arteritis should be distinguished from congenital coarctation of the aorta. The typical features seen with CTA in patients with Takayasu arteritis are obvious concentric thickening of the vessel wall and stenosis of the lumen, which can be observed in thin-layer scanning. In patients with congenital aortic stenosis, the stenotic area is usually located in a limited area without obvious thickening of the vascular wall. Congenital coarctation of the aorta appears as a distal dilatation, even as

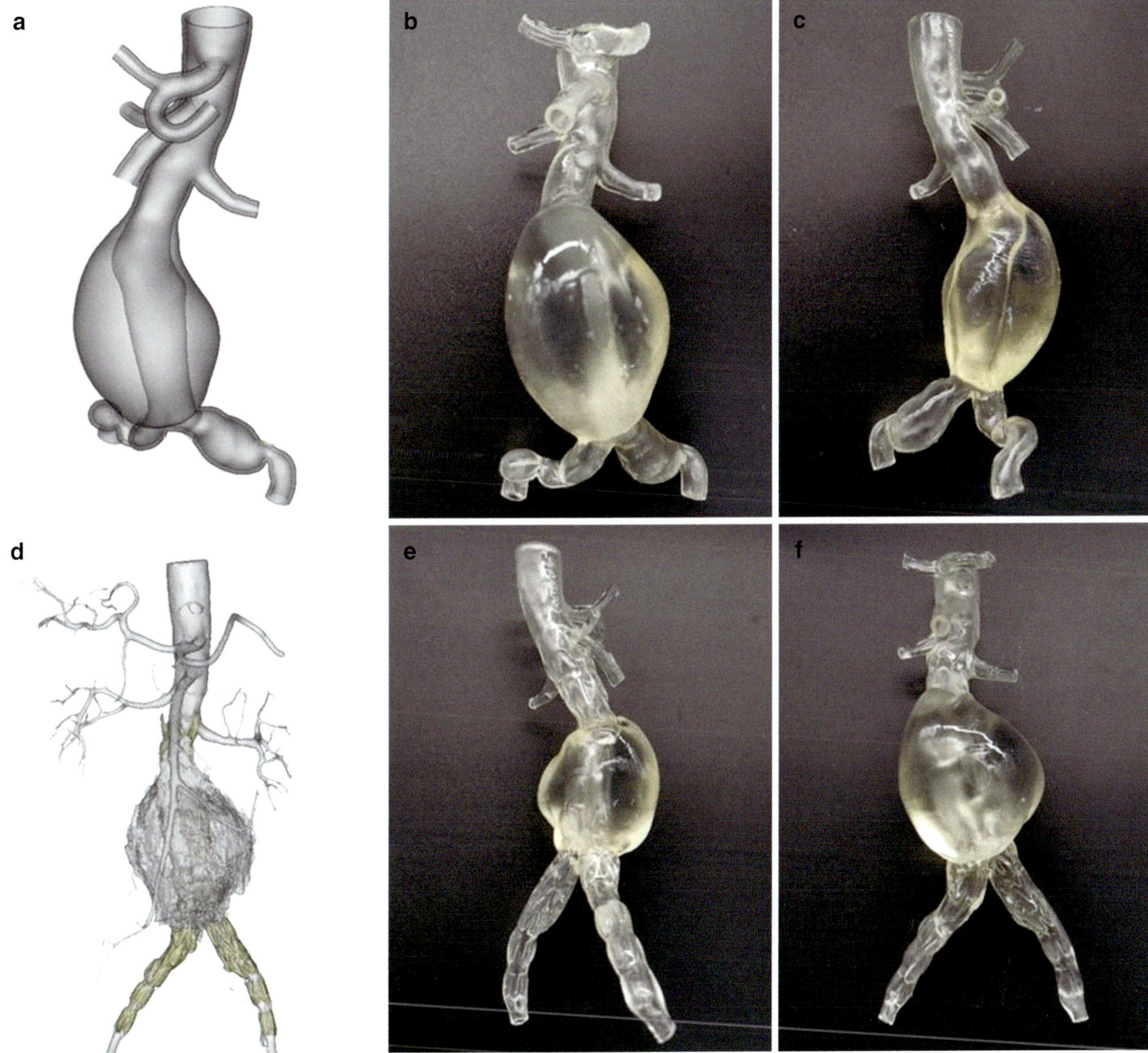

Fig. 11.20 3-Dimensional (3D)-printed images of the abdominal aneurysm after endovascular repair. (**a**) 3D reconstruction of the abdominal aneurysm. (**b**) Front view of the 3D-printed model of the abdominal aneurysm before the procedure. (**c**) Back view of the 3D-printed model of the abdominal aneurysm before the procedure. (**d**) A 3D reconstruction of the abdominal aortic aneurysm. (**e**) Front view of the 3D-printed model of the abdominal aneurysm after the procedure. (**f**) Back view of the 3D-printed model of the abdominal aneurysm after the procedure. Images and 3D-printed model from the Department of Cardiovascular Surgery at Xijing Hospital

an aneurysm. 3D printing can be used to assist in the preoperative planning of the surgical strategy for patients who undergo balloon dilatation and stenting of the area of aortic stenosis. The 3D-printed models can display more directly the location of the coarctation, the lesion of the vessel wall, and the involvement of the surrounding branches. The authors from the Department of Cardiovascular Surgery in Xijing Hospital observed severe stenosis of the left common carotid artery and the subclavian artery in a patient with brachiocephalic Takayasu arteritis based on the CTA images and the 3D-printed model (Fig. 11.21).

Based on the evaluation of the CTA images and the 3D-printed model, the patient underwent ascending aorta to bilateral common carotid artery bypass grafting under general anesthesia. The dizziness and ischemia disappeared after the operation. The CTA showed no restenosis in the graft between the ascending aorta and the bilateral common carotid artery in the 1-year follow-up examination (Fig. 11.22).

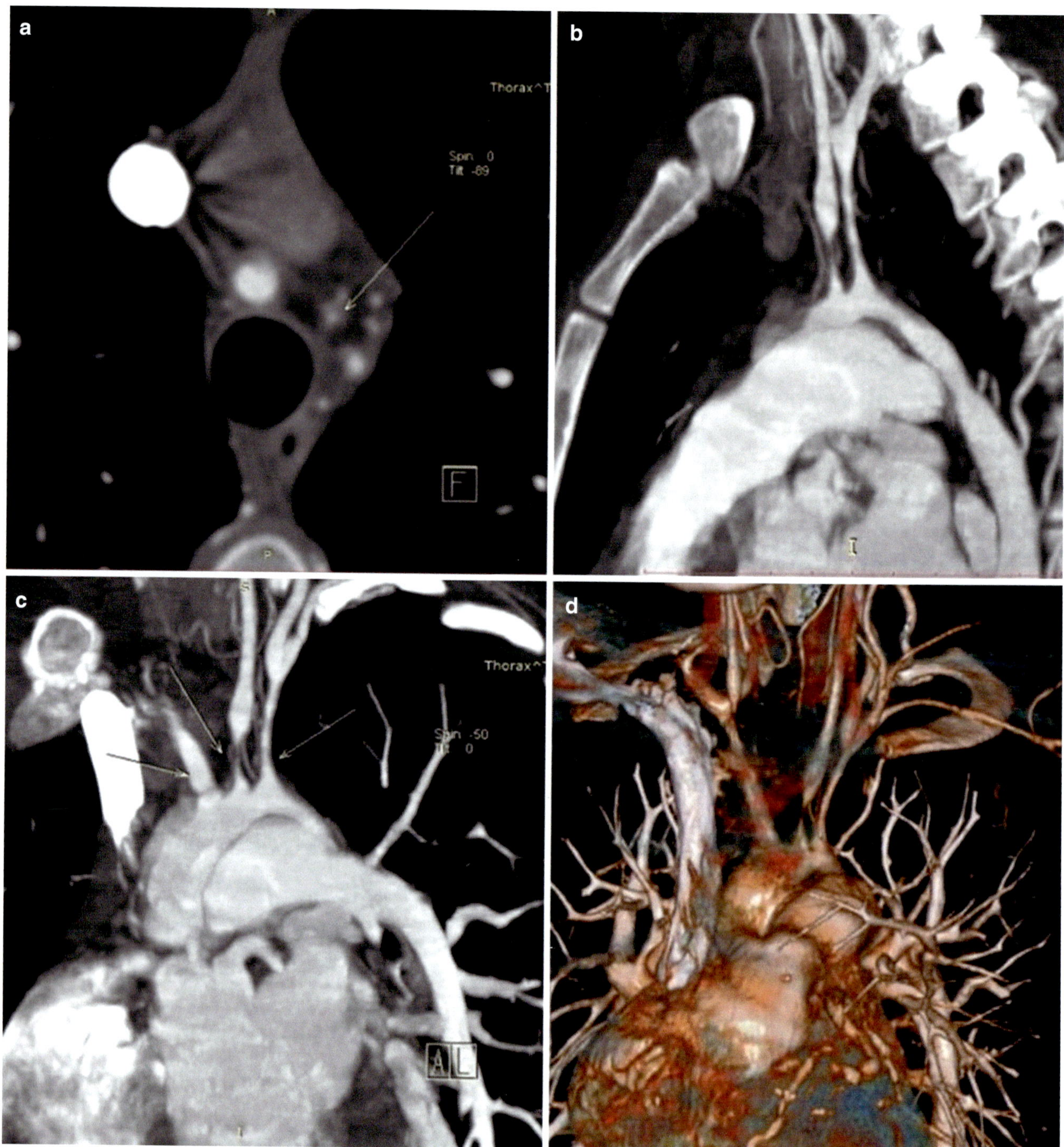

Fig. 11.21 Computed tomography angiographic images of a case of Takayasu arteritis. (**a**) cross-sectional view of the brachiocephalic trunk. The arrow shows severe stenosis of the left common carotid artery and the subclavian artery. (**b**) Sagittal view shows severe stenosis of the left common carotid artery and subclavian artery. (**c**) Arrow shows severe stenosis of the left common carotid artery and the subclavian artery in the tangential view. (**d**) Computer-assisted 3-dimensional reconstruction of the upper brachiocephalic artery in the aortic arch. Images from the Department of Cardiovascular Surgery at Xijing Hospital

Fig. 11.22 Computed tomography angiographic images of a patient with Takayasu arteritis after vascular bypass grafting. (**a**) The 3-dimensional (3D) reconstruction shows that the graft was connected from the ascending aorta to the bilateral common carotid artery in the view from the front. (**b**) The 3D reconstruction image shows the view from the back of the graft connecting the ascending aorta to the bilateral common carotid artery. (**c**) A 3D reconstruction of the arteries after vascular bypass grafting. Images from the Department of Cardiovascular Surgery at Xijing Hospital

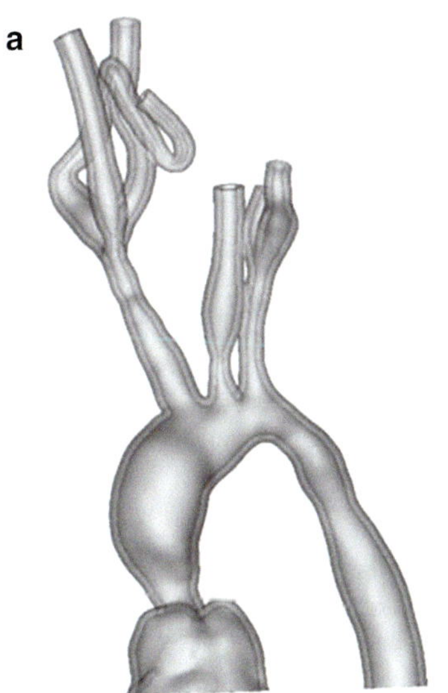
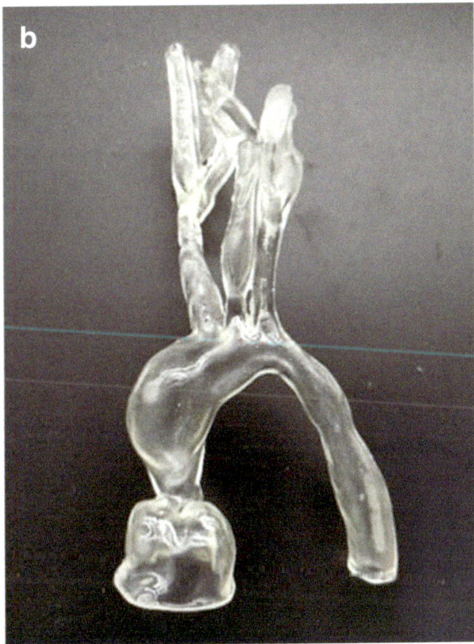
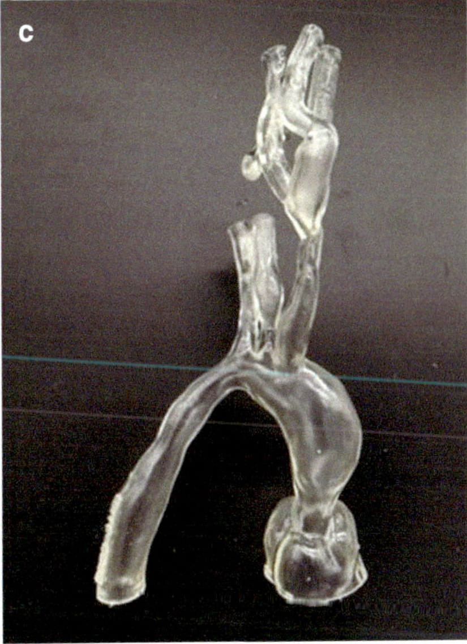

Fig. 11.23 3-Dimensional (3D) printing of a vascular bypass graft in a patient with Takayasu arteritis. (**a**) Preoperative 3D model of a case of Takayasu arteritis. (**b**) Front view of a preoperative 3D-printed model of a case of Takayasu arteritis. (**c**) Back view of a preoperative 3D-printed model of Takayasu arteritis. (**d**) Postoperative 3D model of Takayasu arteritis. (**e**) Front view of a postoperative 3D-printed model of Takayasu arteritis. (**f**) Front view of a postoperative 3D-printed model of Takayasu arteritis. Images from the Department of Cardiovascular Surgery at Xijing Hospital

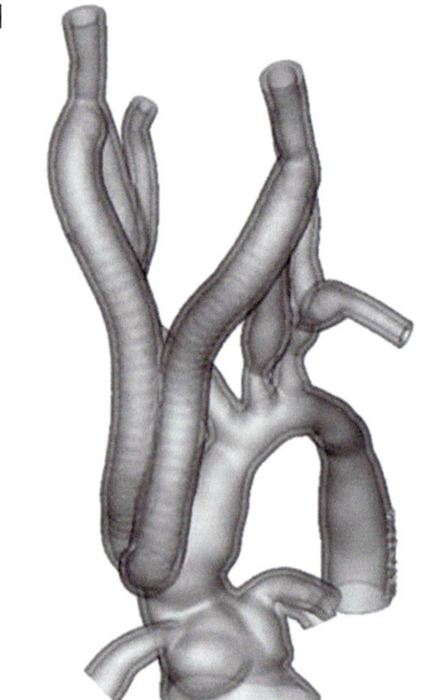

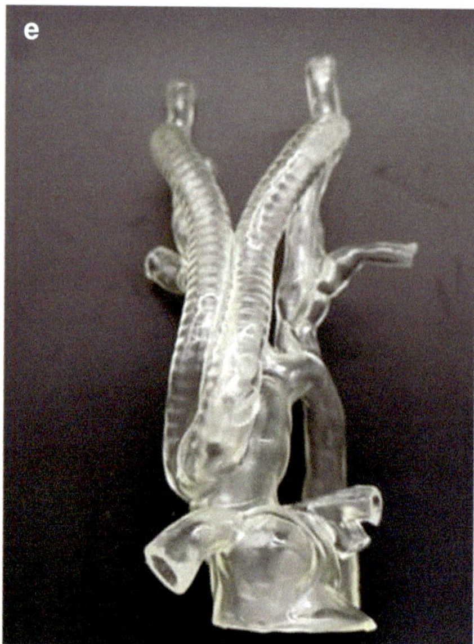

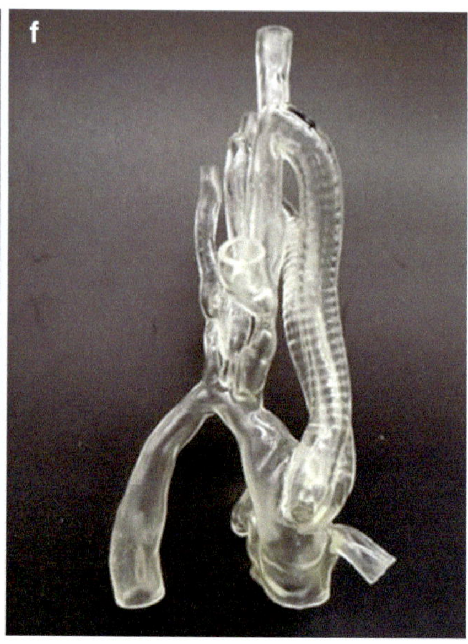

Fig. 11.23 (continued)

Based on 3D reconstruction and a 3D-printed model, the pathological anatomy of Takayasu arteritis can be shown clearly, including the location of the stenosis and the severity and range of the involved branches. It is also useful for the postoperative evaluation of vascular bypass grafting (Fig. 11.23).

For some patients with Takayasu arteritis, if the systemic inflammation is well controlled, balloon dilation and stent implantation can also be adopted [51]. In 1978, Gruntzig first succeeded in conducting balloon dilation of the renal artery, thereby providing a new approach to the treatment of Takayasu arteritis. In recent years, the stent implantation combined with balloon dilation have frequently been adopted to reduce the incidence of restenosis after arteriectasia, where 3D printing is also helpful. However, interventional therapy has its limitations on vessels with the wide range of lesions or severe stenoses. This minimally invasive treatment could not provide reliable outcomes in all patients.

References

Section 11.1

1. Rogers C, Clawson RE. Coarctation of the aorta. JAAPA. 2019;32:46–7.
2. Lemaire A, Cuttone F, Desgue J, Ivascau C, Caprio S, Saplacan V, Belin A, Babatasi G. Late complication after repair of aortic coarctation. Asian Cardiovasc Thorac Ann. 2015;23:423–9.
3. Rosenthal E. Coarctation of the aorta from fetus to adult: curable condition or life long disease process? Heart. 2005;91:1495–502.
4. Tzifa A, Ewert P, Brzezinska-Rajszys G, Peters B, Zubrzycka M, Rosenthal E, Berger F, Qureshi SA. Covered Cheatham-platinum stents for aortic coarctation: early and intermediate-term results. J Am Coll Cardiol. 2006;47:1457–63.
5. Fontes VF, Esteves CA, SLM B, MVD DS, MAP S, JEMR S, JAM DS. It is valid to dilate native aortic coarctation with a balloon catheter. Int J Cardiol. 1990;27:311–6.
6. Ang HL, Lim CW, Hia C, Yip J, Quek SC. Coarctation of the aorta: nonsurgical treatment using stent implantation. Singapore Med J. 2014;55:302–4.
7. Krasemann T, Bano M, Rosenthal E, Qureshi SA. Results of stent implantation for native and recurrent coarctation of the aorta-follow-up of up to 13 years. Catheter Cardiovasc Interv. 2011;78:405–12.
8. Butera G, Dua J, Chessa M, Carminati M. Covered Cheatham-platinum stents for serial dilatation of severe native aortic coarctation. Catheter Cardiovasc Interv. 2010;75:472. author reply 473
9. Bruckheimer E, Dagan T, Amir G, Birk E. Covered Cheatham-platinum stents for serial dilation of severe native aortic coarctation. Catheter Cardiovasc Interv. 2009;74:117–23.
10. Liaw CY, Guvendiren M. Current and emerging applications of 3D printing in medicine. Biofabrication. 2017;9:024102.
11. Ventola CL. Medical applications for 3D printing: current and projected uses. Pharm Ther. 2014;39:704–11.
12. Valverde I, Gomez G, Coserria JF, Suarez-Mejias C, Uribe S, Sotelo J, Velasco MN, Santos De Soto J, Hosseinpour AR, Gomez-Cia T. 3D printed models for planning endovascular stenting in transverse aortic arch hypoplasia. Catheter Cardiovasc Interv. 2015;85:1006–12.
13. Pluchinotta FR, Giugno L, Carminati M. Stenting complex aortic coarctation: simulation in a 3D printed model. EuroIntervention. 2017;13:490.
14. Armillotta A, Bonhoeffer P, Dubini G, Ferragina S, Migliavacca F, Sala G, Schievano S. Use of rapid prototyping models in the planning of percutaneous pulmonary valved stent implantation. Proc Inst Mech Eng H J Eng Med. 2007;221:407–16.

Section 11.2

15. United Kingdom ETI, Greenhalgh RM, Brown LC, Powell JT, Thompson SG, Epstein D, Sculpher MJ. Endovascular versus open repair of abdominal aortic aneurysm. N Engl J Med. 2010;362:1863–71.

16. Sun L, Qi R, Zhu J, Liu Y, Zheng J. Total arch replacement combined with stented elephant trunk implantation: a new "standard" therapy for type a dissection involving repair of the aortic arch? Circulation. 2011;123:971–8.
17. Fattori R, Cao P, De Rango P, Czerny M, Evangelista A, Nienaber C, Rousseau H, Schepens M. Interdisciplinary expert consensus document on management of type b aortic dissection. J Am Coll Cardiol. 2013;61:1661–78.
18. Causey MW, Jayaraj A, Leotta DF, Paun M, Beach KW, Kohler TR, Zierler ER, Starnes BW. Three-dimensional ultrasonography measurements after endovascular aneurysm repair. Ann Vasc Surg. 2013;27:146–53.
19. Nordon IM, Hinchliffe RJ, Manning B, Ivancev K, Holt PJ, Loftus IM, Thompson MM. Toward an "off-the-shelf" fenestrated endograft for management of short-necked abdominal aortic aneurysms: an analysis of current graft morphological diversity. J Endovasc Ther. 2010;17:78–85.
20. Greenberg RK, Haddad F, Svensson L, O'Neill S, Walker E, Lyden SP, Clair D, Lytle B. Hybrid approaches to thoracic aortic aneurysms: the role of endovascular elephant trunk completion. Circulation. 2005;112:2619–26.
21. Nienaber C, Fattori R, Lund G, Dieckmann C, Wolf W, Nicolas V, Pierangeli A, von Kodolitsch Y. Nonsurgical reconstruction of thoracic aortic dissection by stent-graft placement. N Engl J Med. 1999;340:1539–45.
22. Torres IO, De Luccia N. A simulator for training in endovascular aneurysm repair: The use of three dimensional printers. J Vasc Surg. 2017;66:966.
23. Jingbin Z, Xiaopeng Z, Chengyang S, Dong Z. Progress in the application of 3D printing technology in the diagnosis and treatment of Stanford type B aortic dissection. J Vasc Endovasc Surg. 2018;33:169–74.
24. Nienaber CA, Clough RE. Management of acute aortic dissection. Lancet. 2015;385:800–11.
25. Guidong L, Zhongya Y. 3D printing technique for choosing the covered stent in treatment of Stanford A type aortic dissection. Shandong Med J. 2018;58:30–3.
26. Xun Y, Zhongya Y, Yunhua S. Application of rapid proto-typing technology in the treatment of Stanford type A aortic dissection. Acta Universitatis Medicinalis Anhui. 2016;51:748–51.
27. Hossien A, Gelsomino S, Maessen J, Autschbach R. The interactive use of multi-dimensional modeling and 3D printing in preplanning of type A aortic dissection. J Card Surg. 2016;31:441–5.
28. Finotello A, Marconi S, Pane B, Conti M, Gazzola V, Mambrini S, Auricchio F, Palombo D, Spinella G. Twelve-year follow-up post-thoracic endovascular repair in type B aortic dissection shown by three-dimensional printing. Ann Vasc Surg. 2019;55:309 e313–9.

Section 11.3

29. Tam M, Laycock S, Brown J, Jakeways M. 3D printing of an aortic aneurysm to facilitate decision making and device selection for endovascular aneurysm repair in complex neck anatomy. J Endovasc Ther. 2013;20:863–7.
30. Berry E, Marsden A, Dalgarno KW, Kessel D, Scott DJ. Flexible tubular replicas of abdominal aortic aneurysms. Proc I Mech E Part H J Eng Med. 2002;216:211–4.
31. Srinivasa R, Malguria N, Chopra R, Reis S. How to create 3D printable models from CT angiographic images for patient and trainee education. J Vasc Interv Radiol. 2016;27:S230–1.
32. Tam MD, Latham T, Brown JRI, Jakeways M. Use of a 3D printed hollow aortic model to assist EVAR planning in a case with complex neck anatomy: potential of 3D printing to improve patient outcome. J Endovasc Ther. 2014;21:760–2.
33. Matthew D, Tam F, Tom R, Latham F, Mark Lewis F, Kunal Khanna F, Ali Zaman F, Mike Parker C, Iris Q, Grunwald M. A pilot study assessing the impact of 3-D printed models of aortic aneurysms on management decisions in EVAR planning. Vasc Endovascular Surg. 2016;50:4–9.
34. Bangeas P, Voulalas G, Ktenidis K. Rapid prototyping in aortic surgery. Interact Cardiovasc Thorac Surg. 2016;22:513–4.
35. Taher F, Falkensammer J, McCarte J, Strassegger J, Uhlmann M, Schuch P, Assadian A. The influence of prototype testing in three-dimensional aortic models on fenestrated endograft design. J Vasc Surg. 2017;65:1591–7.
36. Mafeld S, Nesbitt C, McCaslin J, Bagnall A, Davey P, Bose P, Williams R. Three-dimensional (3D) printed endovascular simulation models: a feasibility study. Ann Transl Med. 2017;5:42.
37. Torres IO, De Luccia N. A simulator for training in endovascular aneurysm repair: the use of three dimensional printers. Eur J Vasc Endovasc Surg. 2017;54:247–53.
38. Tam C, Chan Y, Law Y, Cheng S. The role of three-dimensional printing in contemporary vascular and endovascular surgery: a systematic review. Ann Vasc Surg. 2018;53:243–54.
39. Eisenmenger L, Kumpati G, Huo E. 3D printed patient specific aortic models for patient education and preoperative planning. J Vasc Interv Radiol. 2016;27:S236–7.
40. Winder RJ, Sun Z, Kelly B, Ellis PK, Hirst D. Abdominal aortic aneurysm and stent graft phantom manufactured by medical rapid prototyping. J Med Eng Technol. 2002;26:75–8.
41. Itagaki MW. Using 3D printed models for planning and guidance during endovascular intervention: a technical advance. Diagn Interv Radiol. 2015;21:338–41.

Section 11.4

42. Yang J, Yang L, Liu J, Zhang J, Zhao H, Yi D. Exceptional survival: acute coronary syndrome in a 56-year-old patient with Takayasu's arteritis. Int J Cardiol. 2009;131:e103–5.
43. Lin YJ, Hwang B, Lee PC, Yang LY, Meng CC. Mid-aortic syndrome: a case report and review of the literature. Int J Cardiol. 2008;123:348–52.
44. Klonaris C, Katsargyris A, Tsekouras N, Alexandrou A, Giannopoulos A, Bastounis E. Primary stenting for aortic lesions: from single Stenoses to total aortoiliac occlusions. J Vasc Surg. 2008;47:310–7.
45. Taketani T, Miyata T, Morota T, Takamoto S. Surgical treatment of a typical aortic coarctation complicating Takayasu's arteritis—experience with 33 cases over 44 years. J Vasc Surg. 2005;41:597–601.
46. Ghazi P, Haji-Zeinali AM, Shafiee N, Qureshi SA. Endovascular abdominal aortic stenosis treatment with the OptiMed self-expandable nitinol stent. Catheter Cardiovasc Interv. 2009;74:634–41.
47. Haji-Zeinali AM, Ghazi P, Alidoosti M. Self-expanding nitinol stent implantation for treatment of aortic coarctation. J Endovasc Ther. 2009;16:224–32.
48. Feugier P, Toursarkissian B, Chevalier J-M, Favre J-P. Endovascular treatment of isolated atherosclerotic stenosis of the infrarenal abdominal aorta: long-term outcome. Ann Vasc Surg. 2003;17:375–85.
49. Yang J, Yang L, Zhang J, Zheng M, Zhao H, Yi D. Patent carotid arteries with nearly occluded aortic arch in Takayasu's arteritis demonstrated by multidetector-row computed tomography. Int J Cardiol. 2007;118:e11–2.
50. Zhongjiu Z. The value of CTA angiography in the diagnosis of arteritis. Modern Med Imagel. 2017;26:1743–4.
51. Yilmaz S, Sindel T, Yegin A, Erdogan A, Luleci E. Primary stenting of focal atherosclerotic infrarenal aortic stenoses: long-term results in 13 patients and a literature review. Cardiovasc Intervent Radiol. 2004;27:121–8.

12 3D Bioprinting in Cardiovascular Disease

Alessandro Fiocco, Francesco Bertelli, Claudia Cattapan, Alvise Guariento, Vladimiro L. Vida, and Jian Yang

12.1 Introduction

Congenital heart defects, valvular heart disease, and coronary artery disease represent the major issues of the cardiovascular panorama, often requiring surgical correction through implantation of a prosthesis/tissue patches or conduits [1]. Unfortunately, current artificial substitutes do not regenerate and are affected by thrombogenicity, calcification, and non-remodeling capacity.

Tissue engineering represents an outstanding innovation giving the promise to solve the limits of the current approaches. Bioprinting is the latter technology landed in the field, representing a real paradigm shift in tissue engineering panorama, allowing both the creation of precise micro-scale resolution scaffolding system and 3D scaffold-free tissue construct, through printable living tissue blocks made of self-assembled cells.

Till today, 3D bioprinting has been employed in several medical fields, generating bone, cartilage, skin, aortic valves, vascular trees, and kidneys [2].

The technologies used for 3D printing of engineered constructs in cardiovascular tissues vary; the most frequently used are inkjet, bioplotting/microextrusion, and laser-assisted printing.

12.2 Technologies

12.2.1 Inkjet

This printing technique is provided by a drop-on-demand ink ejection through pressure generation (Fig. 12.1). The technologies differ also depending on the actuation process: thermal or piezoelectric. Thermal actuation creates a pulse pressure by a localized heating up to 300 °C lasting about two microseconds. Bioink components, such as proteins, cells, and biomolecules, do not receive any damage, despite a significant increment in temperature in the immediate surroundings (usually <10 °C). This technology appears to be not expensive and quite fast; nevertheless, irregular drop sizing and frequent clogging are printed [3].

The piezoelectric system is based on the transformation of a voltage pulse in mechanical force [4]. This technique is superior to the thermal one in terms of virtually non-exposure to heat, avoiding clogging, and uniformity in drop sizing; however, electromagnetic frequencies have been reported to cause cell membrane damage and lysis [5].

Low viscosity is required as bioink property, if printed through inkjet technology, especially if containing cells that cannot survive high pressures. This contrasts with the need for structural integrity and stability of the construct, thus requiring cross-linking mechanisms through chemical and UV exposure that could in turn be cytotoxic and consequently represent an additional concern.

12.2.2 Bioplotting/Microextrusion

This technology is currently the preferred one and the most commonly used in bioprinting [6]. Differently from inkjet technologies, it works by dispensing continuous strands of biomaterial, instead of droplets. This way, high-viscosity inks can be printed, thus allowing the creation of tissues retaining adequate mechanical properties, as well as stability and integrity. Compared to inkjet bioprinters, this technology suffers from less cell viability, apparently directly proportional to extrusion pressure and nozzle gauge. Nevertheless, a vast number of materials can be extruded, from polymers in liquid or melted form to cell spheroid or cell-encapsulated matrices. Besides material's flexibility, microextrusion technique presents several more advantages,

A. Fiocco · F. Bertelli · C. Cattapan · A. Guariento · V. L. Vida
Paediatric and Congenital Cardiac Surgery Unit, Department of Cardiac, Thoracic and Vascular Sciences and Public Health, University of Padua, Padua, Italy

J. Yang (✉)
Department of Cardiovascular Surgery, Xijing Hospital, Xi'an, China

J. Yang et al. (eds.), *Cardiovascular 3D Printing*, https://doi.org/10.1007/978-981-15-6957-9_12

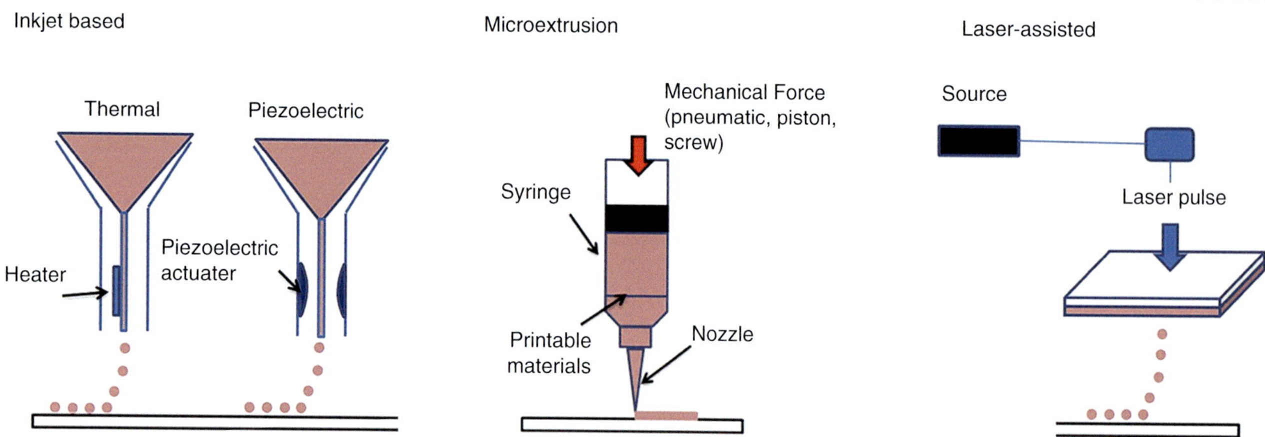

Fig. 12.1 3D bioprinting technologies. (Modified from Duan, Bin. "State-of-the-art review of 3D bioprinting for cardiovascular tissue engineering." Annals of Biomedical Engineering 45.1 (2017): 195–209)

like direct cell inclusion in hydrogel and high cellular densities.

12.2.3 Laser-Assisted

Laser-assisted bioprinting is less commonly used mainly because devices are cumbersome, and the procedure is time-consuming. It is based on the principles of laser-induced forward transfer [7]. It is possible to print cells at a density of 10^8 cells/ml with a microscale resolution of a single cell per drop, allowing precisely population of scaffolds with different cell types and densities [8]. Printed cells are not reported to be damaged by the laser printing procedure. Thus, laser-assisted bioprinting is a promising tool for the ex vivo generation of tissue replacements.

12.3 Materials

Similar to daily-use office printers, ink cartridges are required. This special ink is called "bioink" and can be divided into substrate materials, biomolecules, and cells.

12.3.1 Substrate Materials

Substrate materials, often in hydrogel form, must possess specific properties such as gelling time, swelling and stability, adequate mechanical response, biodegradability, biocompatibility, and, of course, printability. Melted polymers are usually employed to build bio-scaffold because they combine the right mechanical properties with cell-friendly characteristics [9].

Natural polymers like fibrin and alginate hydrogel use cross-linkers to harden the construct during printing time [10]. Hybrid Matrigel™ hydrogel showed coexisting ideal rheological properties for bioprinting and biocompatibility. The agarose element of the hybrid hydrogel system allows the mechanical properties to build 3D-printed structures, whereas Matrigel™ provides essential microenvironments for cell growth [11].

Some natural polymers like hyaluronic acid, gelatin, chitosan, and silk can be mixed to conventional hydrogels to increase mechanical properties of the ink to match the desired requirements [12].

Synthetic polymers, such as polyglycolic acid, polycaprolactone, polylactic acid, and polyethylene glycol, look very appealing because of their strength and easily adaptable mechanical properties [13]. However, they unfortunately show poor biocompatibility and the tendency to degrade into toxic catabolic products. Nevertheless, they remain commonly used [14].

12.3.2 Biomolecules

Biomolecules have paramount importance during cell fate guiding. Growth factors, peptides, and proteins can be included in the gel through functional attachment or simple mixing [15]. Moreover, they can be independently printed with different concentrations on each gel layer. In autologous human tissue fabrication, autologous stem cells may be the only cell source; therefore, the use of growth factors is essential for their precise differentiation and survival [16].

12.3.3 Cells

Successful cardiac cell printing has been reported by several research groups, as well as osteoblasts, pluripotent cells, endothelial cells, and fibro- and osteosarcoma cells [17]. Printing technology has already been used in the medical field to generate a 2D layer for surface treatments, like skin regeneration [18]. 3D printing of cell-containing ink requires a bioink viscosity that is obviously higher than the one used in 2D printing, in order to keep the integrity of the construct [19]. Cell-laden gels have already been used for 3D culture, but they present the inconvenience that cells tend not to fuse easily inside a gel matrix because of cellular low density that prohibits migration and proliferation to a sufficient degree [20]. Other issues are represented by matrix stiffness and lack of vascularization. The use of cell aggregates or spheroids as bioink shows some major advantages over printing single cells or cell-laden gels. This technology provides for the use of printable cellular building blocks, creating a scaffold-free construct [21]. Survival is proven to be higher in cell aggregates compared to cell-laden gels, due to major protection from shear force and damaging [22].

Postprint cell viability and functionality, apoptosis, heat shock, protein denaturation, and pore formation on the cell membrane represent the major concerns.

12.4 Scaffold-Free Bioprinting

In recent years, researchers shifted toward scaffold-free 3D printing, cutting out the catabolic biocompatibility concerns coming from the degradation of the scaffold. A dense cellular slurry is employed as a bioink and printed in the desired structure. After printing, the cells usually start producing their own extracellular matrix, providing mechanical strength without the need for a scaffold (Fig. 12.2). Adding a small quantity of hydrogel into the bioink mixture, together with growth factors and proteins, confers easy printable properties and at the same time can guarantee the required environment for cells to differentiate. Pluronic™, polyethylene glycol, and gelatin (denatured collagen) are often used because of their structural integrity ability [23]. Collagen, fibrin, and hyaluronic acid are directly derived from ECM and therefore act as working matrix for cellular growth.

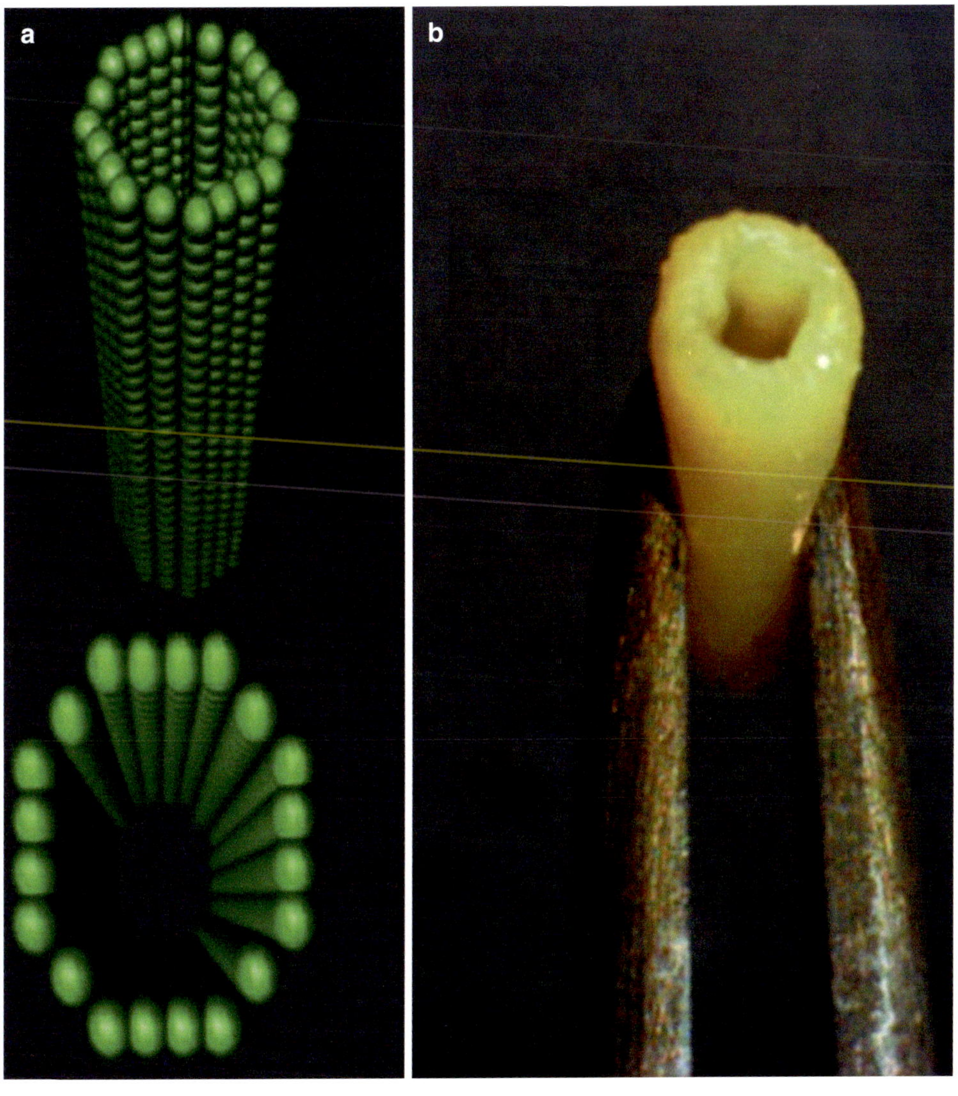

Fig. 12.2 Scaffold-free vascular construct. (**a**) Virtual planning of 3D cell-spheroids disposition. (**b**) Final construct. (Modified from Moldovan, Nicanor I. "Progress in scaffold-free bioprinting for cardiovascular medicine." Journal of Cellular and Molecular Medicine 22.6 (2018): 2964–2969)

12.5 Tissue Engineering and State of the Art

Tissue engineering (TE) uses biodegradable scaffolds that will fully integrate in the host body, degrade over time, and will simultaneously be replaced with autologous tissue, capable of growth and repair. Currently, TE processes can be classified into three main categories: (a) in vitro, (b) in vivo, and (c) in situ approaches. (a) In vitro techniques employ biodegradable constructs seeded with cells, cultured in bioreactors, and surgically implanted in the host body to continue growth processing. (b) In vivo approaches use the human body as a bioreactor: the scaffold is placed subcutaneously, obtaining the growth of a fibrotic matrix that can then be removed and implanted. (c) In situ approach relies on the regenerative capacity of the body to grow new tissue upon implantation of a cell-free construct in the cardiovascular system through recruitment of endogenous cells. These techniques are currently applied in order to build tissue-engineered heart valves (TEHV), tissue-engineered vascular grafts (TEVG), and tissue-engineered myocardial patches (TEMP).

12.5.1 Decellularized Constructs

Decellularized components are currently the most utilized example of tissue engineered grafts, and, in some cases, they have already been translated to a commercially available solution (e.g., CorMatrixTM by CorMatrix Cardiovascular, Inc., Roswell, GA).

Decellularization technology has existed since the end of the twentieth century and is based on the complete removal of cellular nuclei, membranes, and cytoplasmic material from native tissues to leave a 3D structure composed only of extracellular matrix (Fig. 12.3). Several methods of selective cell removal are applied during the process, including mechanical shaking, chemical detergent use, and enzymatic digestion. The selectivity of these processes is the key element for successful decellularization because ECM microstructure, with its biomechanical properties and biological role, must be preserved as much as possible. In fact, extracellular matrix must retain protein signaling, thus allowing tissue-specific cells migration, adhesion, and differentiation.

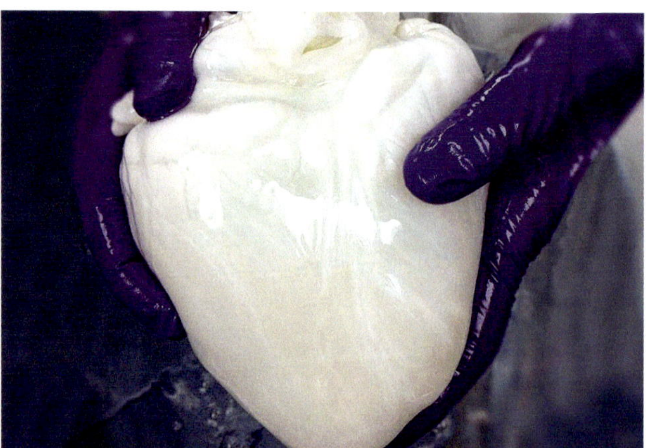

Fig. 12.3 The "ghost heart". Decellularized whole heart. (Open access, adapted from https://steemit.com/medicine/@zezosomo/ghost-heart)

In January 2012, the European Union established the European Clinical Study for the Application of Regenerative Heart Valves (ESPOIR) trial, coordinated by the Hannover Medical School in Germany, and in which our institution participated as a pioneer member. The objective of this study is to evaluate the performance of decellularized pulmonary valve homografts over the long term. These initial results of this prospective study showed an overall freedom from explantation and reintervention rate of 98.3% after an average of 2 years [24]. A twin study of ESPOIR, called ARISE, was started a few years later to determine the feasibility, safety, and efficacy of decellularized aortic valve homografts for aortic valve replacement. The study is again coordinated by the Hannover Medical School, with our institutions among the European centers in partnership, and it is currently obtaining very promising preliminary results with no incidence of explantation thus far [25].

12.5.2 Non Decellularized Tissue-Engineered Constructs

The first attempt at making total artificial scaffolds for potentially growing prostheses was made by Dr. Shinoka and colleagues at the end of the twentieth century, when they successfully created, colonized, and implanted cardiac valve leaflets and extracardiac conduits in lambs. Remarkably, they reported structural organization which resembled that of normal valves and arteries, respectively, as well as satisfactory physiologic function and growth without thrombus formation [26, 27].

This same group started the first human TEVG clinical trial focused on children with CHD [28]. Between 2001 and 2004, 25 patients underwent extracardiac Fontan procedure (total cavopulmonary connection) utilizing an autologous bone-marrow-MNC-seeded TEVG made from PCL/PLLA polymer mixtures on a PGA or PLA backbone. Although many congenital cardiac surgeries have the potential to be impacted significantly by the successful use of TEVGs, the Fontan procedure was chosen because it represents an optimal balance between utility and safety, since the conduits are implanted in a high-flow and low-pressure circulatory system. The midterm results showed no graft-related mortality during the follow-up period of 11 years. There was evidence of valve growth and no evidence of aneurysm formation, graft rupture, graft infection, or calcification. Only seven out of twenty-five patients had asymptomatic graft stenosis and they all underwent successful balloon angioplasty [29].

In Europe in 2017, Bockeria et al. implanted a highly porous conduit, composed of a bioresorbable supramolecular polyester and processed by electrospinning, connecting the inferior vena cava to the pulmonary artery in five pediatric patients with univentricular pathologies. The 12-month follow-up showed graft patency with functional and anatomical stability [30].

Some researchers are currently working on animal models to make a tissue-engineered contractile Fontan conduit, hoping to partially improve the hemodynamic conditions of the Fontan circulation, which include diminished systemic cardiac output and increased systemic-venous pressure [31].

12.5.3 3D-Bioprinted Constructs

3D bioprinting is the newest technological advancement in tissue engineering and promises to revolutionize the regenerative medicine approach. Despite the immense potential of the technique, it is still a nascent technology, and it has yet to be applied in clinical or preclinical settings, except for very rare cases. Major efforts are addressed to engineered heart valves, vascular constructs, and myocardial patch development.

12.5.3.1 Heart Valves

Currently, several valve models/designs have been reported.

Of note, we report the in vitro development of human cell-derived tissue-engineered matrices and their application as tissue-engineered valves, described by Maximilian Emmert research group [32]. Matrices were obtained starting from 3D-printed polyglycolic acid scaffolds. Subsequent culturing in a bioreactor with human neonatal dermal fibroblasts produced a construct covered by dense and shiny extracellular matrix that was retained after decellularization (Fig. 12.4). The engineered valves were evaluated in a pulse duplicator system under physiological pulmonary pressure conditions. In the second phase, transapical delivery was tested for feasibility and safety in a sheep model, reporting good valve performance and early cellular infiltration [32].

Duan et al. created trileaflet valve conduits using a combination of methacrylated hyaluronic acid and methacrylated gelatin with encapsulation of human aortic VIC [33] The encapsulated cells were shown with high viability and matrix remodeling with sulfated GAG deposition. Hockaday et al. used a combination of poly(ethylene glycol) diacrylate (PEGDA) to print valvulated conduits having biomechanical heterogeneity, through combination of more flexibility of the leaflets, with relative rigidness of the root [34]. Both pediatric and adult valve sizes were printed. The same group also generated anatomically derived aortic valve geometric model using a lCT scan of a porcine aortic valve conduit freshly obtained at slaughterhouse. The root and leaflet regions in

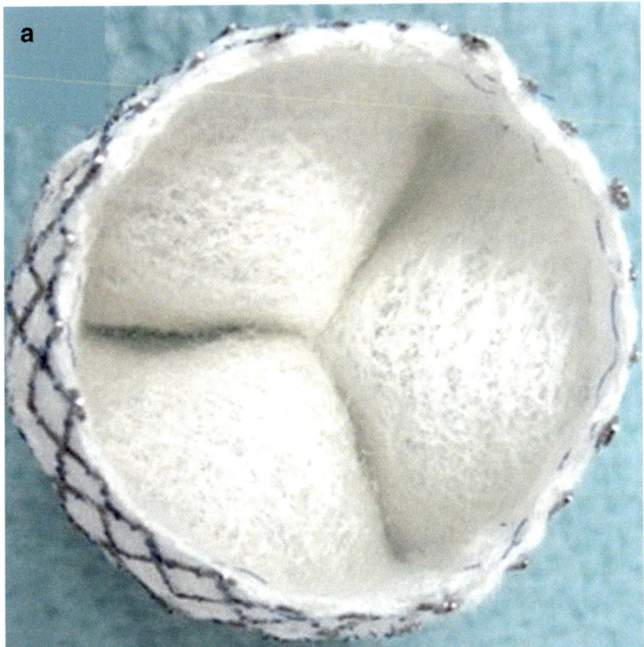

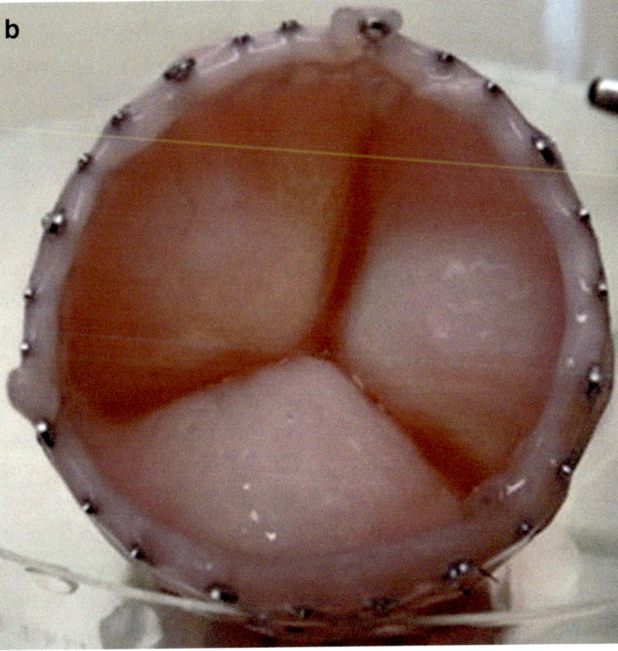

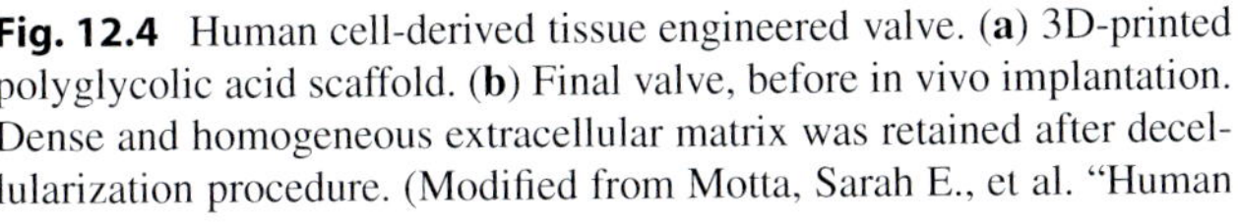

Fig. 12.4 Human cell-derived tissue engineered valve. (**a**) 3D-printed polyglycolic acid scaffold. (**b**) Final valve, before in vivo implantation. Dense and homogeneous extracellular matrix was retained after decellularization procedure. (Modified from Motta, Sarah E., et al. "Human cell-derived tissue-engineered heart valve with integrated Valsalva sinuses: towards native-like transcatheter pulmonary valve replacements." NPJ Regenerative Medicine 4.1 (2019): 1–10

the resulting scanned files and rendered into 3D models into separate stereolithography format of (STL) files were generated. The models maintained many anatomical features of native valves, like ostium and sinus. For heterogeneous bioprinting, first the valve root (SMC laden hydrogel) was deposited, and subsequently the leaflet region (VIC-laden hydrogel) was extruded along its print paths. The aortic valve conduit bioprinted with SMC and VIC encapsulated in the root and leaflet tissue, respectively, exhibited geometry comparable to the original derived valve [35].

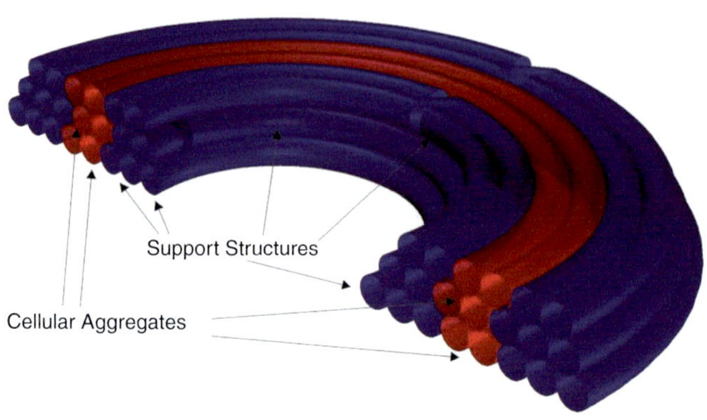

Fig. 12.5 3D bioprinting of biomimetic aortic vascular constructs with self-supporting cells. (Adapted from Kucukgul, Can, et al. "3D bioprinting of biomimetic aortic vascular constructs with self-supporting cells." Biotechnology and Bioengineering 112.4 (2015): 811–821)

12.5.3.2 Vascular Constructs

3D bioprinting technologies can fuse with general tissue engineering approaches to create in vitro vasculature and vascularized constructs. Possible processes can use (a) self-assembly cells to create vascular constructs; (b) inkjet-based bioprinting to generate microvasculatures; and (c) generation of channel-based vascularized constructs.

(a) Cell self-assembly is the autonomous organization of cells in a stable construct. Cell spheroids represent the building blocks that are printed and that fuse into vascular-like products. 3D printing allows the creation of complex multilayered vascular wall by printing multicellular cylinders composed of different cells, e.g., human smooth muscle cells (HSMC) and human skin fibroblasts (HSF). On the negative side of this technology are the time-consuming process and the need for a lot of manual work. The alternative to cell spheroids are cell aggregates. Kucukgul et al. developed a 3D-bioprinted scaffold-free biomimetic macrovascular structure. Computer model mimicking a real human aorta was generated using imaging techniques. An optimized three-dimensional bioprinting path planning was developed. Layer-by-layer 3D bioprinting of mouse embryonic fibroblast (MEF) cell aggregates and support structures (hydrogels) was performed to create an aortic tissue construct (Fig. 12.5) [36]. This approach was relatively efficient, but needed further improvement of the overall resolution and controllability.

(b) Concerning inkjet-based bioprinting, Cui et al. created a microvasculature network by simultaneously printing human microvascular endothelial cells (HMEC) and fibrin [2]. Printed fibrin scaffold retained proper shape after printing and endothelial cells proliferate to form a tubular structure. The printed microvasculature was 21-day-culture, demonstrating improvements in integrity after 21-day culture. The inkjet-based bioprinting allowed multiple cell type deposition, and the use of mesenchymal stem cells or smooth muscle cells supported the formation and maturation of microvasculatures.

(c) Many research groups are printing sacrificial materials to generate channel networks inside engineered tissue constructs. Many of the procedures involves 3D printing of water-soluble material-based networks within the construct. The sacrificial material is then removed, by solution or heat/cold shock. Miller et al. used carbohydrate glass as a cytocompatible sacrificial template to generate cylindrical networks, printing rigid 3D filament. The sugar-glass networks are biocompatible with many types of cell-laden matrices, and the formed channel networks, after removing sugar-glass, can support endothelial cells and pulsatile flow of human blood [37].

12.5.3.3 Myocardium Patches

Cell-based cardiac repair or cellular cardiomyoplasty has made remarkable progress in myocardial tissue regeneration. Myocardial tissue engineering (MTE) requires high density of cardiomyocytes and various supporting cells, efficient vascularization, and oxygen exchange to generate synchronous contractions. 3D bioprinting can pattern and assemble cells with high density, defined distribution, and spatial organization. It also allows the generation of multiple layered constructs with different cell types. Gaetani et al. utilized bioprinted-modified alginate scaffolds with human fetal progenitor cells [38]. They demonstrated that printed constructs had high cell viability, retained their commitment for the cardiac lineage, and showed enhanced gene expression of the early cardiac transcription factors and the sarcomeric proteins. The bioprinted cells were also able to migrate from the constructs and formed tube-like structure on the Matrigel layer. Gaebel et al. applied the laser-induced inkjet bioprinting technique and printed polyester urethane urea cardiac patch with mixed HUVEC and human mesenchymal stem cell (hMSC) [39]. Specific vascular patterns were successfully generated and the cells organized in capillary like pattern. These seeded constructs were cultivated and further transplanted in vivo to the infarcted zone of rat hearts after left anterior descending (LAD) ligation. The same group further bioprinted patch composed of human cardiomyocyte progenitor cell(hCMPC)-laden HA/Gel matrix [40]. Similarly, hCMPCs retained their cardiogenic phenotype in the bioprinted constructs up to 1 month and the construct allowed heart function preservation by improving myocardial viability.

Generation of synergistic contractile force is essential for thick muscle-like tissue bioprinting, together with adequate repairing or replacement of the damaged heart tissue. Major concerns are currently represented by electromechanical and vascular functional integration of the graft and the host tissue.

12.6 Future Perspectives

Despite recent advancements in 3D bioprinting technology and cardiac tissue engineering, we are light years away from daily clinical application. Different issues such as high-resolution imaging, segmentation software, printing speed and resolution, and cost need further advancements. Future development in printing biomaterials will probably reduce the gap between mechanical and physical properties of currently bio-scaffolds and native biologic tissues. The need for engineered vessels and whole organ will keep growing by time with high aging population and rise in chronic illness [41]. The next step will be a further improvement in technologies, moving toward customized tissue engineering. This will allow 3D bioprinting to be potentially utilized in fabricating tailored-made cardiac patches, arteries and vessels, valve, and prosthesis. Of note, stem cell technologies improvement will play an essential role in transferring these thoughts into reality. The iPSC-derived SMCs have shown high proliferation rate, potentially reducing the bioink production time and eliminating the need for harvesting cells from patients or donors [42].

References

1. Goncalves A, Marcos-Alberca P, Almeria C, Feltes G, Ana Hernandez-Antolin R, Rodriguez E, et al. Quality of life improvement at midterm follow-up after transcatheter aortic valve implantation. Int J Cardiol. 2013;162:117–22.
2. Cui X, Boland T.Human microvasculature fabrication using hermal inkjet printing technology. Biomaterials 2009;30(31):6221–7.
3. Cui X, Dean D, Ruggeri ZM, Boland T. Cell damage evaluation of thermal inkjet printed Chinese hamster ovary cells. Biotechnol Bioeng. 2010;106:963–9.
4. de Jong J, de Bruin G, Reinten H, van den Berg M, Wijshoff H, Versluis M, et al. Air entrapment in piezo-driven inkjet printheads. J Acoust Soc Am. 2006;120:1257–65.
5. Seetharam R, Sharma SK. Purification and analysis of recombinant proteins (Biotechnology and bioprocessing). New York: Marcel Dekker; 1991.
6. Maina RM, et al. Generating vascular conduits: from tissue engineering to three-dimensional bioprinting. Innov Surg Sci. 2018;3(3):203–13.
7. Barron JA, Spargo BJ, Ringeisen BR. Biological laser printing of three dimensional cellular structures. Appl Phys A-Mater. 2004a;79:1027–30.
8. Guillotin B, Souquet A, Catros S, Duocastella M, Pippenger B, Bellance S, et al. Laser assisted bioprinting of engineered tissue with high cell density and microscale organization. Biomaterials. 2010;31:7250–6.
9. Ahn S, Kim Y, Lee H, Kim G. A new hybrid scaffold constructed of solid freeform-fabricated PCL struts and collagen struts for bone tissue regeneration: fabrication, mechanical properties, and cellular activity. J Mater Chem. 2012;22:15901–9.
10. Nakamura M, Kobayashi A, Takagi F, Watanabe A, Hiruma Y, Ohuchi K, et al. Biocompatible inkjet printing technique for designed seeding of individual living cells. Tissue Eng. 2005b;11:1658–66.
11. Fan R, Piou M, Darling E, Cormier D, Sun J, Wan J. Bioprinting cell-laden Matrigel–agarose constructs. J Biomater Appl. 2016;31(5):684–92.
12. Ghosh S, Parker ST, Wang XY, Kaplan DL, Lewis JA. Direct-write assembly of microperiodic silk fibroin scaffolds for tissue engineering applications. Adv Funct Mater. 2008;18:1883–9.
13. Ou K-L, Hosseinkhani H. Development of 3D in vitro technology for medical applications. Int J Mol Sci. 2014;15(10):17938–62.
14. Murphy SV, Atala A. 3D bioprinting of tissues and organs. Nat Biotechnol. 2014;32(8):773.
15. Pike DB, Cai S, Pomraning KR, Firpo MA, Fisher RJ, Shu XZ, et al. Heparin-regulated release of growth factors in vitro and angiogenic response in vivo to implanted hyaluronan hydrogels containing VEGF and bFGF. Biomaterials. 2006;27:5242–51.
16. Jana S, Lerman A. Bioprinting a cardiac valve. Biotechnol Adv. 2015;33(8):1503–21.
17. Saunders RE, Gough JE, Derby B. Delivery of human fibroblast cells by piezoelectric drop-on- demand inkjet printing. Biomaterials. 2008;29:193–203.
18. Michael S, Sorg H, Peck CT, Koch L, Deiwick A, Chichkov B, et al. Tissue engineered skin substitutes created by laser-assisted bioprinting form skin-like structures in the dorsal skin fold chamber in mice. PLoS One. 2013a;8:e57741.
19. Birgersdotter A, Sandberg R, Ernberg I. Gene expression perturbation in vitro--a growing case for three-dimensional (3D) culture systems. Semin Cancer Biol. 2005;15:405–12.
20. Boland T, Mironov V, Gutowska A, Roth EA, Markwald RR. Cell and organ printing 2: fusion of cell aggregates in three-dimensional gels. Anat Rec A Discov Mol Cell Evol Biol. 2003;272:497–502.
21. Marga F, Jakab K, Khatiwala C, Shepherd B, Dorfman S, Hubbard B, et al. Toward engineering functional organ modules by additive manufacturing. Biofabrication. 2012;4:022001.
22. Yang X, Mironov V, Wang Q. Modeling fusion of cellular aggregates in biofabrication using phase field theories. J Theor Biol. 2012;303:110–8.
23. Zhang YS, et al. 3D bioprinting for tissue and organ fabrication. Ann Biomed Eng. 2017;45(1):148–63.
24. Boethig D, Horke A, Hazekamp M, et al. A European study on decellularized homografts for pulmonary valve replacement: initial results from the prospective ESPOIR trial and ESPOIR registry data†. Eur J Cardiothorac Surg. 2019;56(3):503–9.
25. Igor T, Alexander H, Samir S, et al. Abstract 19959: aortic valve replacement with decellularized aortic allografts: first clinical results. Circulation. 2014;130(suppl_2):A19959.

26. Mayer JE Jr, Shin'oka T, Shum-Tim D. Tissue engineering of cardiovascular structures. Curr Opin Cardiol. 1997;12(6):528–32.
27. Shoji T, Shinoka T. Tissue engineered vascular grafts for pediatric cardiac surgery. Transl Pediatr. 2018;7(6):188–95.
28. Shin T, Matsumura G, Hibino N, et al. Midterm clinical result of tissue-engineered vascular autografts seeded with autologous bone marrow cells. J Thorac Cardiovasc Surg. 2005 Jun;129(6):1330–8.
29. Sugiura T, Matsumura G, Miyamoto S, Miyachi H, Breuer CK, Shinoka T. Tissue-engineered vascular grafts in children with congenital heart disease: intermediate term followup. Semin Thorac Cardiovasc Surg. 2018;30:175.
30. Bockeria LA, Svanidze O, Kim A, et al. Total cavopulmonary connection with a new bioabsorbable vascular graft: first clinical experience. J Thorac Cardiovasc Surg. 2017;153(6):1542–50.
31. Biermann D, Eder A, Arndt F, et al. Towards a tissue-engineered contractile Fontan-Conduit: the fate of cardiac myocytes in the subpulmonary circulation. PLoS One. 2016;11:1–10.
32. Motta SE, et al. Human cell-derived tissue-engineered heart valve with integrated Valsalva sinuses: towards native-like transcatheter pulmonary valve replacements. NPJ Regenerative Medicine. 2019;4(1):1–10.
33. Duan B, Kapetanovic E, Hockaday LA, Butcher JT. Three-dimensional printed trileaflet valve conduits using biological hydrogels and human valve interstitial cells. Acta Biomater. 2014;10:1836–46.
34. Hockaday LA, Kang KH, Colangelo NW, Cheung PYC, Duan B, Malone E, Wu J, Girardi LN, Bonassar LJ, Lipson H, Chu CC, Butcher JT. Rapid 3D printing of anatomically accurate and mechanically heterogeneous aortic valve hydrogel scaffolds. Biofabrication. 2012;4:035005.
35. Duan B. State-of-the-art review of 3D bioprinting for cardiovascular tissue engineering. Ann Biomed Eng. 2017;45(1):195–209.
36. Kucukgul C, et al. 3D bioprinting of biomimetic aortic vascular constructs with self-supporting cells. Biotechnol Bioeng. 2015;112(4):811–21.
37. Miller JS, Stevens KR, Yang MT, Baker BM, Nguyen DHT, Cohen DM, Toro E, Chen AA, Galie PA, Yu X, Chaturvedi R, Bhatia SN, Chen CS. Rapid casting of patterned vascular networks for perfusable engineered three-dimensional tissues. Nat Mater. 2012;11:768–74.
38. Gaetani R, Doevendans PA, Metz CHG, Alblas J, Messina E, Giacomello A, Sluijtera JPG. Cardiac tissue engineering using tissue printing technology and human cardiac progenitor cells. Biomaterials. 2012;33:1782–90.
39. Gaebel R, Ma N, Liu J, Guan JJ, Koch L, Klopsch C, Gruene M, Toelk A, Wang WW, Mark P. Patterning human stem cells and endothelial cells with laser printing for cardiac regeneration. Biomaterials. 2011;32:9218–30.
40. Gaetani R, Feyen DAM, Verhage V, Slaats R, Messina E, Christman KL, Giacomello A, Doevendans PAFM, Sluijter JPG. Epicardial application of cardiac progenitor cells in a 3D-printed gelatin/hyaluronic acid patch preserves cardiac function after myocardial infarction. Biomaterials. 2015;61:339–48.
41. Prabhakaran D, Anand S, Watkins D, et al. Cardiovascular, respiratory, and related disorders: key messages from disease control priorities, 3rd edition. Lancet. 2018;391(10126):1224–36.
42. Dimitrievska S, Niklason LE. Historical perspective and future direction of blood vessel developments. Cold Spring Harb Perspect Med. 2018;8(2):a025742.

13 Progress and Prospects of Cardiovascular 3D Printing

Yongjian Wu, Vladimiro L. Vida, Minwen Zheng, and Jian Yang

With the development of society and the continuous improvement in requirement of medical safety, medical education has developed rapidly in the twentieth century. Cardiovascular medicine has also undergone tremendous changes. In the field of heart diseases, such as structural heart diseases and cardiac electrophysiology, in vitro surgical simulation and interventional therapy are considered to be important approaches of improving the success rate of treatments and guaranteeing optimal surgical outcomes.

13.1 3D Printing Has Become a Teaching and Simulation Tool for Cardiovascular Surgery and Internal Medicine

3D printing technology has become a powerful tool that can meet the requirements of in vitro surgical simulation and interventional therapy. 3D-printed model can well simulate and describe the relationships among various anatomical structures of the human body, making individualized models possible, which indicates that it can reveal individual anatomical characteristics of patients and allow more comprehensive analysis of complex cardiac anatomical structures and variations, including congenital heart disease, abnormal origin of the coronary artery, pulmonary vascular disease, valvular disease, left atrial appendage (LAA) lesions, etc. 3D printing can also be used to simulate and demonstrate the physiological and pathological activities of patients' hearts.

Doctors must carefully analyze the anatomical characteristics of patients before surgery and, meanwhile, make medical students understand the application of various surgical approaches, such as the treatment of atrial septal defect (ASD) and complex congenital heart diseases, or LAA occlusion. In addressing these problems, 3D-printed model may be an effective tool for interventional therapy or surgical training. For complex interventional surgery, the DSA exposure time can be shortened to the greatest extent by 3D printing guidance.

3D-printed model can also be split into cross sections, which allows students to observe the internal structure of the heart from different angles and is good for students or doctors to understand the anatomical structure of the cardiovascular system and practice their surgical skills. The key to successful intervention, especially for interventional cardiologists or electrophysiologists, is being able to fully understand the cardiac structure (such as the left anterior oblique position, the right anterior oblique position, the lateral head position, and the anterior–posterior projection) in various imaging localizations.

Cardiovascular medicine has increasingly relied on advanced technologies of imaging and 3D printing reconstruction. Frequently used imaging techniques, including computed tomography (CT), magnetic resonance imaging (MRI), and echocardiography, are constantly being improved. The application of 3D printing technology in teaching can enable students to better understand the relationship between cardiac imaging and in vivo anatomy, which is key to cardiovascular interventional surgery. 3D printing technology, which can be easily coupled with imaging tools, such as transesophageal echocardiography (TEE) or intracardiac echocardiography (ICE), and become a complete simulation tool, enables trainees or interventional doctors to match 3D-printed models with images captured using a catheter during actual operation to promote a better understanding of the cardiovascular anatomical structure of patients.

Y. Wu
Fuwai Hospital, Chinese Academy of Medical Sciences, Beijing, China

V. L. Vida
Paediatric and Congenital Cardiac Surgery Unit, Department of Cardiac, Thoracic and Vascular Sciences and Public Health, University of Padua, Padua, Italy

M. Zheng
Xijing Hospital, Xi'an, China

J. Yang (✉)
Department of Cardiovascular Surgery, Xijing Hospital, Xi'an, China

J. Yang et al. (eds.), *Cardiovascular 3D Printing*, https://doi.org/10.1007/978-981-15-6957-9_13

In addition, cardiovascular 3D-printed models can improve students' learning ability and patient safety. As a powerful tool for interventional and surgical operations, 3D printing will play an increasingly important role in the training of complex cardiovascular interventional surgery in the future [1].

13.2 Clinical Application Prospects of 3D Printing in Cardiovascular Diseases

Clinicians have realized individual differences of complex structural heart diseases in the interventional diagnosis and treatment. In the previous chapters, we have discussed the potential application value of 3D printing technology in these patients, including:

1. Preoperative evaluation of transcatheter aortic valve replacement (TAVR), ASD and ventricular septal defect (VSD) occlusion, perivalvular leak (PVL) interventional occlusion, and LAA occlusion. Based on the 3D-printed model of the patient's specific situation, doctors can visualize the intervention, determine the position of the guide wire catheter and the type of implantation device, and thereby select the optimal surgical path and mode [2]. In the future, with the development of 3D printing materials and printing technology, cardiovascular interventional doctors will be able to print customized 3D heart models according to the specific conditions of each patient and optimize the surgical plan [3, 4].
2. Reconstruction of functional models. In clinical practice, cardiovascular doctors often encounter pathological changes such as hemodynamics caused by valvular lesions, which causes challenges to the assessment of severe and complex cases, especially those with severe aortic stenosis (AS) and aortic regurgitation (AR). With multimodal 3D imaging of patients with aortic valve disease and 3D-printed models made of various 3D printing materials combined with dynamic imaging, the spectrum and dysfunction of the aortic valve can be simulated. Recent studies reported that the aortic valves of eight patients with severe degenerative AS were 3D printed with various materials, and each valve was evaluated in a simulated hemodynamic fluid environment in vitro. Each model accurately duplicated the anatomical structure of aortic valves, including calcification points, the location of valve thickening, and the shape of the valve orifice [5]. The results showed that the valve area of the 3D-printed model increased with the flow. Therefore, a patient-specific 3D-printed function model can provide controllable and repeatable tests for different disease states. Similar functional flow models can also be used to test new diagnostic approaches, such as new cardiovascular devices and flow reserve scores. In the future, these patient-specific 3D models may be the cornerstone of preclinical testing of cardiovascular implants. 3D-printed model can reduce the use of experimental animals which are often used in preclinical testing at present and provide more accurate human anatomical and physiological indicators which will lead to additional benefits in the future.
3. The customization of specific implant devices. 3D printing devices have great potential in the application into stomatology and maxillofacial surgery, and there have been many products of such devices [6]. In the future, 3D technology will fulfill the specific needs of more patients under the requirements of medical regulatory bodies for cardiovascular interventional therapy.

13.2.1 Electrophysiological Applications

Radiofrequency ablation is a common method for the treatment of various arrhythmias. In the past two decades, three-dimensional electrophysiological and anatomical mapping and ablation of complex arrhythmias have developed rapidly. Three-dimensional virtual electrophysiological anatomy and real-time visualized catheter have improved the degree of visualization during cardiovascular interventional surgery and have greatly promoted the development of radiofrequency ablation of complex arrhythmias. However, the complexity of cardiac anatomy still causes many challenges to the treatment of arrhythmias. Therefore, patient-specific 3D-printed model can help to better elucidate the mechanism of arrhythmia and have better targetability and repeatability. For example, 3D-printed models of patients with left atrium, pulmonary vein, and LAA are based on the unique anatomical structure of each individual and can help clinicians select the best treatment option, catheter, and ablation technique (endocardium and/or epicardium). Presurgical simulation in vitro using these models is very helpful in improving the success rate of intervention. These models can also help doctors identify ectopic pacing sites in complex anatomical structures such as papillary muscles and the aortic valve apex. Another important electrophysiological application is the establishment of a three-dimensional print model of coronary sinus specificity in cardiac resynchronization therapy to assist in finding the optimal route for entering the coronary sinus. This method can shorten the operation time and reduce radiation exposure and the use of contrast media. In the future, 3D-bioprinted cardiac models will be able to simulate the cardiac conduction system, assist doctors in targeting key parts of arrhythmia (such as AV nodes), and even optimize the pacing position.

13.2.2 Structural Heart Disease

Despite the assistance of multimodal imaging technology, it still remains one of the most difficult problems in cardiology and cardiovascular surgery to realize three-dimensional visualization of complex congenital heart disease and structural heart disease (such as TAVR). For the past decade or so, the development of TAVR in the world has provided new ideas and experiences for the minimally invasive treatment of structural heart diseases, through which many elderly patients with severe valvular diseases have been treated. Therefore, for children or adults with complex structural heart disease, patient-specific 3D-printed models are very important for preoperative selection of the best surgical path and location of defects. In addition, the size, shape, and shunt of patients' main blood vessels are closely related to palliative or corrective surgery, heart transplantation, and ventricular assist device implantation [7]. In the future, the treatment of congenital heart diseases will also be able to be customized according to the patient's age and anatomical structure using special 3D-printed medical devices (such as transplants, occluders, and artificial valves). It can be predicted that because each patient of congenital heart diseases has unique anatomical structure, it will be necessary to develop customized surgical procedures and devices. 3D printing technology will play an increasingly important role in the treatment of congenital heart diseases [8].

13.2.3 Coronary Artery and Vascular Diseases

At present, 3D printing of large vessels and coronary artery models has been realized [9]. For coronary artery diseases, three-dimensional simulation models are helpful for evaluating coronary artery hemodynamics, and the postoperative coronary artery anatomical structure has become a visual and tangible real model. Coronary artery models can be used to assess the in vitro efficacy of noninvasive flow quantification techniques (such as the fraction of blood reserve at the site of coronary artery lesions) and to determine the preoperative surgical options for complex coronary interventions (such as coronary bifurcation stenting).

In the application of systemic large vessels, 3D printing has shown great clinical value in some operations [10]. In patients with Marfan syndrome and aortic aneurysm, the personalized external aortic root support (PEARS) can be an alternative to aortic root replacement. PEARS uses rapid printing technology to reconstruct individualized woven and printed mesh models around the patient's aortic root; it accurately reproduced the shape of the patient's aortic root. Customized external support implants can be surgically implanted to replace the patient's diseased aortic root and valve. Another application of 3D printing is the planning of interventional procedures. The patient's 3D-printed model can assist in selecting the optimal stent size and evaluating the size and location of the aortic arch of the descending aortic aneurysm, especially for simulation of the complex neck and distal anatomical structures of aortic aneurysm. In the future, customized prefenestrated stent grafts for patients will be able to reduce the incidence of complications such as internal leakage.

13.3 Challenges and Future Development of 3D Printing in the Cardiovascular Field

Although 3D printing technology has broad application prospects in cardiovascular diseases, it is still in its infancy. Major breakthroughs need to be made in the following aspects to make full use of the huge potential of 3D printing technology.

13.3.1 Innovation in Acquisition and Postprocessing of Image Is Key to the Application of 3D Printing in the Cardiovascular Field

3D printing in cardiac medicine relies on 3D cardiovascular dynamic or static imaging of the patient's heart structure. Most of the data of the models are from CTA and/or MRI. 3D printing is also applied in the fields of transesophageal three-dimensional echocardiography (TEE), transthoracic echocardiography, and angiography [11]. The ideal 3D printing of cardiovascular imaging is to combine a variety of imaging techniques. For example, cardiac volume can be assessed based on CTA or MRI resolution and the area of the images; on the contrary, echocardiography is very suitable for analyzing the anatomical structure of valves because it can capture images of rapidly moving structures such as valves and papillary muscles based on time resolution. Each imaging technique has its own advantages. Image acquisition and software processing must combine multimodal high-resolution images, and meanwhile minimize artifacts, which is a complex and time-consuming process. Image postprocessing before 3D model printing is also complex, including the use of computer-aided design (CAD) software: reconstruction, compression, segmentation, or clipping, so that anatomical structures can be better displayed and the continuity between tissues can be enhanced.

The acquisition, postprocessing, and 3D printing of multimodal three-dimensional images, which are diverse and complex, need software of image segmentation and CAD modeling. Guidelines and suggestions must be followed to guide, simplify, and standardize the process. Image postprocessing requires commercial software, including a high-end automatic or semi-automatic software of segmenting models, and CAD software aided by medical 3D printing, which simplifies the image postprocessing. In spite of the combined application of a variety of software, the personal factors in the operation of the software will affect the final model printing. Therefore, standardizing image processing is very important for the innovation and long-term development of 3D printing technology.

13.3.2 The Innovation of 3D Printing Materials Is the Driving Force for the Application of 3D Printing in the Cardiovascular Field

To accurately print the heart model, an important factor is to duplicate the heart model with the diversity of heart tissues and physiological functions. This is different from anatomical teaching. Using 3D printing technique to simulate complex surgery or customize medical devices requires advanced modeling with physiological characteristics of the tissues and the accuracy of modeling. For example, these models can accurately simulate the effects of prosthetic valve implantation on the physiological function of heart tissue. In addition, models are needed to confirm the role of aortic stent grafts and coronary stents after implantation. 3D-printed models meet the requirements of replication and functional simulation of cardiovascular tissues and require softer tissue materials that meet the mechanical requirements. With the development of material science, an increasing number of mechanical materials have been manufactured to simulate heart and vascular tissues, and heart extension models with good stiffness and compliance have been manufactured using Tango Plus family materials (Stratasys).

Multimaterial 3D printing technology, e.g., PolyJet, can construct complex anatomical structures by combining materials of various colors and materials. The 3D printer of this kind can use a mixture of very soft (TangoPlus) and hard (VeroPlus) materials to produce high-resolution models with different properties (such as the mitral calcification model). The diversity and plasticity of 3D printing materials are very important for making hemodynamic functional models.

Despite the significant advances in 3D printing materials, currently available materials can only partially replicate the mechanical and physiological properties of cardiovascular tissues. In addition, heart tissue is diverse, and each tissue undergoes complex dynamic changes with age and physiological status (such as heart failure and hypertension). In this new field of material science, the research and development of artificial 3D printing materials with extensive ductility and physiological properties have become a hotspot. In addition, the main problem in 3D printing technology, which is the cost of printing materials and multimaterial 3D printers, also needs to be considered. Therefore, the development of new and cheaper 3D printing materials is very important to maintain the rapid development of 3D printing technology.

In addition to innovations in nonbiological 3D printing materials, the development of biological printing and molecular printing has also had a tremendous impact on the advance of 3D printing technology. In the construction of tissue-engineered bioactive tissue, these techniques can simulate the mechanical and biological properties of the heart tissue structure in patients. New biomimetic materials, including cell suspensions and hydrogels, acellular matrix components, microcarriers that enable cells to quickly attach to surfaces, and scaffold-free cell particles [12, 13], can be used to create heart tissue models with high elasticity and clarity. However, 3D bioprinting still remains a new field of research. 3D printing technology is currently mainly used in vitro. Further research is needed to simulate and replicate complex natural tissues.

Notably, researchers from Tel Aviv University in Israel announced on April 15, 2019, that they had successfully extracted adipose tissue from a patient's own tissue and then separated the cells of the tissue. They reported 3D printing of the world's first "complete" heart containing cells, blood vessels, ventricles, and atria. Although the 3D-printed heart was very small, it can now contract. This significant pioneering achievement is the first reported case of its kind in the world.

One of the greatest challenges in the field of 3D bioprinting is the development of biological tissue structures that can be converted into operational nutrients to maintain long-term cell survival. Molecular 3D printing can also be regarded as an important cornerstone of precision medicine. Molecular 3D-printed models of pathological organs or tissues of patients can reflect the characteristics needed for molecular diagnosis and treatment for specific molecular targets. For example, a patient-specific molecular 3D-printed heart failure model can help test the effects of specific drugs or interventions on cardiac remodeling. Developments in bioprinting require the continuous progress of 3D printing technology and precision medicine tools such as proteomics and genomics.

13.3.3 4D Printing in the Medical Field Will Become a Future Trend

4D bioprinting integrates the fourth dimension of "time" with 3D bioprinting, which can change the shape or state of an individual (such as cell fusion) according to external stimuli. 4D bioprinting can be used to create a model with the characteristics of individual tissue structures that exist in nature, fully simulate the dynamic changes in tissue structure with time, and thus overcome the limitations of 3D bioprinting to a certain extent [14]. In this new field, there is no unified standard for the classification and definition of 4D bioprinting [15]. J. An et al. [16] put forward the classification definition of 4D bioprinting: tissues must take specific forms or tissues on specific basement and be able to self-assemble into specific forms required by growth. The information exchanged between tissues and cells must be induced by certain stimulation, not by natural physiology.

The field of 4D bioprinting of myocardium is still in its infancy, although many notable research studies have been reported [17]. The first method is to print the tissue onto a substrate material (e.g., responsive hydrogel) and fold the tissue into the needed shape under certain stimulation. Researchers in this field are devoted to the development of matrix or support materials that can deform tissues. Kirillova et al. [13] used deformed hydrogels composed of two different biological polymers (alginate and hyaluronate) and made a hollow self-folding tube with a diameter similar to that of the smallest blood vessel to maintain cell survival for 7 days without reducing the cell survival rate. Apsite et al. [14] made porous multilayer scaffolds with thermal responsive polymers. These scaffolds roll automatically to form pipelines with different layers in different temperatures or water environments. By adding collagen, cell viability and adhesion can be changed. In addition, self-heating hydrogels are also used for the treatment and biomedical applications because they can improve the life of functional materials and are similar to human tissue characteristics. Myocardial cells cultured in a 3D fibrinolytic environment can produce contractile force without pacing. Culturing myocardial cells in a hydrogel with different shapes may help to form a more natural 3D structure over time. With the increasing and deepening research on the activity of myocytes in bioprint-stimulated reactive hydrogels and hydrogels, further application of 4D bioprinting technology can improve the ability to control the arrangement and combination of cells and the internal structure of myocardium.

The second method is to promote the self-assembly of tissue cells by stimulating the printing structure. For example, in a mutually perpendicular structure, the printing materials can be accurately positioned in the corresponding structure. Previous studies have reported stimulation and induction of cardiac tissue structure. Kaji et al. [18] analyzed the response of cardiac tissue to chemical stimulation at the single cell level. Under chemical stimulation, cardiac tissue cells conjugate with gap junctions of human tissue cells. Caffeine, as a stimulant, activates gap junction communication, and this process can be reversibly inhibited by 1-octanol. Chin Siang Ong et al. also used specific chemical factors to stimulate the bioprinted cardiac junctions of unsupported materials in order to print better differentiated tissues. Serpooshan et al. [19] used Faraday waves to stimulate hiPSC-CMs to aggregate into pre-customized 3D structures. With the development of 3D bioprinting technology of the heart and the diversification of tissue structure and cell stimulation induction mechanisms, 4D bioprinted myocardium will continue to show further potential for use in new research and development work [13].

13.3.4 Cardiovascular 3D Printing: From Innovation to Clinical Practice

Despite the exciting prospect of 3D printing in cardiovascular medicine, many difficulties need to be overcome for its widespread application in clinical practice, including reducing costs, simplifying the workflow, accumulating additional medical evidence to prove clinical value, and improving the understanding of how 3D printing can change clinical practice. Before clinical transformation, it is necessary to discuss the feasibility, effectiveness, and cost-effectiveness of the application of 3D printing technology in the cardiovascular field. Experts and scholars in this field should start to develop relevant guidelines and recommendations to discuss short-term and long-term goals of cardiovascular 3D printing. Short-term goals include standardizing the 3D printing workflow, selecting the best 3D printing strategy, printing materials for clinical application, establishing 3D printing centers and laboratories, and training doctors, researchers, engineers, and technicians to lead the field. Long-term goals include establishing a sound evidence system and developing guidelines and recommendations for the widespread use of the technology [20]. At first, relevant clinical evidence could be accumulated by integrating different 3D printing technologies and materials, and then, clinical trials should be conducted to examine the application and cost-effectiveness in daily clinical practice. In view of the individual characteristics of 3D printing, innovative and unconventional clinical trials are needed. At the same time, the establishment of excellent 3D printing laboratories and technical centers and the training of outstanding 3D printing technicians are crucial for the development of this field, especially for the transformation to clinical practice [21].

13.3.5 Artificial Intelligence, Network Information Technology, Virtual Reality Technology, and 3D Printing

After 2G, 3G, and 4G, the world' network communication is about to enter the 5G era, with the speed of information dissemination greatly improved in the future. China has taken the lead in the 5G field and various domestic industries are also actively preparing for the arrival of the 5G era. It has become a new research frontier whether 5G communication technology can bring about new breakthroughs and innovations in the field of traditional medicine in the future.

Guangdong Provincial People's Hospital took the lead in combining 5G technology with traditional cardiovascular surgery in China. On the morning of April 3, 2019, Guangdong Provincial People's Hospital and thousand-of-mile-away Gaozhou People's Hospital cooperated to complete the first live broadcast of AI+5G teleoperation using 5G network high-definition transmission systems. The patient was a middle-aged woman who would undergo the repair of an atrial septal defect with thoracoscopy under cardiopulmonary bypass. The specialists who determined the plan were in Guangzhou, while those who are responsible for the actual operation wee in Gaozhou People's Hospital. 5G technology was used for real-time guide for the operation in real time. The anatomical structure was duplicated with 3D printing technology. The preoperative and on-site operation simulation was conducted. A minimally invasive operation of structural heart disease was completed, opening a new chapter of the combination between network information technology and the application of 3D printing technology in the treatment of cardiovascular diseases. This cooperative operation combined virtual reality technology, hybrid reality technology, 3D printing technology, and several other scientific frontier technologies, which embodied the advantages of multidisciplinary integration and presented an AI+5G + 3D medical feast. Thereby, the new technology of AI-aided diagnosis and treatment systems for structural heart diseases will undoubtedly emerge.

In the present, the field of individualized interventional therapy is undergoing internationally technical innovation. In the interventional operating room, the single or joint application of computed tomography coronary angiography (CTA), virtual reality, vascular robots, and 3D printing technology provides precise customized treatment programs for patients and realizes precise treatment. In the preoperative or perioperative period, the use of these techniques to simulate operations can improve the safety of the operation. These new technologies are often first used in teaching centers. A recent study on the incidence of complications in teaching and nonteaching centers of transcatheter aortic valve replacement (TAVR) found a lower incidence of complications in teaching hospitals, which has been confirmed in relevant studies of PCI. Integrating virtual reality technology and 3D printing technology into the training of interventional surgeons may reduce the learning curve effect. The use of virtual reality in learning environment can enhance the cognition and understanding ability of trainees and lead to faster treatment of patients and has already been approved by the Food and Drug Administration (FDA) and the Society for Cardiovascular Angiography and Intervention (SCAI), though the rate of use of these techniques in cardiovascular training programs is still very low. Since Dotter and Judkins first described angioplasty in 1964, the field of cardiovascular intervention has developed rapidly. Virtual reality and 3D printing technology can provide surgical simulation and accurate guidance for complex cardiovascular surgery. More evidence to improve the operational ability of interventional operators is needed, and interventional doctors need to continue to explore interventional training and surgery.

13.4 Summary

The development of 3D printing technology can advance cardiovascular medicine toward customization and a precise medical model. In the communication between patients and doctors, customized 3D-printed models of cardiovascular disease will allow cardiovascular diseases to be explained to patients via three-dimensional visualization of their characteristics. In medical education, the teaching level of cardiovascular anatomy can be improved, and medical students' understanding of physiological and anatomical structure can be deepened. In clinical practice, the formulation of complex interventional procedures and the use of customized printed medical devices can improve the success rate of surgery, reduce complications, and reduce the cost of surgery. It is believed that in the near future, with the development of a 3D printing center and the standardization of technical personnel and guidelines, the relationship between 3D printing technology and cardiovascular medicine will be closer and further developed.

References

1. Schmauss D, Juchem G, Weber S, Gerber N, Hagl C, Sodian R. Three-dimensional printing for perioperative planning of complex aortic arch surgery. Ann Thorac Surg. 2014;97:2160–3.
2. Hermsen JL, Burke TM, Seslar SP, Owens DS, Ripley BA, Mokadam NA, Verrier ED. Scan, plan, print, practice, perform: development and use of a patient-specific 3-dimensional printed model in adult cardiac surgery. J Thorac Cardiovasc Surg. 2017;153:132–40.
3. Giannopoulos AA, Mitsouras D, Yoo SJ, Liu PP, Chatzizisis YS, Rybicki FJ. Applications of 3D printing in cardiovascular diseases. Nat Rev Cardiol. 2016;13:701–18.
4. Little SH, Vukicevic M, Avenatti E, Ramchandani M, Barker CM. 3D printed modeling for patient-specific mitral valve intervention: repair with a clip and a plug. JACC Cardiovasc Interv. 2016;9:973–5.
5. Gosai J, Purva M, Gunn J. Simulation in cardiology: state of the art. Eur Heart J. 2015;36:777–83.
6. Chen J, Zhang Z, Chen X, Zhang C, Zhang G, Xu Z. Design and manufacture of customized dental implants by using reverse engineering and selective laser melting technology. J Prosthet Dent. 2014;112:1088–95.
7. Farooqi KM, Saeed O, Zaidi A, Sanz J, Nielsen JC, Hsu DT, Jorde UP. 3D printing to guide ventricular assist device placement in adults with congenital heart disease and heart failure. JACC Heart failure. 2016;4:301–11.
8. Sodian R, Weber S, Markert M, Rassoulian D, Kaczmarek I, Lueth TC, Reichart B, Daebritz S. Stereolithographic models for surgical planning in congenital heart surgery. Ann Thorac Surg. 2007;83:1854–7.

9. Modi BN, Ryan M, Chattersingh A, Eruslanova K, Ellis H, Gaddum N, Lee J, Clapp B, Chowienczyk P, Perera D. Optimal application of fractional flow reserve to assess serial coronary artery disease: a 3D-printed experimental study with clinical validation. J Am Heart Assoc. 2018;7:e010279.
10. Pluchinotta FR, Giugno L, Carminati M. Stenting complex aortic coarctation: simulation in a 3D printed model. EuroIntervention. 2017;13:490.
11. Mahmood F, Owais K, Taylor C, Montealegre-Gallegos M, Manning W, Matyal R, Khabbaz KR. Three-dimensional printing of mitral valve using echocardiographic data. J Am Coll Cardiol Img. 2015;8:227–9.
12. Wang Y, Adokoh CK, Narain R. Recent development and biomedical applications of self-healing hydrogels. Expert Opin Drug Deliv. 2018;15:77–91.
13. Kirillova A, Maxson R, Stoychev G, Gomillion CT, Ionov L. 4D biofabrication using shape-morphing hydrogels. Adv Mater. 2017;29:1703443.
14. Apsite I, Stoychev G, Zhang W, Jehnichen D, Xie J, Ionov L. Porous stimuli-responsive self-folding electrospun mats for 4D biofabrication. Biomacromolecules. 2017;18:3178–84.
15. Khoo ZX, Teoh JEM, Liu Y, Chua CK, Yang S, An J, Leong KF, Yeong WY. 3D printing of smart materials: a review on recent progresses in 4D printing. Virtual Phys Prototyp. 2015;10:103–22.
16. An J, Chua CK, Mironov V. A perspective on 4D bioprinting. Int J Bioprinting. 2016;2:3–5.
17. Gao B, Yang Q, Zhao X, Jin G, Ma Y, Xu F. 4D bioprinting for biomedical applications. Trends Biotechnol. 2016;34:746–56.
18. Kaji H, Takii Y, Nishizawa M, Matsue T. Pharmacological characterization of micropatterned cardiac myocytes. Biomaterials. 2003;24:4239–44.
19. Serpooshan V, Chen P, Wu H, Lee S, Sharma A, Hu DA, Venkatraman S, Ganesan AV, Usta OB, Yarmush M, Yang F, Wu JC, Demirci U, Wu SM. Bioacoustic-enabled patterning of human IPSC-derived cardiomyocytes into 3D cardiac tissue. Biomaterials. 2017;131:47–57.
20. Bartel T, Rivard A, Jimenez A, Mestres CA, Müller S. Medical three-dimensional printing opens up new opportunities in cardiology and cardiac surgery. Eur Heart J. 2018;39:1246–54.
21. Vukicevic M, Mosadegh B, Min JK, Little SH. Cardiac 3D printing and its future directions. J Am Coll Cardiol Img. 2017;10:171–84.

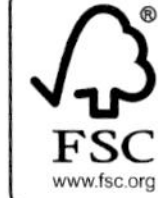

MIX
Papier aus verantwortungsvollen Quellen
Paper from responsible sources
FSC® C105338

If you have any concerns about our products,
you can contact us on
ProductSafety@springernature.com

In case Publisher is established outside the EU,
the EU authorized representative is:
Springer Nature Customer Service Center GmbH
Europaplatz 3, 69115 Heidelberg, Germany

Printed by Libri Plureos GmbH
in Hamburg, Germany